Air Fryer Coo For Beginners 2022

A Cookbook With Detailed Information On The Usage Of Air Fryer And Its Benefits With 800 Amazing Recipes

By

CAMILLE HURLBUTT

Table of Contents

Introduction

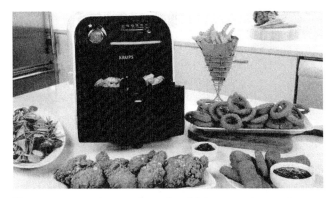

Do you want to produce healthier versions of your favorite treats like fries, chicken wings, mozzarella sticks, and more?

It may sound too wonderful to be true, but air fryer fans claim that their beloved device can do just that. The device has been popping up on work surfaces all across the country, offering a quick and easy way to prepare crispy, tasty fried food without all the calories.

The Air Fryer is a technological advancement that has made many lives much easier. It has ushered in a new way of cooking that is full of health benefits. As a consequence of marketing activities, it appears that new kitchen products and small appliances appear on the horizon on a daily basis, seemingly out of nowhere. Every new "must-have" item is extolled as the best. The Air Fryer is one example of a small device that has taken the culinary world by storm. The Air Fryer has not only earned a place on every cook's counter, but it's still as useful and important today as it was when the fryers first appeared on supermarket shelves in 2010. It's no surprise that most people juggle the need for tasty, nutritious, and convenient meals seven days a week. The quickest dinner options, on the other hand, have always been unhealthy and high in salt and oil. As our lives move at significantly faster speeds, many consumers struggle to strike a balance between quick, delicious, and simple meals. As a solution to the problem, the Philips Electronics Corporation introduced the world to the Air Fryer, a truly unique appliance. This ingenious piece of machinery solved all facets of mealtime problems.

Air fryers are small ovens with a concentrated source of heat and a strong fan that pumps the hot air to fry up fries, wings, veggies, and other oil-free dishes. They provide your food a fantastic "fried" finish that your oven can't duplicate, as well as cooking results that blow the traditional microwave out of the sea. In addition, an air fryer uses very little oil to achieve crunchy results with a less fraction of the calories and fat present in traditional cooking methods like deep-frying.

This book is a detailed guide for beginners to get to know the art of cooking in air fryers.

Apart from the know-how of the machine, this book comprises various recipes that can be easily made in air fryer devices.

What is an Air Fryer?

Air fryers are rectangular or egg-shaped machines that sit on your countertop and are roughly the size of a coffeemaker. In a slide-out basket, you place the food you want to fry. You can give it a light coat of oil if you desire.

A fan circulates hot air (up to 400 degrees Fahrenheit) over the food. It works in a similar way as a convection oven.

The rotating air cooks the exterior of the goods first, resulting in a crispy brown coating on the surface and a soft interior, similar to deep-fried dishes. A container beneath the basket collects any grease that drips as the food cooks.

Air fryers produce the crispy, chewy delicacies that customers crave without the use of a lot of oil.

Is it healthy to eat air-fried food?

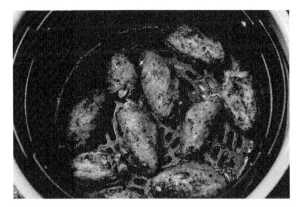

Air-fried food, on the other hand, might be argued to be healthier than deep-fried food because it requires less oil. In comparison to deep-fried French fries, which have a whopping 17 grams of fat per serving, frozen French fries heated in an air fryer have between 4 and 6 grams of fat per serving.

Is it worthwhile to invest in an air fryer?

With so many variants on the market, the price of this popular appliance has dropped in recent years—many models are around $200, and others are under $100. Still, buying an air fryer is probably only worthwhile if you frequently prepare fried dishes (frozen or homemade).

What Air Fryer size does one need?

Basket-style air fryers can't hold a lot of food. If you accept this, you and your air fryer will have a lot better relationship.

An air fryer with a capacity of 1.75 to 3 quarts is suitable for cooking meals for one or two people. Also, don't anticipate any leftovers.

Even a big air fryer (four to five quarts) frequently requires batch cooking. You'll probably need to cook a recipe in more than one batch if it serves more than two people.

Consumer Reports discovered that several air fryers' capacity was somewhat less than what manufacturers advertised. This may sound tedious, but keep in mind that air fryers cook food quickly.

Tips to consider while purchasing an air fryer

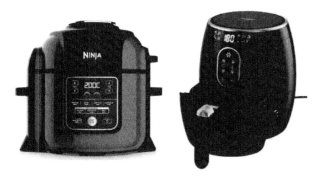

There are a few things to consider while selecting the ideal air fryer for your kitchen:

Cost
They can cost anything from around $100 to over $500. Pricier models include more functionality, such as pressure cooking or grilling, so you may save money on other kitchen equipment in the long term.

Size
While the size of the air fryer you purchase will be determined by the amount of counter space you have available; and you should also assess how many people you'll be cooking for.

Style
Oven-style and basket-style air fryers are the two most common types. Although the oven takes up more counter space, it is more useful and can cook larger amounts of food. Although it normally has fewer functions, the basket drawer type allows you to shake rather than spin the food to scatter it.

Cleaning
Do you despise cleaning the dishes? We recommend choosing a smaller basket because there are fewer parts to wash, and they are easy to clean.

After considering the above, you can select your desired air fryer from a wide range of air fryers that are on the market.

Benefits of an Air Fryer

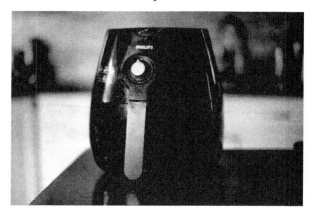

Air fryers have enjoyed a recent rebound in sales, owing to a greater awareness of nutritional content and a continuing desire for fried foods. Potatoes are consumed more than any other vegetable in the United States, with frozen items such as fries accounting for 40% of total consumption.

When compared to dishes prepared in other ways, deep-fried foods include a lot more fat.

Because air fryers utilize a fraction of the oil that deep fryers use, people can enjoy a healthier supper with the same flavors and textures.

This is perfect because cutting down on one's oil use might be beneficial to one's health. According to studies, dietary fat from vegetable oil has been linked to a range of health risks, including an increased risk of heart disease and higher rates of inflammation.

This isn't to say that air-fried chicken is better for you than roasted, slow-cooked, grilled, or pan-seared chicken. There is a wealth of supplementary equipment available to produce wholesome and delectable meals. They simply do not have the same fried, crunchy texture as air fryers.

The following are some of the benefits of air frying: -

Healthy eating and weight loss
Consumption of fried foods has been related to an increased risk of obesity. This is due to deep-fried foods' high fat and calorie content.

Weight loss can be improved by switching from deep-fried to air-fried foods and avoiding the use of unhealthy oils on a daily basis.

The air fry is fast and convenient
Deep-frying foods necessitates the use of a big

container filled with hot oil. This might be dangerous. Although air fryers do get hot, there really is no danger of splashing, spilling, or touching boiling oil by accident. To maintain safety, individuals must use frying equipment carefully and follow the instructions properly.

The air fried food has the same taste as deep fry food

Air fryers eliminate moisture from foods by heating air containing fine oil droplets, according to studies. As a result, air-fried food has similar properties to fried food but with far lower fat levels.

The Maillard effect is a chemical reaction that occurs when food is air-fried, as it does in many other culinary operations, and it enhances the colour and flavour of the dish.

Use less fat and oil

Air fryers use less oil and fat to cook the same food that would require a lot of oil if cooked in the usual manner.

Air fryers pump hot air over a food item to generate the same crispiness as traditional fried foods. Air fryers are able to achieve this by removing high-calorie oil from the food preparation process.

By using only one tablespoon of oil instead of many cups, a person can accomplish the same outcomes as a deep fryer but consuming a fraction of the fat and calories.

Ease and versatility

Air fryers are easy to use. The manufactures provide a step-by-step user manual for the individuals to use the air fryer without any hassle and with ease.

Air fryers are versatile, and it's not restricted to air frying only. One can bake, hydrate, steam, heat and cook a lot many things using the air fryer.

There are a variety of brands in the market that provide the users with a plethora of additional functions and cooking techniques that can be carried out by an air frying device.

Reduce the risk of diseases

The development of harmful compounds such as acrylamide can occur when food is fried in oil. This chemical emerges in some meals when high-heat cooking techniques, such as deep-frying, are used.

Endometrial cancer, breast cancer, pancreatic cancer, ovarian cancer, and esophageal cancer have all been related to acrylamide. Additional research has indicated a link between dietary acrylamide and kidney, endometrial, and ovarian cancers, while the evidence is still ambiguous.

By switching to air frying, people can lower their risk of acrylamide contamination in their food.

Cooking with oil and eating fried foods on a regular basis has been related to a number of health issues. To reduce the danger of these outcomes, deep frying can be replaced with alternate cooking methods.

Automatic cooking programs

With air fryers, one doesn't have to learn and follow different methods in order to cook different types of food with different cooking methods. Air fryers have various automatic programs that are meant for cooking different types of foods. One doesn't need to be a professional in order to cook food in an air fryer. It has an automatic system that lets you cook your food by just selecting the function, temperature and time.

Saves the nutritional values of the food

Air frying the food also saves the nutritional value of the food. In an air, fryer less amount of oil and fat is used, and food is prepared by the hot air that is pumped into the device. Although the food prepared is not always of less calorific value, but the nutrients of the food are not destroyed in an air fryer. The food cooked is healthy and nutritious. While in the traditional way of cooking, the food that was supposed to be delicious was overcooked on direct heat that is resulting in destroying the nutritional value of the food, whereas in an air fryer, the food is cooked indirectly, just like in case of a convection oven and is not overcooked which in the end preserves the nutritional content of the food.

Steps on how to use an Air Fryer

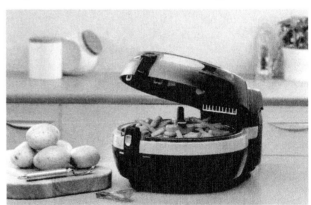

Set the air fryer

The frying basket is sealed into the drawer inside the Air Fryer body when it is shipped. To open the frying

basket drawer, grab the handle firmly; then pull the drawer from the device and lay it on a firm, clear work surface

Push the clear basket lock forth to reveal the basket eject button, which will release and detach the frying basket from the drawer.

Pull the frying basket up straight and out of the drawer while pressing the basket release switch.

Remove all packing materials and labels from the Air Fryer's interior and exterior. Make sure the frying basket and drawer don't have any packaging underneath or around them.

In warm soap water, wash the frying basket and drawer. The air fryer should not be submerged in water. Wipe the body of the Air Fryer with a moist towel. Thoroughly dry all components.

Place the cleaned frying basket in the drawer and close it. On each side of the handle, there are two tabs. Insert the two grip tabs into the grooves on the basket drawer's top. The frying basket lever locks firmly into place with an audible click.

Set your device and make a note of the following-

The plug on this appliance is polarized. This plug will only fit in a polarized outlet one way to prevent the risk of electric shock. Rotate the plug if it does not fit completely into the socket. If it still doesn't fit, hire a professional electrician. Make no changes to the plugin anyway.

To avoid getting tangled in or stumbling over a larger power supply cord, use the specified short power supply cord. This product should not be used with an extension cord. Always connect to a wall outlet or receptacle.

Placemats or non-plastic coasters between the appliance and the finish of the countertop or tabletop to prevent Plasticizers from spreading to the surface of the countertop or tabletop or other furniture. Neglect to do so may cause the finish to discolor, resulting in permanent flaws or stains.

Choose recipes
After successfully setting up the air fryer, it is pertinent to choose the recipes beforehand.

Prepare the ingredients
After choosing the recipes, prepare the ingredients. Whether you want to cook meats or vegetables, you are supposed to prepare them before cooking them. Wash the vegetables and meat and pat them dry. It is crucial for the food to be dry before placing them in the food basket.

Place food in the basket
The basket may accommodate anywhere from two to ten quarts, depending on the size of your air fryer.

Make sure that you do not overcrowd the basket. In most circumstances, either one or two teaspoons of oil will be needed to help the dish get crunchy.

Setting temperature and time
If the Air Fryer is cold, set the timer to the specified air frying duration plus three minutes for warming. The blue heat on light and the red power light will both activate, signaling that the Air Fryer is ready to use.

When the set temperature is attained, the blue heat on the light will turn off.

Depending on the item you're cooking, air fryer cooking durations and temperatures range from 5 to 25 minutes at 350° to 400°F.

According to the food you're preparing, adjust the temperature timer and gauge on the air fryer. Non-vegetarian meals need at least 15 minutes to fry, whereas veggies take about 10 minutes. However, the fryer's user manual will also have pre-programmed settings for various cuisines.

Check food during cooking
To assist the food crisping up evenly, you may need to toss or turn it midway throughout the cooking period.

Pull the basket drawer midway during the cooking period to check for even cooking/browning. To turn or shake things in the frying basket, remove it from the frying basket drawer. Put the frying basket in the frying basket drawer when finished. If necessary, adjust the temperature. When the drawer is opened, the timer will resume to count down, but the Air Fryer will stop warming until the drawer is reinstalled.

Cleaning and maintenance for the air fry
Because a build-up of oil might cause the air fryer to smoke, it's critical to clean it after each usage. In certain cases, a paper towel will suffice to clean the drawer and grate. Assume they're filthy and wash your hands. Check your manual to see whether any parts of your model are dishwasher safe.

Follow the following instructions in order to clean your device: -

Remove the Air Fryer from the outlet. Take the frying basket out of the drawer and set it aside. Before cleaning the frying, basket drawer and frying basket, make sure they are fully cooled.

In warm soap water, rinse the basket drawer and frying basket. Metal kitchen utensils, as well as caustic cleaners and cleaning agents, can harm the non-stick coating.

The drawer and the frying basket are dishwasher-safe. Place in the top rack of your dishwasher to clean for the best results.To clean the Air Fryer, use a soft, non-abrasive moist cloth.

Chapter 1~Air Fried Breakfast Recipes

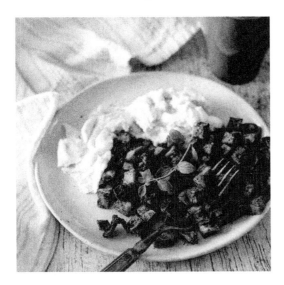

Artichoke Frittata

Preparation Time-10 minutes | Cook Time-15 minutes | Servings-2 | Difficulty-Easy

Nutritional Facts- Calories-138 | Fats-6g |Carbohydrates-12.9g |Proteins-7.8g

Ingredients

- One canned artichokes heart, drained and chopped
- One tablespoon of olive oil
- Half teaspoon of dried oregano
- Salt and black pepper to the taste
- Two eggs

Instructions

- In a bowl, mix artichokes with oregano, salt, pepper and eggs and whisk well.
- Add the oil to your air fryer's pan, add eggs, mix and cook at 320 degrees F for 15 minutes.
- Divide frittata among plates and serve for breakfast.
- Enjoy!

Asparagus Frittata

Preparation Time-10 minutes | Cook Time-30 minutes | Servings-2 | Difficulty-Moderate

Nutritional Facts- Calories-273 | Fats-8.19g|Carbohydrates-6.9g |Proteins-14.1g

Ingredients

- Four whisked eggs
- Two tablespoons of parmesan, grated
- Four tablespoons of milk
- Salt and black pepper to the taste
- Ten asparagus tips, steamed
- Cooking spray

Instructions

- In a bowl, mix eggs with parmesan, milk, salt and pepper and whisk well.
- Heat up the air fryer at 400 degrees F and spray it with oil.
- Add asparagus, add eggs, mix, toss a bit and cook for 5 minutes.
- Divide frittata among plates and serve for breakfast.
- Enjoy!

Avocado Taco Fry

Preparation Time- 5 minutes| Cook Time- 20 minutes| Servings-2 | Difficulty-Easy

Nutritional Facts- Calories-140 | Fats-8.7g|Carbohydrates-12g |Proteins-6g

Ingredients

- One peeled and sliced avocado
- One beaten egg
- Half cup of panko bread crumbs
- Salt
- Tortillas and toppings

Instructions

- Using a bowl, add in the egg.
- Using a separate bowl, set in the breadcrumbs.
- Dip the avocado into the bowl with the beaten egg and coat with the breadcrumbs. Sprinkle the coated wedges with a bit of salt.
- Arrange them in the cooking basket in a single layer.
- Set the Air Fryer to 392 degrees F and cook for 15 minutes. Shake the basket halfway through the cooking process.
- Put them on tortillas with your preferred toppings.

Bacon and Egg Breakfast Biscuit Bombs

Preparation Time-10 minutes | Cook Time-40 minutes | Servings-2 | Difficulty-Moderate

Nutritional Facts- Calories-200 | Fats-10.8g |Carbohydrates-9.9g |Proteins-15g

Ingredients

- A quarter teaspoon of pepper
- Two ounces of sharp cheddar cheese, cut into ten 3/4-inch cubes
- Four slices of bacon, cut into 1/2-inch pieces
- One tablespoon of water
- Two beaten eggs
- Five biscuits
- One egg
- One tablespoon of butter

Instructions

- Cut two 8-inch rounds of parchment paper for cooking. Set one round at the bottom of the basket of the air fryer. Spray with cooking spray.
- In a nonstick 10-inch skillet, cook bacon until crisp over medium-high heat.
- Place on a paper towel; remove from the pan. Wipe the skillet carefully with a paper towel. To the skillet, add butter and melt over medium heat. Add two beaten eggs and pepper to the skillet; cook until the eggs are thickened, stirring frequently but still moist. Remove from the heat; add bacon and stir. Cool for five minutes.
- Meanwhile, divide the dough into five biscuits; separate the two layers of each biscuit. Press into a 4-inch round each. Then spoon one onto the center of each round heaping tablespoon full of the egg mixture. Top it with one of the cheese pieces. Fold the edges gently up and over the filling; pinch to seal. Beat the remainder of the egg and water in a small bowl. Brush the biscuits with egg wash on all sides.
- Place 5 of the biscuit bombs on the parchment in the air fryer basket, seam side down. With cooking spray, spray both sides of the second round of parchment. Top the biscuit bombs in the basket with the second parchment, then top with the remaining five biscuit bombs.
- Set to 325 ° F; cook for eight minutes. Remove the top of the round parchment; use tongs to carefully turn the biscuits and place them in a single layer in the basket. Cook 4 to 6 minutes longer or (at least 165°F) until cooked through.

Bacon BBQ

Preparation Time-2 minutes | Cook Time- 8 minutes| Servings-2 | Difficulty-Easy

Nutritional Facts- Calories-112.4 | Fats-7.2g |Carbohydrates-5.88g |Proteins-4.89g

Ingredients

- One tablespoon of dark brown sugar
- One teaspoon of chili powder
- Half teaspoon of ground cumin
- Half teaspoon of cayenne pepper
- Four slices of halved bacon

Instructions

- Mix seasonings until well combined.
- Dip the bacon in the dressing until it is completely covered. Leave aside.
- Adjust the air fryer to 356 degrees F.
- Place the bacon in the preheated air fryer
- Select the Bacon option and press Start/Pause. Serve.

Baked Oatmeal

Preparation Time-15 minutes| Cook Time-35 minutes| Servings-2 | Difficulty-Easy

Nutritional Facts- Calories-235 | Fats-13.2g |Carbohydrates-28.5g |Proteins-4.89g

Ingredients

- One cup of original oats
- One banana
- A quarter cup of pecans
- Half cup of milk
- One tablespoon of flax meal
- Two teaspoons of olive oil
- Two teaspoons of maple syrup
- Half teaspoon of baking powder
- Half teaspoon of ground cinnamon & salt
- Half teaspoon of vanilla extract

Instructions

- Preheat the Air Fryer Grill at 350 degrees F on the baking setting.

- Make a batter with mashed banana and all the ingredients
- Grease a 7x5-inch dish and pour your batter into it. Bake it for 25-35 minutes.

Bell Peppers Frittata

Preparation Time-10 minutes | Cook Time-20 minutes | Servings-2 | Difficulty-Easy

Nutritional Facts- Calories-178 | Fats-9g |Carbohydrates-15.9g |Proteins-9g

Ingredients

- Two tablespoons of olive oil
- A quarter pounds chicken sausage, casings removed and chopped
- One chopped sweet onion
- One chopped red bell pepper
- One chopped orange bell pepper
- One chopped green bell pepper
- Salt and black pepper to the taste
- Four whisked eggs
- A quarter cup of shredded mozzarella cheese
- Two teaspoons of chopped oregano

Instructions

- Add One tablespoon of oil to your air fryer, add sausage, heat up at 320 degrees F and brown for 1 minute.
- Add the rest of the oil, onion, red bell pepper, orange and green one, stir and cook for 2 minutes more.
- Add oregano, salt, pepper and eggs, stir and cook for 15 minutes.
- Add mozzarella, leave frittata aside for a few minutes, divide among plates and serve.
- Enjoy!

Biscuits Casserole

Preparation Time-10 minutes | Cook Time-20 minutes | Servings-2 | Difficulty-Moderate

Nutritional Facts- Calories-213 | Fats-7.8g |Carbohydrates-12.9g |Proteins-4.8g

Ingredients

- Six ounces biscuits, quartered
- One and a half tablespoons of flour
- A quarter chopped pound sausage

A pinch of salt and black pepper
One and a quarter cups of milk
Cooking spray

Instructions

- Grease your air fryer with cooking spray and heat it over 350 degrees F.
- Add biscuits to the bottom and mix with sausage.
- Add flour, milk, salt and pepper, toss a bit and cook for 15 minutes.
- Divide among plates and serve for breakfast.
- Enjoy!

Blackberry French Toast

Preparation Time-10 minutes | Cook Time-20 minutes | Servings-2 | Difficulty-Easy

Nutritional Facts- Calories-215 | Fats-7.8g |Carbohydrates-13.8g |Proteins-6.9g

Ingredients

- One cup of blackberry jam, warm
- Four ounces of cubed bread loaf
- Two ounces of cubed cream cheese, cubed
- Two eggs
- One teaspoon of cinnamon powder
- Two cups of half and half
- Half cup of brown sugar
- One teaspoon of vanilla extract
- Cooking spray

Instructions

- Grease your air fryer with cooking spray and heat it up at 300° F.
- Add blueberry jam to the bottom, layer half of the bread cubes, then add cream cheese and top with the rest of the bread.
- In a bowl, mix eggs with half and half, cinnamon, sugar and vanilla, whisk well and add over bread mix.
- Cook for 20 minutes, divide among plates and serve for breakfast.
- Enjoy!

Breakfast Bread Rolls

Preparation Time-10 minutes | Cook Time-15 minutes | Servings-2 | Difficulty-Easy

Nutritional Facts- Calories-143 | Fats-6.9g

|Carbohydrates-12.9g |Proteins-6.9g

Ingredients

- Five potatoes, boiled, peeled and mashed
- Four bread slices, white parts only
- One chopped coriander bunch
- Two chopped green chilies
- One chopped small yellow onion
- Half teaspoon of turmeric powder
- Two curry leaf springs
- Half teaspoon of mustard seeds
- Two tablespoons of olive oil
- Salt and black pepper to the taste

Instructions

- Heat up a pan with one teaspoon of oil, add mustard seeds, onions, curry leaves and turmeric, stir and cook for a few seconds.
- Add mashed potatoes, salt, pepper, coriander and chilies, stir well, take off the heat and cool it down.
- Divide potatoes mix into four parts and shape ovals using your wet hands.
- Wet bread slices with water, press in order to drain excess water and keep one slice in your palm.
- Add a potato oval over the bread slice and wrap it around it.
- Repeat with the remaining potato mix and bread.
- Heat up the air fryer at 400 degrees F, add the rest of the oil, add bread rolls, cook them for 12 minutes.
- Divide bread rolls among plates and serve for breakfast.
- Enjoy!

Breakfast Burger

Preparation Time-10 minutes | Cook Time-45 minutes | Servings-2 | Difficulty-Moderate

Nutritional Facts- Calories-176 | Fats-7.8g |Carbohydrates-15.9g |Proteins-9.9g

Ingredients

- Half pound ground beef
- One chopped yellow onion
- One teaspoon of tomato puree
- One teaspoon of minced garlic

- One teaspoon of mustard
- One teaspoon of dried basil
- One teaspoon of chopped parsley
- One tablespoon of grated cheddar cheese
- Salt and black pepper to the taste
- Two bread buns, for serving

Instructions

- In a bowl, mix beef with onion, tomato puree, garlic, mustard, basil, parsley, cheese, salt and pepper, stir well and shape two burgers out of this mix.
- Heat up the air fryer at 400 degrees F, add burgers and cook them for 25 minutes.
- Reduce temperature to 350 degrees F and bake burgers for 20 minutes more.
- Arrange them on bread buns and serve them for a quick breakfast.
- Enjoy!

Breakfast Burritos

Preparation Time-5 minutes | Cook Time-15 minutes | Servings-2 | Difficulty-Easy

Nutritional Facts- Calories-160 | Fats-7.8g |Carbohydrates-9.9g |Proteins-12g

Ingredients

- Two scrambled eggs
- A quarter minced bell pepper
- Two medium flour tortillas
- A quarter cup of shredded cheese
- A quarter lb. of grounded sausage
- 1/3 cup of bacon bits
- oil for spraying

Instructions

- Combine in a big bowl scrambled eggs, bell pepper, cooked sausage, bacon bits & cheese. Stir to blend.
- A half-cup of the mixture is spooned into the middle of a flour tortilla.
- Fold the sides and then roll.
- For the remaining ingredients, you have to repeat the same process.
- Put filled burritos in the basket of the air fryer & liberally spray with oil.
- Cook for 5 minutes at 330 degrees F.

Breakfast Cheese Bread Cups

Preparation Time-6 minutes | Cook Time-15 minutes| Servings-2 | Difficulty-Easy

Nutritional Facts- Calories- 162| Fats-7.8g|Carbohydrates-9.9g|Proteins-10.8g

Ingredients

- Two eggs
- Two tablespoons of grated cheddar cheese
- Salt and pepper
- One ham slice cut into two pieces
- Four bread slices flat with a rolling pin

Instructions

- Spray both sides of the ramekins with cooking spray.
- Place two slices of bread into each ramekin.
- Add the ham slice pieces into each ramekin.
- Crack an egg in each ramekin, then sprinkle with cheese.
- Season with salt and pepper.
- Place the ramekins into the air fryer at 300Fahrenheit for 15-minutes.
- Serve warm.

Breakfast Doughnuts

Preparation Time-10 minutes | Cook Time-12 minutes | Servings-2 | Difficulty-Easy

Nutritional Facts- Calories-164 | Fats-7.8g |Carbohydrates-15g |Proteins-7.8g

Ingredients

- Two tablespoons of softened butter
- Half teaspoon of baking powder
- One and a quarter cups of white flour
- A quarter cup of sugar
- A quarter cup of caster sugar
- One teaspoon of cinnamon powder
- One egg yolk
- A quarter cup of sour cream

Instructions

- In a bowl, mix Two tablespoons of butter with simple sugar and egg yolks and whisk well.
- Add half of the sour cream and stir.
- In another bowl, mix flour with baking powder, stir and also add to eggs mix.

- Stir well until you obtain a dough, transfer it to a floured working surface, roll it out and cut big circles with smaller ones in the middle.
- Brush doughnuts with the rest of the butter, heat up your air fryer at 360 degrees F, place doughnuts inside and cook them for 8 minutes.
- In a bowl, mix cinnamon with caster sugar and stir.
- Arrange doughnuts among plates and dip them in cinnamon and sugar before serving.
- Enjoy!

Breakfast Egg Bowls

Preparation Time-10 minutes | Cook Time-20 minutes | Servings-2 | Difficulty-Easy

Nutritional Facts- Calories-238 | Fats-4g |Carbohydrates-13.8g |Proteins-6.9g

Ingredients

- Two dinner rolls top cut off, and insides scooped out
- Two tablespoons of heavy cream
- Two eggs
- Two tablespoons of mixed chives and parsley
- Salt and black pepper to the taste
- Four tablespoons of grated parmesan

Instructions

- On a baking sheet, arrange dinner rolls and crack an egg into each one.
- In each roll, divide the heavy cream and mixed herbs and season with pepper and salt.
- Sprinkle parmesan cheese on top of the rolls before placing them in your air fryer and cooking for 20 minutes at 350 degrees F.
- Serve your bread bowls for breakfast by dividing them among plates.
- Enjoy!

Breakfast Egg Rolls

Preparation Time-5 minutes| Cook Time-20 minutes| Servings-2 | Difficulty-Easy

Nutritional Facts- Calories-185| Fats-9g|Carbohydrates-12g|Proteins-13.8g

Ingredients

- Two eggs

- Two tablespoons of milk
- Pepper
- Salt
- Half cup of shredded cheddar cheese
- Two sausage patties or any other additional stir-ins
- Four egg roll wrappers
- One tablespoon of olive oil
- Water

Instructions

- Cook or replace the sausage in a small skillet according to the packet. It should be removed from the pan and sliced into small pieces.
- Whisk the eggs, sugar, a pinch of pepper and salt together. Over medium/low heat, add a teaspoon of oil or a little pat of butter to a pan. Pour in the mixture of eggs and cook for a few minutes, stirring regularly to produce scrambled eggs. Stir the sausage in. And put aside.
- Place the egg roll wrapper with points that create a diamond shape on a working surface. Then place roughly one tablespoon of the cheese at the bottom third of the wrapper. Cover with a mixture of eggs.
- Wet a finger or pastry brush and brush all the sides of the egg roll wrapper, helping it to seal.
- The egg roll wrapper should be folded up and over the filling, trying to get it as secure as you can. Then, fold the sides together to make an envelope-looking shape. Place the seam side down and start assembling the remaining rolls.
- Preheat an air fryer for 5 minutes to 400 F.
- Rub rolls with oil or spray them with a misto if you have one. Put in the preheated basket. Set for 8 minutes to 400 F.
- Flip the eggs over after 5 minutes. For another 3 minutes, return the egg rolls to the air fryer.
- Serve and Enjoy.

Breakfast Fish Tacos

Preparation Time-10 minutes | Cook Time-15 minutes | Servings-2 | Difficulty-Easy

Nutritional Facts- Calories-192 | Fats-9.9g | Carbohydrates-15g | Proteins-12.9g

Ingredients

- Two big tortillas

- Half chopped red bell pepper
- Half chopped yellow onion
- One cup of corn
- Two white fish fillets, skinless and boneless
- Half cup of salsa
- A handful mixed spinach, romaine lettuce and radicchio
- Two tablespoons of grated parmesan

Instructions

- Place the fish fillets in your air fryer and cook for 6 minutes at 350 degrees F.
- Meanwhile, heat a pan over medium-high heat, add the onion, bell pepper, and corn, and cook for 1-2 minutes, stirring occasionally.
- Arrange tortillas on a work surface, divide fish fillets, put salsa on top, split mixed vegetables and mixed greens, and finish with parmesan.
- Roll your tacos, set them in the preheated air fryer, and cook for another 6 minutes at 350 degrees F.
- Serve fish tacos for breakfast by dividing them among plates.
- Enjoy!

Breakfast Frittata

Preparation Time-5 minutes | Cook Time-30 minutes | Servings-2 | Difficulty-Easy

Nutritional Facts- Calories-227 | Fats-10.8g | Carbohydrates-12g | Proteins-20g

Ingredients

- Four lightly beaten eggs
- Quarter pound of breakfast sausage fully cooked and crumbled
- One pinch of cayenne pepper (Optional)
- Cooking spray
- Two tablespoons of diced red bell pepper
- One chopped green onion
- A half-cup of shredded Cheddar-Monterey Jack cheese blend

Instructions

- Mix well in small bowl eggs, sausage, cheddar cheese, cayenne, bell pepper and onion.
- Heat the air fryer to 360 degrees F.
- Next, spray with a cooking spray a nonstick pan.

- Put the egg in the pan.
- Then cook it in the air for eighteen to twenty minutes.

Breakfast Muffins

Preparation Time-10 minutes | Cook Time-10 minutes| Servings-2 | Difficulty-Easy

Nutritional Facts- Calories- 276| Fats-12g |Carbohydrates-10.2g |Proteins-17.4g

Ingredients

- Two whole-wheat English muffins
- Four slices of bacon
- Pepper
- Two eggs

Instructions

- Crack an egg each into ramekins, then season with pepper.
- Place the ramekins in your preheated air fryer at 390 F.
- Allow cooking for 6-minutes with the bacon and muffins alongside.
- Remove the muffins from the air fryer after a few minutes and split them.
- When the bacon and eggs are done cooking, add two pieces of bacon and one egg to each egg muffin. Serve when hot.

Breakfast Mushroom Quiche

Preparation Time-10 minutes | Cook Time-10 minutes | Servings-2 | Difficulty-Easy

Nutritional Facts- Calories-206 | Fats-6.9g |Carbohydrates-19g |Proteins-9g

Ingredients

- One tablespoon of flour
- One tablespoon of softened butter
- 9-inch pie dough
- One chopped button mushroom
- One tablespoon of chopped ham
- Two eggs
- One chopped small yellow onion
- A quarter cup of heavy cream
- A pinch of nutmeg, ground
- Salt and black pepper to the taste
- Half teaspoon of dried thyme

- A quarter cup of Swiss cheese, grated

Instructions

- Dust a working surface with the flour and roll the pie dough.
- Press it into the bottom of the pie pan your air fryer has.
- In a bowl, mix butter with mushrooms, ham, onion, eggs, heavy cream, salt, pepper, thyme and nutmeg and whisk well.
- Add this over pie crust, spread, sprinkle Swiss cheese all over and place the pie pan in your air fryer.
- Cook your quiche at 400 degrees F for 10 minutes.
- Slice and serve for breakfast.
- Enjoy!

Breakfast Pea Tortilla

Preparation Time-10 minutes | Cook Time-7 minutes | Servings-2 | Difficulty-Easy

Nutritional Facts- Calories-143 | Fats-6.9g |Carbohydrates-12.9g |Proteins-6.9g

Ingredients

- A quarter-pound of baby peas
- One tablespoon of butter
- Half cup of yogurt
- Two eggs
- Two tablespoons of chopped mint
- Salt and black pepper to the taste

Instructions

- Heat up a pan that fits your air fryer with the butter over medium heat, add peas, stir and cook for a couple of minutes.
- Meanwhile, in a bowl, mix half of the yogurt with salt, pepper, eggs and mint and whisk well.
- Pour this over the peas, toss, introduce in your air fryer and cook at 350 degrees F for 7 minutes.
- Spread the rest of the yogurt over your tortilla, slice and serve.
- Enjoy!

Breakfast Pizza

Preparation Time-10 minutes | Cook Time-15 minutes | Servings-2 | Difficulty-Easy

Nutritional Facts- Calories-311 | Fats-10.8g |Carbohydrates-43g |Proteins-9.9g

Ingredients

- Half pound of bacon
- Four ounces of crescent dinner rolls
- One cup of cheddar cheese
- Three eggs

Instructions

- Place the rolls on the pizza pan.
- Mix cheese, eggs, and bacon in a bowl.
- Pour the mixture over the crust.
- Place the pan in the Air Fryer Grill.
- Set the Air Fryer Grill to the pizza function.
- Cook for 15 minutes at 370F.
- Serve immediately

Breakfast Pizzas with English Muffins

Preparation Time-5 minutes| Cook Time-35 minutes| Servings-2 | Difficulty-Easy

Nutritional Facts- Calories-283| Fats-15g|Carbohydrates-13.8g|Proteins-23g

Ingredients

- Olive Oil Spray
- One Pound of cooked ground Sausage
- Three English Muffins, Sliced in half
- Six Eggs, Cooked & Scrambled
- Fennel Seed (Optional)
- A half-cup of Shredded Colby Jack Cheese

Instructions

- First, ensure that eggs and sausage are properly cooked.
- Spray the oil cooking spray into the air fryer's basket.
- You will have to fill it in 2 batches, with each batch containing three or more.
- Spray with a light coat of olive oil spray the English muffins. Then top them with cooked sausage and cooked eggs.

- Next, the cheese is added to the top of each one. Moreover, you can also use fennel seed, but it is usually not required.
- Cook for five minutes at 355 degrees F.
- Remove the muffins cautiously and repeat the process for the additional muffins.

Breakfast Potatoes

Preparation Time-10 minutes| Cook Time- 55 minutes| Servings-2 | Difficulty-Moderate

Nutritional Facts-Calories-156| Fats-7.8g|Carbohydrates-15.9g|Proteins-4.8g

Ingredients

- Half teaspoon of salt
- A quarter chopped onion
- Two minced garlic cloves
- A quarter teaspoon of pepper
- One and a half pounds of potatoes
- Half teaspoon of paprika
- One chopped green bell pepper
- One tablespoon of olive oil

Instructions

- Wash the potatoes and bell pepper.
- Dice the potatoes and boil them for 30 minutes in water. Pat, it dry after 30 minutes.
- Then onion, bell pepper and potatoes are to be chopped. Use minced garlic.
- Apply all the ingredients and mix them together in a dish. Put it into an air-fryer.
- Cook in an air fryer for 10 minutes at 390-400 degrees F. Shake the basket and cook for another 10 minutes, then shake the basket again and cook for another 5 minutes, for a total of 25 minutes.
- Serve and enjoy.

Breakfast Sausage

Preparation Time- 5 minutes| Cook Time-15 minutes| Servings-2-4 | Difficulty-Easy

Nutritional Facts- Calories-270 | Fats-12.9g|Carbohydrates-7.8g|Proteins-30g

Ingredients

- Half pound ground pork
- Half pound ground turkey
- One teaspoon of fennel seeds

- One teaspoon of dry-rubbed sage
- One teaspoon of garlic powder
- One teaspoon of paprika
- One teaspoon of sea salt
- One teaspoon of dried thyme
- One tablespoon of real maple syrup

Instructions

- Start by combining in a wide bowl the pork and turkey together. Mix the rest of the ingredients together in a small bowl: fennel, sage, salt, powdered garlic, paprika and thyme. Mix spices into the meat and keep combining until the spices are thoroughly blended.
- Spoon (about 2-3 teaspoons of meat) into balls and then flatten into patties. You would actually have to do this in two batches.
- Fix the temperature and cook for 10 minutes at 370 degrees F. Remove and repeat for the leftover sausage in the air fryer.

Breakfast Sausage Casserole

Preparation Time-10 minutes| Cook Time-30 minutes| Servings-2 | Difficulty-Easy

Nutritional Facts- Calories-244 | Fats-12g|Carbohydrates-13.8g|Proteins-20g

Ingredients

- One pound of hash browns
- One pound of ground breakfast sausage
- One diced yellow bell pepper
- A quarter cup of diced sweet onion
- Four eggs
- One diced green bell pepper
- One diced red bell pepper

Instructions

- Line with a foil the air fryer's basket.
- At the bottom, put the hash browns.
- Top with uncooked sausage.
- The onions and peppers should be uniformly placed on top.
- Cook for 10 minutes at 355 degrees F.
- Open the air fryer and, if necessary, mix the casserole a little.
- Crack eggs in a bowl, then pour on the casserole top.

- Cook for another ten minutes at 355 degrees F. Enjoy with pepper and salt as per your taste.

Breakfast Scramble Casserole

Preparation Time-25 minutes | Cook Time-11 minutes | Servings-2 | Difficulty-Easy

Nutritional Facts- Calories-348 | Fats-26g|Carbohydrates-4g|Proteins-30g

Ingredients

- Four slices of bacon
- Cooking oil
- Salt
- Four eggs
- Pepper
- Half cup of chopped red bell pepper
- Half cup of chopped green bell pepper
- Half cup of chopped onion
- 1/3 cup of shredded Cheddar cheese

Instructions

- In a pan, cook the bacon, 5 to 7 minutes, flipping to evenly crisp. Dry out on paper towels, crumble, and set aside. In a medium bowl, whisk the eggs. Add salt and pepper to taste.
- Spray a barrel pan with cooking oil. Make sure to cover the bottom and sides of the pan. Add the beaten eggs, crumbled bacon, red bell pepper, green bell pepper, and onion to the pan. Place the pan in the air fryer. Cook for 6 minutes. Open the air fryer and sprinkle the cheese over the casserole. Cook for an additional 2 minutes. Cool before serving.

Breakfast Strata

Preparation Time- 15 minutes| Cook Time-Three hours | Servings-2 | Difficulty-Hard

Nutritional Facts- Calories-140 | Fats-4.8g |Carbohydrates-6g|Proteins-15.9g

Ingredients

- Four eggs
- Half packs of croutons
- A quarter pack of cheddar
- Salt and pepper
- A quarter pack of chopped spinach
- One cup of milk

- One cup of chopped ham
- Half jar of Red Peppers

Instructions

- Preheat the Air Fryer Grill to 135 C or 275 F.
- Spray the pan with a non-stick spray.
- Spread layers of ham, spinach, cheese, and croutons, and red peppers.
- Pour eggs mixed with milk and seasoning in the pan and refrigerate.
- Bake for two hours and leave to rest for a quarter-hour.

Breakfast Stuffed Peppers

Preparation Time-18 minutes | Cook Time-15 minutes | Servings-2 | Difficulty-Easy

Nutritional Facts- Calories-139 | Fats-6.9g | Carbohydrates-4.8g | Proteins-13.8g

Ingredients

- Four eggs
- One teaspoon of olive oil
- One medium-sized bell pepper halved and deseeded
- One pinch of pepper and salt
- One pinch of Sriracha flakes for a bit of spice, optional

Instructions

- Bell peppers should be cut in half lengthwise and the seeds and center removed, but the sides should be left intact like bowls.
- Apply a small amount of olive oil to the exposed edges with your finger (where it was cut).
- In each bell pepper half, crack two eggs. Season with the spices of your choice.
- Place them on a trivet straight in your air fryer of choice.
- Close your air fryer's lid.
- Turn the machine on and set the temperature to 390 degrees Fahrenheit for 13 minutes.
- Alternatively, if you'd like your bell pepper and egg to be less brown on the outside, add just one egg to your pepper and cook for 15 minutes at 330°F in the air fryer. (for a hard-boiled egg consistency)

Breakfast Tomato Quiche

Preparation Time-10 minutes | Cook Time-30 minutes | Servings-2 | Difficulty-Moderate

Nutritional Facts- Calories-241 | Fats-7.8g | Carbohydrates-16.8g | Proteins-7.8g

Ingredients

- Four tablespoons of chopped yellow onion
- Four eggs
- Half cup of milk
- One cup of shredded gouda cheese
- Half cup of chopped tomatoes
- Salt and black pepper to the taste
- Cooking spray

Instructions

- Grease a ramekin with cooking spray.
- Crack eggs, add onion, milk, cheese, tomatoes, salt and pepper and stir.
- Add this to your air fryer's pan and cook at 340 degrees F for 30 minutes. Serve hot.
- Enjoy!

Breakfast Veggie Mix

Preparation Time-10 minutes | Cook Time-25 minutes | Servings-2 | Difficulty-Easy

Nutritional Facts- Calories-231 | Fats-9g | Carbohydrates-12.9g | Proteins-20g

Ingredients

- Half sliced yellow onion
- Half chopped red bell pepper
- Half chopped gold potato
- Two tablespoons of olive oil
- Three ounces of brie, trimmed and cubed
- Four ounces of cubed sourdough bread
- Two ounces of grated parmesan
- Four eggs
- Two tablespoons of mustard
- One cup of milk
- Salt and black pepper to the taste

Instructions

- Heat up your air fryer at 350 degrees F, add oil, onion, potato and bell pepper and cook for 5 minutes.

- In a bowl, mix eggs with milk, salt, pepper and mustard and whisk well.
- Add bread and brie to your air fryer, add half of the eggs, mix and add half of the parmesan as well.
- Add the rest of the bread and parmesan, toss just a little bit and cook for 20 minutes.
- Divide among plates and serve for breakfast.
- Enjoy!

Broccoli Quiche

Preparation Time- 10 minutes | Cook Time-10 minutes | Servings-2 | Difficulty-Easy

Nutritional Facts- Calories-173 | Fats-12.9g | Carbohydrates-6.9g | Proteins-9.9g

Ingredients

- Two eggs
- Two tablespoons of grated cheddar cheese
- Eight broccoli florets
- Six tablespoons of heavy cream

Instructions

- Spray 5-inch quiche dish with cooking spray.
- In a bowl, whisk the egg with cheese, cream, pepper, and salt. Add broccoli and stir well.
- Pour egg mixture into the quiche dish.
- Place dish into the air fryer basket and cook at 325 F for 10 minutes.

Buttermilk Breakfast Biscuits

Preparation Time-10 minutes | Cook Time-10 minutes | Servings-2 | Difficulty-Easy

Nutritional Facts- Calories-192 | Fats-7.8g | Carbohydrates-13.8g | Proteins-12g

Ingredients

- One cup of white flour
- Half cup of self-rising flour
- A quarter teaspoon of baking soda
- Half teaspoon of baking powder
- One teaspoon of sugar
- Two tablespoons of cold and cubed butter plus One tablespoon of melted butter
- 3/4 cup of buttermilk
- Maple syrup for serving

Instructions

- In a bowl, mix white flour with self-rising flour, baking soda, baking powder and sugar and stir.
- Add cold butter and stir using your hands.
- Add buttermilk, stir until you obtain a dough and transfer to a floured working surface.
- Roll your dough and cut five to six pieces using a round cutter.
- Arrange biscuits in your air fryer's cake pan, brush them with melted butter and cook at 400 degrees F for 8 minutes.
- Serve them for breakfast with some maple syrup on top.
- Enjoy!

Cheese Air Fried Bake

Preparation Time-10 minutes | Cook Time-20 minutes | Servings-2 | Difficulty-Moderate

Nutritional Facts- Calories-214 | Fats-7.8g | Carbohydrates-12.9g | Proteins-13.8g

Ingredients

- Two bacon slices, crumbled and cooked
- Two cups of milk
- Two cups of shredded cheddar cheese
- Half pound of breakfast sausage, chopped and casings removed
- Two eggs
- Half teaspoon of onion powder
- Black pepper and salt to the taste
- Two tablespoons of chopped parsley
- Cooking spray

Instructions

- In a bowl, mix eggs with cheese, milk, onion powder, pepper salt, and parsley and whisk well.
- Spray your air fryer with cooking spray, preheat to 320°F, then add the sausage and bacon.
- Cook for 20 minutes after adding the eggs, mixing them up well.
- Serve by dividing the mixture among plates.
- Enjoy!

Cheesy Tater Tot Breakfast Bake

Preparation Time-5 minutes| Cook Time-20 minutes| Servings-2 | Difficulty-Easy

Nutritional Facts- Calories-518 | Fats-30g|Carbohydrates-31g |Proteins-30g

Ingredients

- Two eggs
- One cup of milk
- One teaspoon of onion powder
- Salt
- Pepper
- Cooking oil
- Twelve ounces of ground chicken sausage
- One pound of frozen tater tots
- 1/3 cup of shredded Cheddar cheese

Instructions

- In a medium bowl, whisk the eggs. Add the milk, onion powder, and salt and pepper to taste. Stir to combine.
- Spray a skillet with cooking oil and set over medium-high heat. Add the ground sausage. Using a spatula or spoon, break the sausage into smaller pieces. Cook the sausage is brown. Remove from heat and set aside.
- Spray a barrel pan with cooking oil. Make sure to cover the bottom and sides of the pan.
- Place the tater tots in the barrel pan. Cook for 6 minutes
- Open the air fryer and shake the pan, then add the egg mixture and cooked sausage. Cook for an additional 6 minutes. Open the air fryer and sprinkle the cheese over the tater tot bake. Cook for another 2 to 3 minutes
- Cool before serving.

Cherries Risotto

Preparation Time-10 minutes | Cook Time-12 minutes | Servings-2 | Difficulty-Easy

Nutritional Facts- Calories-158 | Fats-7.8g |Carbohydrates-13.8g |Proteins-7.8g

Ingredients

- One and a quarter cups of Arborio rice
- One teaspoon of cinnamon powder
- A quarter cup of brown sugar

- A pinch of salt
- Two tablespoons of butter
- One apple cored and sliced
- One cup of apple juice
- One and a half cups of milk
- A quarter cup of dried cherries

Instructions

- Heat up a pan that fist your air fryer with the butter over medium heat, add rice, stir and cook for 4-5 minutes.
- Add sugar, apples, apple juice, milk, cinnamon and cherries, stir, introduce in your air fryer and cook at 350 degrees F for 8 minutes.
- Divide into bowls and serve for breakfast.
- Enjoy!

Cinnamon and Cheese Pancake

Preparation Time- 10 minutes| Cook Time- 20 minutes | Servings-2 | Difficulty-Easy

Nutritional Facts- Calories-140 | Fats-10.5g |Carbohydrates-5.4g |Proteins-22.5g

Ingredients

- Two eggs
- Two cups of reduced-fat cream cheese
- Half teaspoon of cinnamon
- One pack of Stevia

Instructions

- Adjust the Air Fryer to 330 degrees F.
- In a blender, mix cream cheese, cinnamon, eggs, and stevia.
- Set a quarter of the mixture into the air fryer basket. Cook for 2 minutes on all sides. Repeat the process with the remaining portion of the mixture. Serve.

Cinnamon and Cream Cheese Oats

Preparation Time-10 minutes | Cook Time-25 minutes | Servings-2 | Difficulty-Easy

Nutritional Facts- Calories-158 | Fats-7.8g |Carbohydrates-13.8g |Proteins-7.8g

Ingredients

- One cup of steel oats
- One and a half cups of milk

- One tablespoon of butter
- 3⁄4 cup of raisins
- One teaspoon of cinnamon powder
- A quarter cup of brown sugar
- Two tablespoons of white sugar
- Two ounces cream cheese, soft

Instructions

- Heat up a pan that fits your air fryer with the butter over medium heat, add oats, stir and toast them for 3 minutes.
- Add milk and raisins, stir, introduce in your air fryer and cook at 350 degrees F for 20 minutes.
- Meanwhile, in a bowl, mix cinnamon with brown sugar and stir.
- In a second bowl, mix white sugar with cream cheese and whisk.
- Divide oats into bowls and top each with cinnamon and cream cheese.
- Enjoy!

Creamy Breakfast Tofu

Preparation Time-15 minutes | Cook Time-20 minutes | Servings-2 | Difficulty-Moderate

Nutritional Facts- Calories-110 | Fats-4.8g |Carbohydrates-7.8g |Proteins-9g

Ingredients

Half a block firm tofu, pressed and cubed
One teaspoon of rice vinegar
Two tablespoons of soy sauce
- Two teaspoons of sesame oil
- One tablespoon of potato starch
- One cup of Greek yogurt

Instructions

- In a bowl, mix tofu cubes with vinegar, soy sauce and oil, toss, and leave aside for 15 minutes.
- Dip tofu cubes in potato starch, toss, transfer to your air fryer, heat up at 370 degrees F and cook for 20minutes shaking halfway.
- Divide into bowls and serve for breakfast with some Greek yogurt on the side.
- Enjoy!

Creamy Hash Browns

Preparation Time-10 minutes | Cook Time-20 minutes | Servings-2 | Difficulty-Easy

Nutritional Facts- Calories-261 | Fats-10.8g |Carbohydrates-15.9g |Proteins-19g

Ingredients

- One pound of hash browns
- Half cup of whole milk
- Two chopped bacon slices
- Two ounces of cream cheese
- One chopped yellow onion
- One cup of shredded cheddar cheese
- Two chopped green onions
- Salt and black pepper to the taste
- Two eggs
- Cooking spray

Instructions

- Heat up your air fryer at 350 degrees F and grease it with cooking spray.
- In a bowl, mix eggs with milk, cream cheese, cheddar cheese, bacon, onion, salt and pepper and whisk well.
- Add hash browns to your air fryer, add eggs, mix over them and cook for 20 minutes.
- Divide among plates and serve.
- Enjoy!

Dates and Millet Pudding

Preparation Time-10 minutes | Cook Time-15 minutes | Servings-2 | Difficulty-Easy

Nutritional Facts- Calories-158 | Fats-7.8g |Carbohydrates-13.8g |Proteins-7.8g

Ingredients

- Seven ounces of milk
- Three ounces of water
- 2/3 cup of millet
- Two pitted dates
- Honey for serving

Instructions

- Put the millet in a pan that fits your air fryer, add dates, milk and water, stir, introduce in your air fryer and cook at 360 degrees F for 15 minutes.
- Divide among plates, drizzle honey on top and

serve for breakfast.

- Enjoy!

Delicious Potato Frittata

Preparation Time-10 minutes | Cook Time-30 minutes | Servings-2 | Difficulty-Moderate

Nutritional Facts- Calories-198 | Fats-12.9g | Carbohydrates-34g | Proteins-12g

Ingredients

- Two ounces of chopped jarred roasted red bell peppers
- Four whisked eggs
- Half cup of grated parmesan
- Three minced garlic cloves
- One tablespoon of chopped parsley
- Salt and black pepper to the taste
- Two tablespoons of chopped chives
- Four potato wedges
- Three tablespoons of ricotta cheese
- Cooking spray

Instructions

- In a bowl, mix eggs with red peppers, garlic, parsley, salt, pepper and ricotta and whisk well.
- Heat up your air fryer at 300 degrees F and grease it with cooking spray.
- Add half of the potato wedges to the bottom and sprinkle half of the cheese (parmesan) all over.
- Add half of the egg mix, add the rest of the potatoes and the rest of the parmesan.
- Add the rest of the eggs, mix, sprinkle chives and cook for 20 minutes.
- Divide among plates and serve for breakfast.
- Enjoy!

Delicious Tofu and Mushrooms

Preparation Time-10 minutes | Cook Time-10 minutes | Servings-2 | Difficulty-Easy

Nutritional Facts- Calories-142 | Fats-4g | Carbohydrates-7.8g | Proteins-12g

Ingredients

- One tofu block pressed and cut into medium pieces
- One cup of panko bread crumbs
- Salt and black pepper to the taste
- Half tablespoon of flour
- One egg
- One tablespoon of minced mushrooms

Instructions

In a bowl, mix egg with mushrooms, flour, salt and pepper and whisk well.

Dip tofu pieces in egg mix, then dredge them in panko bread crumbs, place them in your air fryer and cook at 350 degrees F for 10 minutes.

Serve them for breakfast right away. Enjoy!

Egg Muffins

Preparation Time-10 minutes | Cook Time-15 minutes | Servings-2 | Difficulty-Easy

Nutritional Facts- Calories-251 | Fats-6g | Carbohydrates-9g | Proteins-30g

Ingredients

- One egg
- Two tablespoons of olive oil
- Three tablespoons of milk
- Two ounces of white flour
- One tablespoon of baking powder
- One ounce of grated parmesan
- A splash of Worcestershire sauce

Instructions

- Combine egg, flour, baking powder, oil, milk, Worcestershire, and parmesan in a mixing dish, whisk well, and divide among four silicon muffin cups.
- Place cup of in the frying basket of your air fryer, cover, and cook for 15 minutes at 392 degrees F.
- For breakfast, serve warm.
- Enjoy!

Egg White Omelet

Preparation Time-10 minutes | Cook Time-15 minutes | Servings-2 | Difficulty-Easy

Nutritional Facts- Calories-134 | Fats-6g | Carbohydrates-12g | Proteins-7.8g

Ingredients

- One cup of egg whites
- A quarter cup of chopped tomato

- Two tablespoons of skim milk
- A quarter cup of chopped mushrooms
- Two tablespoons of chopped chives
- Salt and black pepper to the taste

Instructions

- In a bowl, mix egg whites with tomato, milk, mushrooms, chives, salt and pepper, whisk well and pour into your air fryer's pan.
- Cook at 320 degrees F for 15 minutes, cool omelet down, slice, divide among plates and serve.
- Enjoy!

Eggs Casserole

Preparation Time-10 minutes | Cook Time-30 minutes | Servings-2 | Difficulty-Moderate

Nutritional Facts- Calories-300 | Fats-4.8g |Carbohydrates-12.9g |Proteins-9g

Ingredients

- Half pound of ground turkey
- One tablespoon of olive oil
- Half teaspoon of chili powder
- Four eggs
- Half cubed sweet potato
- One cup of baby spinach
- Salt and black pepper to the taste
- One chopped tomato for serving

Instructions

- In a bowl, mix eggs with salt, pepper, chili powder, potato, spinach, turkey and sweet potato and whisk well.
- Heat up your air fryer at 350 degrees F, add oil and heat it up.
- Add eggs, mix, spread into your air fryer, cover and cook for 25 minutes.
- Divide among plates and serve for breakfast.
- Enjoy!

Espresso Oatmeal

Preparation Time-10 minutes | Cook Time-20 minutes | Servings-2 | Difficulty-Easy

Nutritional Facts- Calories-161 | Fats-7.8g |Carbohydrates-15g |Proteins-7.8g

Ingredients

- Half cup of milk
- Half cup of steel-cut oats
- One and a half cups of water
- One tablespoon of sugar
- One teaspoon of espresso powder
- Two teaspoons of vanilla extract

Instructions

- In a pan that fits your air fryer, mix oats with water, sugar, milk and espresso powder, stir, introduce in
- your air fryer and cook at 360 degrees F for 17 minutes.
- Add vanilla extract, stir, leave everything aside for 5 minutes, divide into bowls and serve for breakfast.
- Enjoy!

Fast Eggs and Tomatoes

Preparation Time-5 minutes | Cook Time-10 minutes | Servings-2 | Difficulty-Easy

Nutritional Facts- Calories-198 | Fats-7.8g |Carbohydrates-12g |Proteins-13.8g

Ingredients

- Two eggs
- One ounce of milk
- One tablespoon of grated parmesan
- Salt and black pepper to the taste
- Four cherry tomatoes halved
- Cooking spray

Instructions

- Grease your air fryer with cooking spray and heat it up at 200 degrees F.
- In a bowl, mix eggs with cheese, milk, salt and pepper and whisk.
- Add this mix to your air fryer and cook for 6 minutes.
- Add tomatoes, cook your scrambled eggs for 3 minutes, divide among plates and serve.
- Enjoy!

Fried Egg

Preparation Time- 5 minutes| Cook Time- 5 minutes| Servings-2 | Difficulty-Easy

Nutritional Facts- Calories-90 | Fats-6.9g |Carbohydrates-6g|Proteins-13g

Ingredients

- Two pastured eggs
- One teaspoon of salt
- Two teaspoons of cracked black pepper

Instructions

- Grease the fryer pan with olive oil, then crack the egg in it.
- Insert the fryer pan into the air fryer, close the lid. Then adjust the fryer to 370°F.
- After 3minutes, open the air fryer to check if the egg needs more cooking. If yes, leave it for an extra 1 minute.
- Serve the egg. Add salt and black pepper to season it.

Garlic Potatoes with Bacon

Preparation Time-10 minutes | Cook Time-20 minutes | Servings-2 | Difficulty-Easy

Nutritional Facts- Calories-185 | Fats-9g |Carbohydrates-15g |Proteins-13.8g

Ingredients

- Two potatoes, peeled and cut into medium cubes
- Three minced garlic cloves
- Two chopped bacon slices
- One chopped rosemary spring
- One tablespoon of olive oil
- Salt and black pepper to the taste
- Two eggs

Instructions

- In your air fryer's pan, mix oil with potatoes, garlic, bacon, rosemary, salt, pepper and eggs and whisk.
- Cook potatoes at 400 degrees F for 20 minutes, divide everything among plates and serve for breakfast.
- Enjoy!

Grilled Cheese

Preparation Time- 5 minutes| Cook Time- 10 minutes| Servings-2 | Difficulty-Easy

Nutritional Facts- Calories-214 | Fats-11.1g |Carbohydrates-17g |Proteins-13.2g

Ingredients

- Four slices of brown bread
- Half cup of shredded sharp cheddar cheese
- A quarter cup of melted butter

Instructions

- Adjust your air fryer to 360F.
- In separate bowls, place cheese and butter.
- Melt butter and brush it onto the four slices of bread.
- Place cheese on two sides of bread slices.
- Put sandwiches together and place them into the cooking basket.
- Cook for 5 minutes and serve warm.

Ham Breakfast

Preparation Time-10 minutes | Cook Time-15 minutes | Servings-2 | Difficulty-Easy

Nutritional Facts- Calories-200 | Fats-6.9g |Carbohydrates-12.9g |Proteins-15g

Ingredients

- Two cups of cubed French bread
- Two ounces of chopped green chilies
- Three and a half ounces of cubed ham
- Two ounces of shredded cheddar cheese
- One cup of milk
- Two eggs
- One tablespoon of mustard
- Salt and black pepper to the taste
- Cooking spray

Instructions

- Heat up your air fryer at 350 degrees F and grease it with cooking spray.
- In a bowl, mix eggs with milk, cheese, mustard, salt and pepper and stir.
- Add bread cubes in your air fryer and mix with chilies and ham.
- Add eggs, mix, spread and cook for 15 minutes.
- Divide among plates and serve.

- Enjoy!

Ham Breakfast Pie

Preparation Time-10minutes | Cook Time-25minutes | Servings-2 | Difficulty-Moderate

Nutritional Facts- Calories-387 | Fats-27g |Carbohydrates-21.9g |Proteins-20g

Ingredients

- Five ounces of crescent rolls dough
- One whisked egg
- One cup of grated cheddar cheese
- One tablespoon of grated parmesan
- One cup of cooked and chopped ham
- Salt and black pepper to the taste
- Cooking spray

Instructions

- Cooking spray the bottom of your air fryer pan and press half of the crescent roll dough on it.
- In a mixing dish, whisk together the eggs, cheddar cheese, parmesan cheese, salt, and pepper. Pour over the dough.
- Spread ham on top, then cut the remaining of the crescent roll dough into strips, stack them over the ham, and bake for 25 minutes at 300 degrees F.
- It can be served as breakfast by slicing the pie.
- Enjoy!

Ham Rolls

Preparation Time-10 minutes | Cook Time-10 minutes | Servings-2 | Difficulty-Easy

Nutritional Facts- Calories-180 | Fats-7.8g |Carbohydrates-15.9g |Proteins-12.9g

Ingredients

- One sheet puff pastry
- Two handfuls of grated gruyere cheese
- Four teaspoons of mustard
- Four ham slices, chopped

Instructions

- Roll out puff pastry on a working surface, divide cheese, ham and mustard, roll tight and cut into medium rounds.

- Place all rolls in the air fryer and cook for 10 minutes at 370 degrees F.
- Divide rolls among plates and serve.
- Enjoy!

Hard-Boiled Eggs

Preparation Time-10 minutes | Cook Time-15 minutes | Servings-2 | Difficulty-Easy

Nutritional Facts- Calories-105| Fats-7.8g |Carbohydrates-2.1g|Proteins-30g

Ingredients

- Two eggs
- Salt and pepper to taste

Instructions

- Preheat the air fryer to 270°F.
- Cook the eggs in the air fryer for 15-17 minutes, preferably on a wire rack.
- Place the eggs in a bowl of cold water and ice for at least 5 minutes to chill.
- Eggs can be peeled and seasoned with salt and pepper, or they can be refrigerated for up to a week.

Homemade Cherry Breakfast Tarts

Preparation Time-15 minutes| Cook Time-20 minutes | Servings-2 | Difficulty-Easy

Nutritional Facts- Calories-119 | Fats-4g |Carbohydrates-19g |Proteins-1.5g

Ingredients

For the frosting

A quarter cup of vanilla yogurt

- A half-ounce of cream cheese
- One teaspoon of stevia
- Rainbow sprinkles

For the tarts

- One refrigerated pie crust
- A quarter cup of cherry preserves
- One teaspoon of cornstarch
- Cooking oil

Instructions

To make the tarts

- On a flat surface, place the piecrusts. Cut each pie

crust into three rectangles with a knife or pizza cutter, for a total of six.

- Combine the preserves and cornstarch in a small bowl. Mix thoroughly.
- One tablespoon of the preserves mixture should be spooned onto the top half of each pie crust.
- To close the tart, fold the bottoms of each piece up. Using the back of a fork, press along the sides of each tart to seal it.
- Place the breakfast tarts in the air fryer after sprinkling them with cooking oil. It's not a good idea to pile the breakfast tarts on top of one other. If heaped together, they will stick together. It's possible that you'll have to cook them in two batches. 10 minutes in the oven
- Before removing the breakfast tarts from the air fryer, let them cool completely.

To make the frosting

- Combine the cream cheese, yogurt, and stevia in a small mixing dish. Mix thoroughly.
- Serve the breakfast tarts with a layer of icing and sprinkles on top.

Long Beans Omelet

Preparation Time-10 minutes | Cook Time-10 minutes | Servings-2 | Difficulty-Easy

Nutritional Facts- Calories-161 | Fats-7.8g |Carbohydrates-15g |Proteins-7.8g

Ingredients

- Half teaspoon of soy sauce
- One tablespoon of olive oil
- Two eggs
- A pinch of salt and black pepper
- Two garlic cloves, minced
- Two long beans, trimmed and sliced

Instructions

- In a bowl, mix eggs with a pinch of salt, black pepper and soy sauce and whisk well.
- Heat up your air fryer at 320 degrees F, add oil and garlic, stir and brown for 1 minute.
- Add long beans and eggs, mix, spread and cook for 10 minutes.
- Divide omelet among plates and serve for breakfast.

- Enjoy!

Low Carb Air Fryer Baked Eggs

Preparation Time-5 minutes | Cook Time-15 minutes | Servings-2 | Difficulty-Easy

Nutritional Facts- Calories-146 | Fats-6g|Carbohydrates-12g|Proteins-10.8g

Ingredients

- Black pepper, to taste
- One tablespoon of milk
- Two to Four teaspoons of grated cheese
- Two large eggs
- Cooking Spray for ramekins or muffin cups
- Two tablespoons of sautéed fresh spinach or thawed frozen spinach
- Salt, to taste

Instructions

- Spray with oil spray inside of the ramekin or silicone muffin cup.
- Add the muffin or ramekin cup with egg, cream, cheese and spinach.
- Then season with pepper and salt. Gently mix the egg whites with the ingredients without separating the yolk.
- Air Fry for roughly around 10 to 12 minutes at 330 ° F.
- It may need a little longer to cook in the ramekin. Cook for less time if you like runny yolks. After 5 minutes, keep testing the eggs to ensure that the egg is of your desired texture.

Low-Carb Breakfast Casserole Air Fryer

Preparation Time-10 minutes | Cook Time-45 minutes | Servings-2 | Difficulty-Moderate

Nutritional Facts- Calories-159 | Fats-6.9g|Carbohydrates-12g|Proteins-12g

Ingredients

- One teaspoon of fennel seed
- A quarter-pound of ground sausage
- A quarter cup of diced white onion
- A half-cup of shredded Colby Jack Cheese
- One diced Green Bell Pepper
- Two whole Eggs, Beaten
- A half teaspoon of Garlic Salt

Instructions

- Sauté the sausages in the skillet inserted in the air fryer.
- Insert the onion and pepper and simmer until the vegetables are soft and the sausage is cooked, along with the ground sausage.
- Spray an 8.75 inches pan or the air fryer with the cooking spray.
- Place the mixture of ground sausages on the bottom of the pan.
- Cover with cheese uniformly.
- Pour the beaten eggs uniformly over the sausage and cheese.
- Over the eggs, add fennel seed and garlic salt uniformly.
- In the air fryer, put the dish straight into the air fryer's basket and cook at 390 degrees F for 15 minutes.
- Remove and serve wisely.

Mushroom Oatmeal

Preparation Time-10 minutes | Cook Time-20 minutes | Servings-2 | Difficulty-Easy

Nutritional Facts- Calories-161 | Fats-7.8g |Carbohydrates-15g |Proteins-7.8g

Ingredients

- Half chopped small yellow onion
- Half cup of steel-cut oats
- Two minced garlic cloves
- Two tablespoons of butter
- Half cup of water
- Seven ounces of canned chicken stock
- Two chopped thyme springs
- Two tablespoons of extra virgin olive oil
- A quarter cup of grated gouda cheese
- Four ounces of sliced mushroom
- Salt and black pepper to the taste

Instructions

- Heat up a pan that fits your air fryer with the butter over medium heat, add onions and garlic, stir and cook for 4 minutes.
- Add oats, water, salt, pepper, stock and thyme, stir, introduce in your air fryer and cook at 360 degrees F for 16 minutes.

- Meanwhile, heat up a pan with the olive oil over medium heat, add mushrooms, cook them for 3 minutes, add to oatmeal and cheese, stir, divide into bowls and serve for breakfast.
- Enjoy!

Oatmeal Casserole

Preparation Time-10 minutes | Cook Time-20 minutes | Servings-2 | Difficulty-Moderate

Nutritional Facts- Calories-288 | Fats-4.8g |Carbohydrates-12.9g |Proteins-9.9g

Ingredients

- One cup of rolled oats
- One teaspoon of baking powder
- A quarter cup of brown sugar
- One teaspoon of cinnamon powder
- A quarter cup of chocolate chips
- A quarter cup of blueberries
- Half banana, peeled and mashed
- One cup of milk
- One egg
- One tablespoon of butter
- Half teaspoon of vanilla extract
- Cooking spray

Instructions

- In a bowl, mix sugar with baking powder, cinnamon, chocolate chips, blueberries and banana and stir.
- In a separate bowl, mix eggs with vanilla extract and butter and stir.
- Heat up your air fryer at 320 degrees F, grease with cooking spray and add oats on the bottom.
- Add cinnamon mix and eggs mix, toss and cook for 20 minutes.
- Stir one more time, divide into bowls and serve for breakfast.
- Enjoy!

Olives, Kale, and Pecorino Baked Eggs

Preparation Time-10 minutes | Cook Time- 12 minutes| Servings-2 | Difficulty-Easy

Nutritional Facts- Calories-119 | Fats-4g |Carbohydrates-19g |Proteins-1.5g

Ingredients

- One cup of roughly chopped kale leaves, stems and center ribs removed
- A quarter cup of grated pecorino cheese
- A quarter cup of olive oil
- One peeled garlic clove
- Three tablespoons of whole almonds
- Kosher salt and ground black pepper to flavor
- Four large eggs
- Two tablespoons of heavy cream
- Three tablespoons of chopped pitted mixed olives

Instructions

- Place the kale, pecorino, olive oil, garlic, almonds, salt, and pepper in a small blender and blitz until well incorporated.
- One at a time, crack the eggs in a baking pan. Drizzle the kale pesto on top of the egg whites. Top the yolks with the cream and swirl together the yolks and the pesto.
- Bring the pan into the air fryer oven. Press the Power Button. Cook at 300°F (150°C) for 11 minutes.
- When cooked, the top should be browned, and the eggs should be set.
- Set the eggs to cool for 5 minutes. Scatter the olives on top and serve warm.

Omelet Frittata

Preparation Time-10 minutes | Cook Time-8 minutes| Servings-2 | Difficulty-Easy

Nutritional Facts- Calories-160 | Fats-9.9g|Carbohydrates-4g|Proteins-12g

Ingredients

- Three lightly beaten eggs
- Two tablespoons of cheddar cheese, shredded
- Two tablespoons of heavy cream
- Two sliced mushrooms
- A small quarter onion, chopped
- A quarter bell pepper, diced
- Pepper
- Salt

Instructions

- In a bowl, whisk eggs with cream, vegetables, pepper, and salt.

- Preheat the air fryer to 400 F.
- Pour egg mixture into the air fryer pan. Place pan in air fryer basket and cook for 5 minutes
- Add shredded cheese on top of the frittata and cook for 1 minute more.
- Serve and enjoy.

Onion Frittata

Preparation Time-10 minutes | Cook Time-20 minutes | Servings-2 | Difficulty-Easy

Nutritional Facts- Calories-189 | Fats-9g |Carbohydrates-16.8g |Proteins-9.9g

Ingredients

- Four whisked eggs
- One tablespoon of olive oil
- One pound of chopped small potato
- One chopped yellow onion
- Salt and black pepper to the taste
- A half-ounce of grated cheddar cheese
- A quarter cup of sour cream

Instructions

- In a large bowl, mix eggs with potatoes, onions, salt, pepper, cheese and sour cream and whisk well.
- Grease your air fryer's pan with the oil, add eggs mix, place in the air fryer and cook for 20 minutes at 320 degrees F.
- Slice frittata, divide among plates and serve for breakfast.
- Enjoy!

Peanut Butter-Pumpkin Muffins

Preparation Time-10 minutes | Cook Time-25 minutes | Servings-2 | Difficulty-Moderate

Nutritional Facts- Calories-525 | Fats-25g |Carbohydrates-34g |Proteins-41g

Ingredients

- Two tablespoons of powdered peanut butter
- Two tablespoons of finely ground flaxseeds
- Two tablespoons of coconut flour
- One tablespoon of dried cranberries
- One teaspoon of pumpkin pie spice
- Half teaspoon of baking powder
- Half cup of water

- One cup of canned pumpkin
- Two large eggs
- Half teaspoon of vanilla extract
- Cooking spray

Instructions

- In a bowl, use together with the powdered peanut butter, flaxseeds, coconut flour, dried cranberries, pumpkin pie spice, baking powder and water.
- In another bowl, stir together the pumpkin and eggs until smooth.
- Add the pumpkin mixture to the peanut butter mixture. Stir to combine. Add the vanilla extract to the bowl. Mix well.
- Spritz 2 ramekins with cooking spray. Set half of the batter into each ramekin. Place the ramekins on a sheet pan.
- Bring the pan into the air fryer oven. Press the Power Button. Cook at 356 degrees Fahrenheit for 25 minutes.
- When cooking is complete, a toothpick inserted in the center should come out clean. Serve immediately.

Peppered Maple Bacon Knots

Preparation Time-5 minutes | Cook Time-8 minutes | Servings-2 | Difficulty-Easy

Nutritional Facts- Calories-384 | Fats-23g |Carbohydrates-10.5g |Proteins-34.2g

Ingredients

- Half pound of maple smoked center-cut bacon
- A quarter cup of maple syrup
- A quarter cup of brown sugar
- Coarsely cracked black peppercorns to taste

Instructions

- On a clean work surface, tie each bacon strip in a loose knot.
- Stir together the maple syrup and brown sugar in a bowl. Generously brush this mixture over the bacon knots.
- Place the bacon knots in the airflow racks and sprinkle with the coarsely cracked black peppercorns.

- Slide the racks into the air fryer oven. Press the Power Button. Cook at 390F (199C) for 8 minutes.
- After 5 minutes, remove the racks from the air fryer oven and flip the bacon knots. Return the racks to the air fryer oven and continue cooking for 2 to 3 minutes more.
- When cooking is processed, the bacon should be crisp. Detach from the air fryer oven to a paper towel-lined plate. Let the bacon knots cool for a few minutes and serve warm.

Quick Air Fryer Breakfast Pockets

Preparation Time-10 minutes | Cook Time-20 minutes | Servings-2 | Difficulty-Easy

Nutritional Facts- Calories-170 | Fats-9g |Carbohydrates-12g |Proteins-10.2g

Ingredients

- Three eggs
- A half-cup of sausage crumbles, cooked
- Half cup of bacon, cooked
- Half box puff pastry sheets
- A half-cup of shredded cheddar cheese

Instructions

- Cook eggs in the form of regular scrambled eggs. If desired, add meat to the egg mixture while you are cooking.
- Spread puff pastry sheets on a cutting board and use a cookie cutter or knife to cut out rectangles, making sure they are all uniform, so they fit together nicely.
- Spoon half of the pastry rectangles with the preferred combination of egg, meat, and cheese.
- Place a rectangle of pastry on top of the mixture and press the edges together with a sealing fork.
- Spray with spray oil if a shiny, smooth pastry is desired, but it is really optional.
- Place breakfast pockets in the air-fryer basket and cook at 370 degrees F for 8-10 minutes.
- Carefully watch and check for desired doneness every 2-3 minutes.

Rice, Almonds and Raisins Pudding

Preparation Time-5 minutes | Cook Time-10 minutes | Servings-2 | Difficulty-Easy

Nutritional Facts- Calories-158 | Fats-7.8g |Carbohydrates-13.8g |Proteins-7.8g

Ingredients

- Half cup of brown rice
- A quarter cup of coconut chips
- Half cup of milk
- One cup of water
- A quarter cup of maple syrup
- A quarter cup of raisins
- A pinch of cinnamon powder
- A quarter cup of almonds

Instructions

- Place the rice in an air fryer-compatible pan, add the water, and heat on the stove over medium-high heat until the rice is mushy. Drain.
- Stir together the milk, cinnamon, almonds, coconut chips, raisins, and maple syrup, then pour into your air fryer and cook for 8 minutes at 360 degrees F.
- Serve rice pudding in individual dishes.
- Enjoy!

Rustic Breakfast

Preparation Time-10 minutes | Cook Time-15 minutes | Servings-2 | Difficulty-Easy

Nutritional Facts- Calories-312 | Fats-6g |Carbohydrates-15g |Proteins-4.8g

Ingredients

- Four ounces of baby spinach
- Four halved chestnuts mushrooms
- Four halved tomatoes
- One minced garlic clove
- Two chipolatas
- Two chopped bacon slices
- Salt and black pepper to the taste
- Two eggs
- Cooking spray

Instructions

- Add the garlic, tomatoes, and mushrooms to a frying pan that has been greased with oil.

- Add the bacon and chipolatas at the end, as well as the spinach and cracked eggs.
- Season with salt and pepper, then place the pan in the air fryer's frying basket and cook for 13 minutes at 350°F.
- Serve for breakfast by dividing the mixture among dishes.
- Enjoy!

Sausage and Cheese Quiche

Preparation Time-5 minutes | Cook Time-25 minutes | Servings-2 | Difficulty-Easy

Nutritional Facts- Calories-333 | Fats-13.8g |Carbohydrates-27g |Proteins-24g

Ingredients

- Six large eggs
- One cup of heavy cream
- Salt and black pepper, to taste
- Six ounces of sugar-free breakfast sausage
- One cup of shredded Cheddar cheese
- Cooking spray

Instructions

- Coat a casserole dish with cooking spray.
- Beat together the eggs, heavy cream, salt and pepper in a large bowl until creamy. Stir in the breakfast sausage and Cheddar cheese.
- Pour the sausage mixture into the prepared casserole dish.
- Slide the dish into the air fryer oven. Press the Power Button. Cook at 375F (190C) for 25 minutes.
- When done, the top of the quiche should be golden brown, and the eggs will be set.
- Detach from the air fryer oven and let sit for 5 to 10 minutes before serving.

Sausage and Egg Breakfast Burrito

Preparation Time-8 minutes | Cook Time-32 minutes | Servings-2 | Difficulty-Easy

Nutritional Facts- Calories-236 | Fats-12.9g |Carbohydrates-15.9g |Proteins-11.1g

Ingredients

- Salt
- Cooking oil

- Half cup of chopped green bell pepper
- Half cup of salsa
- Half cup of shredded Cheddar cheese
- Two eggs
- Pepper
- Half cup of chopped red bell pepper
- Four ounces of ground chicken sausage
- Two medium (8-inch) flour tortillas

Instructions

- Whisk the eggs in a medium mixing bowl. Season to taste with salt and pepper.
- Preheat a skillet to medium-high. Cooking oil is sprayed over the surface. Toss in the eggs. Scramble the eggs for 2 to 3 minutes, or until they are light and fluffy. Set the eggs aside after removing them from the skillet.
- More oil can be sprayed into the skillet if necessary. Add the red and green bell peppers, chopped. Once the peppers are tender, cook for another 2 to 3 minutes.
- In the same skillet, add the ground sausage. Using a spatula or spoon, break the sausage into smaller pieces. Cook until the sausage has turned a golden brown color.
- Combine the salsa and scrambled eggs in a mixing bowl. To blend, stir everything together. Turn off the heat in the skillet.
- Using a spoon, evenly distribute the mixture onto the tortillas.
- Fold the sides of each tortilla in toward the center and then roll up from the bottom to make the burritos. A toothpick can be used to secure each burrito. Alternatively, a small bit of water can be used to moisten the tortilla's exterior edge.
- Place the burritos in the air fryer after spraying them with cooking oil. Do not stack the items. If the burritos don't all fit in the basket, cook them in batches. 8 minutes in the oven
- Flip the burritos in the air fryer. Heat it for another 2 minutes, or until it's crisp.
- Cheddar cheese should be strewn over the burritos. Allow cooling before serving.

Sausage, Eggs and Cheese Mix

Preparation Time-12 minutes | Cook Time-22 minutes | Servings-2 | Difficulty-Moderate

Nutritional Facts- Calories-320 | Fats-12g |Carbohydrates-12.9g |Proteins-13.8g

Ingredients

- One cup of shredded cheddar cheese
- Four whisked eggs
- Salt and black pepper to the taste
- Five ounces of cooked and crumbled sausages
- One cup of shredded mozzarella cheese
- One cup of milk
- Cooking spray

Instructions

- Whisk together sausages, mozzarella, cheese, eggs, salt, milk, and pepper in a mixing bowl.
- Preheat your air fryer to 380°F, coat it with cooking oil, and add the eggs and sausage mixture. Cook for 20 minutes.
- Serve by dividing the mixture among plates.
- Enjoy!

Scrambled Egg

Preparation Time- 5 minutes| Cook Time-10 minutes| Servings-2 | Difficulty-Easy

Nutritional Facts- Calories-105| Fats-7.8g |Carbohydrates-2.1g|Proteins-6.4g

Ingredients

- Two eggs
- One chopped tomato
- Dash of salt
- One teaspoon of butter
- A quarter cup of cream

Instructions

- Put the eggs in a bowl, then add salt and cream. Whisk until fluffy.
- Adjust the air fryer to 300 degrees F.
- Add butter to the baking pan and place it into the preheated air fryer.
- Add the egg mixture to the baking pan once the butter has melted.
- Cook for 10-minutes. Serve warm.

Shrimp Frittata

Preparation Time-10 minutes | Cook Time-10 minutes | Servings-2 | Difficulty-

Nutritional Facts- Calories-192 | Fats-9.9g

|Carbohydrates-15g |Proteins-12.9g

Ingredients

Two eggs

- Half teaspoon of dried basil
- Cooking spray
- Salt and black pepper to the taste
- A quarter cup of cooked rice
- A quarter cup of shrimp, cooked, peeled, deveined and chopped
- A quarter cup of chopped baby spinach
- A quarter cup of grated Monterey jack cheese

Instructions

- In a bowl, mix eggs with salt, pepper and basil and whisk.
- Grease your air fryer's pan with cooking spray and add rice, shrimp and spinach.
- Add eggs mix, sprinkle cheese all over and cook in your air fryer at 350 degrees F for 10 minutes.
- Divide among plates and serve for breakfast.
- Enjoy!

Simple Egg Soufflé

Preparation Time-5 minutes | Cook Time-8 minutes | Servings-2 | Difficulty-Easy

Nutritional Facts- Calories-116 | Fats-10.5g |Carbohydrates-1g |Proteins-6g

Ingredients

- Two eggs
- A quarter teaspoon of chili pepper
- Two tablespoons of heavy cream
- A quarter teaspoon of pepper
- One tablespoon of chopped parsley
- Salt

Instructions

- Whisk the eggs with the remaining ingredients in a mixing bowl.
- Using cooking spray, coat two ramekins.
- Fill the ramekins with the egg mixture and place them in the air fryer basket.

- Soufflé should be cooked at 390°F for 8 minutes.
- Serve and have fun.

Smoked Air Fried Tofu Breakfast

Preparation Time-10 minutes | Cook Time-15 minutes | Servings-2 | Difficulty-

Nutritional Facts- Calories-172 | Fats-1g |Carbohydrates-13.8g |Proteins-12g

Ingredients

- One tofu block pressed and cubed
- Salt and black pepper to the taste
- One tablespoon of smoked paprika
- A quarter cup of cornstarch
- Cooking spray

Instructions

- Grease your air fryer's basket with cooking spray and heat the fryer at 370 degrees F.
- In a bowl, mix tofu with salt, pepper, smoked paprika and cornstarch and toss well.
- Add tofu to your air fryer's basket and cook for 12 minutes, shaking the fryer every 4 minutes.
- Divide into bowls and serve for breakfast.
- Enjoy!

Smoked Sausage Breakfast Mix

Preparation Time-10 minutes | Cook Time-30 minutes | Servings-2 | Difficulty-Moderate

Nutritional Facts- Calories-312 | Fats-10.8g |Carbohydrates-30g |Proteins-16.8g

Ingredients

- One pound of chopped and browned smoked sausage,
- A pinch of salt and black pepper
- One and a half cups of grits
- Two and a half cups of water
- Eight ounces of shredded cheddar cheese
- One cup of milk
- A quarter teaspoon of garlic powder
- One teaspoon of chopped thyme
- Cooking spray
- Two whisked eggs

Instructions

- Put the water in a pot, bring to a boil over

medium heat, add grits, stir, cover, cook for 5 minutes and take off the heat.

- Add cheese, stir until it melts and mix with milk, thyme, salt, pepper, garlic powder and eggs and whisk really well.
- Heat up your air fryer at 300 degrees F, grease with cooking spray and add browned sausage.
- Add grits, mix, spread and cook for 25 minutes.
- Divide among plates and serve for breakfast.
- Enjoy!

Spanish Omelet

Preparation Time-10 minutes | Cook Time-10 minutes | Servings-2 | Difficulty-Easy

Nutritional Facts- Calories-160 | Fats-7.8g | Carbohydrates-12.9g | Proteins-9g

Ingredients

- Two eggs
- Half chopped chorizo, chopped
- One peeled and cubed potato
- A quarter cup of corn
- One tablespoon of olive oil
- One tablespoon of chopped parsley
- One tablespoon of crumbled feta cheese
- Salt and black pepper to the taste

Instructions

- Heat up your air fryer at 350 degrees F and add oil.
- Add chorizo and potatoes, stir and brown them for a few seconds.
- In a bowl, mix eggs with corn, parsley, cheese, salt and pepper and whisk.
- Pour this over chorizo and potatoes, spread and cook for 5 minutes.
- Divide omelet among plates and serve for breakfast.
- Enjoy!

Special Corn Flakes Breakfast Casserole

Preparation Time-10 minutes | Cook Time-10 minutes | Servings-2 | Difficulty-Easy

Nutritional Facts- Calories-214 | Fats-4.8g | Carbohydrates-12g | Proteins-4.8g

Ingredients

- A quarter cup of milk
- Two teaspoons of sugar
- One whisked egg
- 1/8 teaspoon of ground nutmeg
- A quarter cup of blueberries
- Two tablespoons of whipped cream cheese
- One cup of crumbled corn flakes
- Two bread slices

Instructions

- In a bowl, mix eggs with sugar, nutmeg and milk and whisk well.
- In another bowl, mix cream cheese with blueberries and whisk well.
- Put corn flakes in a third bowl.
- Spread blueberry mix on each bread slice, then dip in eggs mix and dredge in corn flakes at the end.
- Place bread in your air fryer's basket, heat up at 400 degrees F and bake for 8 minutes.
- Divide among plates and serve for breakfast.
- Enjoy!

Spinach and Bacon English Muffins

Preparation Time-5 minutes | Cook Time-10 minutes | Servings-2 | Difficulty-Easy

Nutritional Facts- Calories-233 | Fats-9g | Carbohydrates-34g | Proteins-4g

Ingredients

- Two whole-grain English muffins, split
- A quarter ripe pear, peeled and thinly sliced
- Two strips of turkey bacon
- One cup of fresh baby spinach, long stems detached
- Four slices of Provolone cheese

Instructions

In the airflow racks, place the turkey bacon strips.

- Place the racks in the air fryer oven and close the door. Toggle the Power Button on and off. Cook for 6 minutes at 390°F (199°C).
- Midway through the cooking time, remove the strips from the oven.
- The bacon should be crisp when finished cooking.

- Remove the air fryer from the oven and drain on paper towels.
- In the airflow racks, place the muffin halves.
- For two minutes in the oven, cook it. Return the racks to the air fryer oven. The muffin halves will be gently toasted after processing.
- Remove the air fryer from the oven. Place a quarter of the baby spinach, several pear pieces, a strip of turkey bacon, and a slice of cheese on each muffin half.
- Toggle the Power Button on and off. Cook for 2 minutes at 360°F (182°C). Return the racks to the air fryer oven. The cheese will have melted by the time you're done.
- Warm the dish before serving.

Spinach and Bacon Roll-ups

Preparation Time-5 minutes | Cook Time-10 minutes | Servings-2 | Difficulty-Easy

Nutritional Facts- Calories-348 | Fats-26g |Carbohydrates-1g |Proteins-12g

Ingredients

- Two slices of cheese
- Two slices of turkey bacon
- Two flour tortillas
- One cup of spinach leaves

Instructions

- On a clean work area, a quarter cup of spinach and layer one slice of cheese on each tortilla, then roll them up tightly.
- Wrap a strip of turkey bacon around each tortilla and fasten with a toothpick.
- Place the roll-ups in the airflow racks with enough room between them.
- In the air fryer oven, slide the racks in. Toggle the Power Button on and off. Cook for 8 minutes at 390°F (199°C).
- Remove the air fryer oven after 4 minutes. Toss the roll-ups in the pan with tongs for more even frying. Return to the air fryer oven and cook for a further 4 minutes.
- The bacon should be crisp when finished cooking. Remove the air fryer from the oven. Before serving, set aside for 5 minutes and remove the toothpicks.

Spinach Breakfast Parcels

Preparation Time-10 minutes | Cook Time-5 minutes | Servings-2 | Difficulty-Easy

Nutritional Facts- Calories-168 | Fats-7.8g |Carbohydrates-13.8g |Proteins-12g

Ingredients

Four sheets of filo pastry
- One pound of roughly chopped baby spinach leaves
- Half pound of ricotta cheese
- Two tablespoons of pine nuts
- One egg
- Zest from one lemon
- Greek yogurt for serving
- Salt and black pepper to the taste

Instructions

- In a bowl, mix spinach with cheese, egg, lemon zest, salt, pepper and pine nuts and stir.
- Arrange filo sheets on a working surface, divide spinach mix, fold diagonally to shape your parcels and place them in your preheated air fryer at 400 degrees F.
- Bake parcels for 4 minutes, divide them among plates and serve them with Greek yogurt on the side.
- Enjoy!

Spinach Frittata

Preparation Time-5 minutes | Cook Time-10 minutes | Servings-2 | Difficulty-Easy

Nutritional Facts- Calories-384 | Fats-24g |Carbohydrates-10.8g |Proteins-34.2g

Ingredients

- Four eggs
- Two cups of chopped spinach
- One small minced onion
- Two tablespoons of grated mozzarella cheese
- Pepper
- Salt

Instructions

- Preheat the air fryer to 350 degrees Fahrenheit. Coat the inside of the air fryer pan with cooking spray.

- In a mixing bowl, whisk together the eggs and the remaining ingredients until thoroughly incorporated.
- Place the prepared pan in the air fryer basket and pour the egg mixture into it.
- Cook for 8 minutes or until the frittata is set. Serve and have fun.

Spinach, Leek and Cheese Frittata

Preparation Time-10 minutes | Cook Time-25 minutes | Servings-2 | Difficulty-Easy

Nutritional Facts- Calories-518 | Fats-30g |Carbohydrates-30g |Proteins-30g

Ingredients

- Four ounces of mushrooms
- Half cup of shredded Cheddar cheese
- A quarter cup of halved grape tomatoes
- A quarter teaspoon of dried oregano
- Half teaspoon of kosher salt
- Cooking spray
- Four large eggs
- One cup of spinach, divided
- 1/3 cup of chopped leek, white part only
- One tablespoon of 2% milk
- A quarter teaspoon of garlic powder
- Freshly ground black pepper, to taste

Instructions

- Set aside a baking dish that has been sprayed with cooking spray.
- In a large mixing basin, whisk the eggs until foamy. Combine the mushrooms, cheese, baby spinach, leek, milk, tomatoes, oregano, salt, garlic powder, and pepper in a blender and blend until smooth. Place the mixture in the baking dish that has been prepared.
- In the air fryer, place the baking dish. Toggle the Power Button on and off. Cook for 22 minutes at 300°F (150°C).
- The center will inflate up, and the top will be golden brown after processing.
- Allow 5 minutes for the frittata to cool before slicing to serve.

Sweet Breakfast Casserole

Preparation Time-10 minutes | Cook Time-30 minutes | Servings-2 | Difficulty-Moderate

Nutritional Facts- Calories-214 | Fats-4.8g |Carbohydrates-12g |Proteins-4.8g

Ingredients

- Three tablespoons of brown sugar
- Four tablespoons of butter
- Two tablespoons of white sugar
- Half teaspoon of cinnamon powder
- Half cup of flour

For the casserole

- Two eggs
- Two tablespoons of white sugar
- Two and a half cups of white flour
- One teaspoon of baking soda
- One teaspoon of baking powder
- Two eggs
- Half cup of milk
- Two cups of buttermilk
- Four tablespoons of butter
- Zest from one lemon
- One and 2/3 cup of blueberries

Instructions

- In a bowl, mix eggs with Two tablespoons of white sugar, two and a half cups of white flour, baking powder, baking soda, two eggs, milk, buttermilk, four tablespoons of butter, lemon zest and blueberries, stir and pour into a pan that fits your air fryer.
- In another bowl, mix three tablespoons of brown sugar with two tablespoons of white sugar, Four tablespoons of butter, a half cup of flour and cinnamon; stir until you obtain a crumble and spread over blueberries mix.
- Place in the preheated air fryer and bake at 300 degrees F for 30 minutes.
- Divide among plates and serve for breakfast.
- Enjoy!

Tomato and Bacon Breakfast

Preparation Time-10 minutes | Cook Time-30 minutes | Servings-2 | Difficulty-Moderate

Nutritional Facts- Calories-231 | Fats-9g |Carbohydrates-12.9g |Proteins-20g

Ingredients

- Half pound of cubed white bread
- Half pound of chopped and cooked smoked bacon
- A quarter cup of olive oil
- One chopped yellow onion
- Twelve ounces of canned tomatoes, chopped
- Half teaspoon of crushed red pepper
- A quarter-pound of shredded cheddar
- Two tablespoons of chopped chives
- A quarter-pound of shredded Monterey jack
- Two tablespoons of stock
- Black pepper and salt as per taste
- Four whisked eggs

Instructions

- Heat the oil in your air fryer to 350 degrees Fahrenheit.
- Stir in the bread, onion, red pepper, bacon, tomatoes, and stock.
- Cook for 20 minutes with the eggs, cheddar, and Monterey jack cheeses.
- Serve by dividing among dishes and garnishing with chives.
- Enjoy!

Turkey Breakfast Sausage Patties

Preparation Time-5 minutes | Cook Time-10 minutes | Servings-2 | Difficulty-Easy

Nutritional Facts- Calories-236 | Fats-12.9g |Carbohydrates-15.9g |Proteins-19g

Ingredients

One tablespoon of chopped fresh sage
- One teaspoon of chopped fennel seeds
- Half teaspoon of onion powder
- 1/8 teaspoon of crushed red pepper flakes
- One tablespoon of chopped fresh thyme
- One and a quarter teaspoon of kosher salt
- 1/3 teaspoon of smoked paprika
- Half teaspoon of garlic powder
- 1/8 teaspoon of freshly ground black pepper
- Half cup of finely minced sweet apple (peeled)
- One pound of 93% lean ground turkey

Instructions

- In a medium mixing bowl, whisk together the thyme, salt, sage, fennel seeds, onion powder, paprika, red pepper flakes, garlic powder, and black pepper.
- Stir in the ground turkey and apple until completely combined. Cut the ingredients into eight equal amounts and form each into quarter-inch thick, 3-inch diameter patties using your hands.
- In the airflow racks, place the patties.
- Place the racks in the air fryer oven and close the door. Toggle the Power Button on and off. Cook for 10 minutes at 400 degrees Fahrenheit (205 degrees Celsius).
- Halfway through the cooking time, turn the patties.
- When the patties are through frying, they should be well browned and cooked through. Transfer to a platter and serve warm from the air fryer oven.

Veggie Burritos

Preparation Time-10 minutes | Cook Time-10 minutes | Servings-2 | Difficulty-Easy

Nutritional Facts- Calories-143 | Fats-6.9g |Carbohydrates-12.9g |Proteins-6.9g

Ingredients

- One tablespoon of cashew butter
- One tablespoon of tamari
- One tablespoon of water
- One tablespoon of liquid smoke
- Two rice papers
- A quarter cup of sweet potatoes, steamed and cubed
- Half small broccoli head, florets separated and steamed
- Four asparagus stalks
- Four chopped roasted red peppers
- A handful of chopped kale

Instructions

- In a bowl, mix cashew butter with water, tamari and liquid smoke and whisk well.

- Wet rice papers and arrange them on a working surface.
- Divide sweet potatoes, broccoli, asparagus, red peppers and kale, wrap burritos and dip each in cashew mix.
- Arrange burritos in your air fryer and cook them at 350 degrees F for 10 minutes.
- Divide veggie burritos among plates and serve.
- Enjoy!

Veggie Frittata

Preparation Time-10 minutes | Cook Time-15 minutes | Servings-2 | Difficulty-Easy

Nutritional Facts- Calories-5o9 | Fats-28.9g |Carbohydrates-28.9g |Proteins-30g

Ingredients

- Half cup of chopped red bell pepper
- 1/3 cup of grated carrot
- 1/3 cup of minced onion
- One teaspoon of olive oil
- One egg
- Four egg whites
- 1/3 cup of 2% milk
- One tablespoon of shredded Parmesan cheese

Instructions

- Mix the red bell pepper, carrot, onion, and olive oil in a baking pan and stir to combine.
- Bring the pan into the air fryer oven. Press the Power Button. Cook at 356 degrees Fahrenheit for 12 minutes.
- After 3 minutes, remove from the air fryer oven. Stir the vegetables. Bring to the air fryer oven and continue cooking.
- Meantime, whisk together the egg, egg whites, and milk in a medium bowl until creamy.
- After 3 minutes, remove from the air fryer oven. Pour the egg mixture over the top and scatter with the Parmesan cheese. Bring to the air fryer oven and continue cooking for additional 6 minutes.
- When cooking is complete, the eggs will be set, and the top will be golden around the edges.
- Set the frittata to cool for 5 minutes before slicing and serving.

Wake Up Air Fryer Avocado Boats

Preparation Time-5 minutes | Cook Time-10 minutes | Servings-2 | Difficulty-Easy

Nutritional Facts- Calories-122 | Fats-6g |Carbohydrates-7.8g |Proteins-10.8g

Ingredients

- A quarter cup of diced red onion
- Two plums seeded and diced tomatoes
- One tablespoon of lime juice
- A quarter teaspoon of black pepper
- One tablespoon of finely diced jalapeno
- Two avocados halved and pitted
- Half teaspoon of salt
- Two tablespoons of chopped fresh cilantro
- Four eggs

Instructions

- Scoop the avocado pulp out of the skin with a spoon, keeping the shell intact. Dice the avocado and put it in a medium bowl. Combine the tomatoes, cilantro, onion, jalapeno, salt, lime juice, and pepper; if needed, cover and refrigerate the mixture of avocado until ready for use.
- The air fryer is preheated to 350 degrees F.
- Place them on a foil ring to make sure that avocado shells do not lose their shape or break while cooking. Simply roll two three-inch-wide strips of foil into rope shapes to make them, and form each into a three-inch circle. In an air fryer basket, place each avocado shell on a foil ring. Break one egg into each shell of avocado and fry for 6 to 8 minutes or until the required doneness is achieved.
- Remove from the basket; top with salsa the avocado and serve.

Walnuts and Pear Oatmeal

Preparation Time-10 minutes | Cook Time-20 minutes | Servings-2 | Difficulty-Easy

Nutritional Facts- Calories-161 | Fats-7.8g |Carbohydrates-15g |Proteins-7.8g

Ingredients

- Half cup of water
- One tablespoon of softened butter
- A quarter cup of brown sugar

- Half teaspoon of cinnamon powder
- One cup of rolled oats
- A quarter cup of chopped walnuts
- One cup of peeled and chopped pear,
- A quarter cup of raisins

Instructions

- In a heat-proof dish that fits your air fryer, mix milk with sugar, butter, oats, cinnamon, raisins, pears and walnuts, stir, introduce in your fryer and cook at 360 degrees F for 12 minutes.
- Divide into bowls and serve.
- Enjoy!

Western Omelet

Preparation Time-5 minutes | Cook Time-20 minutes | Servings-2 | Difficulty-Easy

Nutritional Facts- Calories-525 | Fats-15g |Carbohydrates-34g |Proteins-41g

Ingredients

A quarter cup of chopped bell pepper, green or red
- A quarter cup of chopped onion
- A quarter cup of diced ham
- One teaspoon of butter
- Four large eggs
- Two tablespoons of milk
- 1/8 teaspoon of salt
- 1/3 cup of shredded sharp Cheddar cheese

Instructions

- Put the bell pepper, onion, ham, and butter in a baking pan and mix well.
- Bring the pan into the air fryer oven. Press the Power Button. Cook at 390°F (199°C) for 5 minutes.
- After 1 minute, remove from the air fryer oven. Stir the mixture. Set to the air fryer oven and continue to cook for another 4 minutes.
- When done, the veggies should be softened.
- Whisk together the eggs, milk, and salt in a bowl. Whisk the egg mixture over the veggie mixture.
- Place the pan in the air fryer oven. Press the Power Button. Cook at 360F (182C) for 15 minutes.
- After 14 minutes, remove from the air fryer oven. Scatter the omelet with the shredded cheese. Set

to the air fryer oven and continue to cook for another 1 minute.
- When cooking is complete, the top will be lightly golden browned, the eggs will be set, and the cheese will be melted.
- Set the omelet to cool for 5 minutes before serving.

Zucchini Breakfast Patties

Preparation Time-10 minutes | Cook Time-15 minutes | Servings-2 | Difficulty-

Nutritional Facts- Calories-51 | Fats-4g |Carbohydrates-1g|Proteins-4g

Ingredients

- Half cup of zucchini, shredded and squeeze out all liquid
- Two tablespoons of minced onion
- One lightly beaten eggs
- A quarter teaspoon of red pepper flakes
- A quarter cup of parmesan cheese, grated

Instructions

- Add all ingredients into the bowl and mix until well combined.
- Make small patties from the zucchini mixture and place them into the air fryer basket.
- Cook at 400 degrees F for 15 minutes.

Chapter 2-Air Fried Lunch Recipes

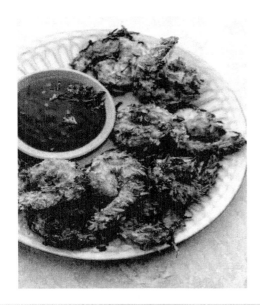

Almond Coconut Shrimp

Preparation Time-10 minutes| Cook Time-10 minutes | Servings-2 | Difficulty-Easy

Nutritional Facts- Calories-200 | Fats-6.9g |Carbohydrates-4g |Proteins-27.9g

Ingredients

- Eight ounces shrimp, peeled
- Half cup of almond flour
- One egg white
- A quarter teaspoon of cayenne pepper
- Half cup of unsweetened shredded coconut
- Half teaspoon of salt

Instructions

- Preheat the air fryer to 400 F.
- Spray air fryer basket with cooking spray.
- Whisk egg whites in a shallow dish.
- In a bowl, merge together the shredded coconut, almond flour, and cayenne pepper.
- Set shrimp into the egg mixture, then coat with coconut mixture.
- Place coated shrimp into the air fryer basket and cook for 5 minutes.
- Serve and enjoy.

Asian Halibut

Preparation Time-30 minutes | Cook Time-10 minutes | Servings-2 | Difficulty-Easy

Nutritional Facts- Calories-285 | Fats-7.8g |Carbohydrates-16.8g |Proteins-23g

Ingredients

- One pound halibut steaks
- 2/3 cup of soy sauce
- A quarter cup of sugar
- Two tablespoons of lime juice
- Half cup of mirin
- A quarter teaspoon of crushed red pepper flakes
- A quarter cup of orange juice
- A quarter teaspoon of grated ginger
- Two minced garlic cloves

Instructions

- Put soy sauce in a pan, heat up over medium heat, add mirin, sugar, lime and orange juice, pepper flakes, ginger and garlic, stir well, bring to a boil and take off the heat.
- Transfer half of the marinade to a bowl, add halibut, toss to coat and leave aside in the fridge for 30 minutes.
- Transfer halibut to your air fryer and cook at 390 degrees F for 10 minutes, flipping once. Divide halibut steaks among plates, drizzle the rest of the marinade all over and serve hot.
- Enjoy!

Asian Sirloin Steaks

Preparation Time-10 minutes | Cook Time-20 minutes | Servings-2 | Difficulty-Easy

Nutritional Facts- Calories-342 | Fats-9.9g |Carbohydrates-4.8g |Proteins-52g

Ingredients

- Twelve ounces of sirloin steaks
- One tablespoon of minced garlic
- One tablespoon of grated ginger
- Half tablespoon of Worcestershire sauce
- One and a half tablespoons of soy sauce
- Two tablespoons of Erythritol
- Pepper
- Salt

Instructions

- Add steaks in a large zip-lock bag along with the remaining ingredients. Shake well and place in the refrigerator overnight.
- Spray air fryer basket with cooking spray.
- Place marinated steaks in an air fryer basket and cook at 400 F for 10 minutes.
- Turn steaks to another side and cook for 10-15 minutes more.
- Serve and enjoy.

Bacon and Garlic Pizzas

Preparation Time-10 minutes | Cook Time- 10 minutes | Servings-2 | Difficulty-Easy

Nutritional Facts- Calories-217 | Fats-13.8g |Carbohydrates-21g |Proteins-12g

Ingredients

- Two frozen dinner rolls
- Two minced garlic cloves
- Half teaspoon of dried oregano
- Half teaspoon of garlic powder
- One cup of tomato sauce
- Four cooked and chopped bacon slices
- One cup of grated cheddar cheese
- Cooking spray

Instructions

- Place dinner rolls on a working surface and press them to obtain four ovals.
- Spray each oval with cooking spray, transfer them to your air fryer and cook them at 370 degrees F for 2 minutes.
- Spread tomato sauce on each oval, divide garlic, sprinkle oregano and garlic powder and top with bacon and cheese.
- Return pizzas to your heated air fryer and cook them at 370 degrees F for 8 minutes more.
- Serve them warm for lunch.
- Enjoy!

Bacon Pudding

Preparation Time-10 minutes | Cook Time- minutes | Servings-2 | Difficulty-Easy

Nutritional Facts- Calories-266 | Fats-9.9g |Carbohydrates-23g |Proteins-12g

Ingredients

- Two cooked and chopped bacon strips
- One tablespoon of softened butter
- One cup of corn
- One chopped yellow onion
- A quarter cup of chopped celery
- Half cup of chopped red bell pepper
- One teaspoon of chopped thyme
- Two teaspoons of minced garlic
- Salt and black pepper to the taste
- Half cup of heavy cream
- One and a half cups of milk
- Two whisked eggs
- Two cups of cubed bread
- Two tablespoons of grated parmesan
- Cooking spray

Instructions

- Grease your air fryer's pan with cooking spray.
- In a bowl, mix bacon with butter, corn, onion, bell pepper, celery, thyme, garlic, salt, pepper, milk, heavy cream, eggs and bread cubes, toss, pour into greased pan and sprinkle cheese all over
- Add this to your preheated air fryer at 320 degrees and cook for 30 minutes.
- Divide among plates and serve warm for a quick lunch.
- Enjoy!

Basil Parmesan Shrimp

Preparation Time-10 minutes | Cook Time-10 minutes | Servings-2 | Difficulty-Easy

Nutritional Facts- Calories-290 | Fats-9.9g |Carbohydrates-1g |Proteins-40g

Ingredients

- One lb. of peeled and deveined shrimp
- One teaspoon of basil
- Half teaspoon of oregano
- One teaspoon of pepper
- 2/3 cup of grated parmesan cheese
- Two minced garlic cloves
- Two tablespoons of olive oil
- One teaspoon of onion powder

Instructions

- Add all ingredients into the bowl and toss well.
- Spray air fryer basket with cooking spray.
- Transfer shrimp into the air fryer basket and cook at 350 F for 10 minutes.
- Serve and enjoy.

BBQ Cheddar Stuffed Chicken Breasts

Preparation Time-10 minutes | Cook Time-35 minutes | Servings-2 | Difficulty-Moderate

Nutritional Facts- Calories-375 | Fats-19g |Carbohydrates-13g |Proteins-37.8g

Ingredients

- Three strips bacon
- Two four ounces chicken breast skinless and boneless
- Two ounces of cubed cheddar cheese
- A quarter cup of BBQ sauce
- One pinch of salt and black pepper

Instructions

- Place one strip of bacon in a crisper tray and air fry for 2 minutes. Cut the bacon into small pieces.
- Line the crisper tray with parchment paper.
- Make a 1 inch cut on the chicken horizontally such that you create an internal pouch.
- Stuff each chicken breast with cooked bacon and cheese mixture, and then wrap the breasts with bacon.
- Set the chicken with BBQ sauce and place them on the lined crisper tray. Place the crisper tray on the pizza rack and select air fry.
- Set temperature of the Air Fryer to 380 F and the time for 20 minutes. Press start.
- Turn the chicken breasts when halfway cooked. The internal chicken temperature should be 165 F when fully cooked. Serve.

Beef and Asparagus

Preparation Time-40 minutes | Cook Time-15 minutes | Servings-2 | Difficulty-Moderate

Nutritional Facts- Calories-523 | Fats-7.8g |Carbohydrates-34g |Proteins-41g

Ingredients

- Two New York strips steaks, sliced into cubes

For Marinade

- One teaspoon of olive oil
- One teaspoon of steak seasoning
- Half teaspoon of dried onion powder
- Half teaspoon of dried garlic powder
- Salt and pepper to taste
- Pinch cayenne pepper

For Asparagus

- One lb. of asparagus
- Salt to taste
- One teaspoon of olive oil

Instructions

- Warm your air fryer to 400 degrees F.
- Combine marinade ingredients in a bowl.
- Stir in steak cubes.
- Cover and marinate for 30 minutes.
- Air fry at 5 minutes.
- Coat asparagus with oil.
- Season with salt.
- Add asparagus to the air fryer.
- Toss to combine.
- Cook for another 3 to 5 minutes.

Beef and Cabbage Mix

Preparation Time-10 minutes | Cook Time- 40 minutes | Servings-2 | Difficulty-Moderate

Nutritional Facts- Calories-352 | Fats-15.9g |Carbohydrates-27g |Proteins-24g

Ingredients

- Two pounds of beef brisket
- One cup of beef stock
- Two bay leaves
- Three chopped garlic cloves
- Two chopped carrots
- One cabbage head, cut into medium wedges
- Salt and black pepper to the taste
- Two turnips, cut into quarters

Instructions

- Put beef brisket and stock in a large pan that fits your air fryer, season beef with salt and pepper, add garlic and bay leaves, carrots, cabbage, potatoes and turnips, toss, introduce in your air fryer and cook at 360 degrees F and cook for 40 minutes.

- Divide among plates and serve.
- Enjoy!

Beef and Green Beans

Preparation Time-15 minutes | Cook Time-25 minutes | Servings-2 | Difficulty-Easy

Nutritional Facts- Calories-199 | Fats-12g |Carbohydrates-13.8g |Proteins-12g

Ingredients

Beef and green beans

- Half lb. of thinly sliced flank steak
- A quarter cup of cornstarch
- Half lb. of trimmed, sliced and steamed green beans

Sauce

- Two teaspoons of vegetable oil
- Half teaspoon of ginger
- One tablespoon of minced garlic
- Half cup of soy sauce
- Half cup of water
- 1/3 cup of brown sugar

Instructions

- Coat steak strips with cornstarch.
- Select air fry setting.
- Cook at 390 degrees F for 5 to 7 minutes per side.
- Add sauce ingredients to a pan over medium heat.
- Simmer for 10 minutes.
- Dip the steaks in the sauce.
- Serve with green beans.

Beef Curry

Preparation Time-10 minutes | Cook Time- 45 minutes | Servings-2 | Difficulty-Moderate

Nutritional Facts- Calories-398 | Fats-15.9g |Carbohydrates-24g |Proteins-25g

Ingredients

- Two pounds of cubed beef steak
- Two tablespoons of olive oil
- Two cubed potatoes
- One tablespoon of wine mustard

- Two and a half tablespoons of curry powder
- Two chopped yellow onions
- Two minced cloves of garlic
- Ten ounces of canned coconut milk
- Two tablespoons of tomato sauce
- Salt and black pepper to the taste

Instructions

- Heat up a pan that fits your air fryer with the oil over medium-high heat, add onions and garlic, stir and cook for 4 minutes.
- Add potatoes and mustard, stir and cook for 1 minute.
- Add beef, curry powder, salt, pepper, coconut milk and tomato sauce, stir, transfer to your air fryer and cook at 360 degrees F for 40 minutes.
- Divide into bowls and serve.
- Enjoy!

Beef Fillet with Garlic Mayo

Preparation Time-10 minutes | Cook Time-40 minutes | Servings-2 | Difficulty-Moderate

Nutritional Facts- Calories-400 | Fats-12g |Carbohydrates-26g |Proteins-19g

Ingredients

- One lb. beef fillet
- A quarter cup of mayonnaise
- One tablespoon of Dijon mustard
- 1/3 cup of sour cream
- A quarter cup of chopped tarragon
- Two tablespoons of chopped chives
- Two minced garlic cloves
- Black pepper and salt as per taste

Instructions

- Preheat the air fryer to 370 degrees F.
- Season beef using salt and pepper, transfer to the air fryer and cook for 20 minutes. Remove and set aside.
- In a bowl, whisk the mustard and tarragon. Add the beef and toss, return to the air fryer and cook for 20 minutes.
- In a separate bowl, mix the garlic, sour cream, mayonnaise, chives, salt, and pepper. Whisk and set aside.
- Serve the beef with the garlic-mayo spread.

Beef Lunch Meatballs

Preparation Time-10 minutes | Cook Time- 15 minutes | Servings-2 | Difficulty-Easy

Nutritional Facts- Calories-333 | Fats-23g |Carbohydrates-12g |Proteins-23g

Ingredients

- Half pound chopped Italian sausage
- Half teaspoon of onion powder
- Half cup of grated cheddar cheese
- Half pound ground beef
- Half teaspoon of garlic powder
- Salt and black pepper to the taste
- Mashed potatoes for serving

Instructions

- Combine beef, pepper, garlic powder, onion powder, sausage, salt, and cheese in a mixing bowl, stir well, and form 16 meatballs from the mixture.
- Cook the meatballs in your air fryer for 15 minutes at 370 degrees F.
- Serve your meatballs alongside some mashed potatoes.
- Enjoy!

Beef Mac and Cheese

Preparation Time-30 minutes | Cook Time-35 minutes | Servings-2 | Difficulty-Easy

Nutritional Facts- Calories-166 | Fats-4g |Carbohydrates-7.8g |Proteins-25g

Ingredients

- Half lb. of elbow macaroni
- Half cup of chicken broth
- Two cups of milk
- Eight ounces of shredded cheddar cheese
- Four tablespoons of cream cheese
- Four tablespoons of butter
- One cup of cooked ground beef
- Salt and pepper to taste
- One teaspoon of dry mustard
- Pinch cayenne pepper
- Grated nutmeg
- One cup of shredded mozzarella cheese

Instructions

- Set a pot filled with water, cook the pasta according to package directions.
- Drain and set aside.
- In a pan over medium heat, mix the broth, milk, cheese, cream cheese and butter.
- Simmer for 5 minutes.
- Pour broth mixture into a baking pan.
- Stir in the pasta and the rest of the ingredients except the mozzarella cheese.
- Top with the mozzarella cheese.
- Cover with foil.
- Choose bake setting.
- Cook at 400 F for 30 minutes.

Beef Roast

Preparation Time-10 minutes | Cook Time-35 minutes | Servings-2 | Difficulty-Moderate

Nutritional Facts- Calories-238 | Fats-12.9g |Carbohydrates-1g |Proteins-25g

Ingredients

- One lb. of beef roast
- One tablespoon of olive oil
- One teaspoon of thyme
- Two teaspoons of garlic powder
- A quarter teaspoon of pepper
- One tablespoon of kosher salt

Instructions

- Coat roast with olive oil.
- Mix together thyme, garlic powder, pepper, and salt and rub all over roast.
- Place roast into the air fryer basket and cook at 400 F for 20 minutes.
- Spray roast with cooking spray and cook for 15 minutes more.
- Slice and serve.

Beef Roast with Wine Sauce

Preparation Time-10 minutes | Cook Time-45 minutes | Servings-2 | Difficulty-Moderate

Nutritional Facts- Calories-302 | Fats-20g |Carbohydrates-27g |Proteins-31.8g

Ingredients

- Eight ounces of beef stock
- Two ounces of red wine
- Half teaspoon of chicken salt
- Half teaspoon of smoked paprika
- One chopped yellow onion
- Four minced garlic cloves
- Two chopped carrots
- Three chopped potatoes
- Salt and black pepper to the taste
- Two pounds of beef roast

Instructions

- In a bowl, mix salt, pepper, chicken salt and paprika, stir, rub the beef with this mix and put it in a big pan that fits your air fryer.
- Add onion, garlic, stock, wine, potatoes and carrots, introduce in your air fryer and cook at 360 degrees F for 45 minutes.
- Divide everything among plates and serve.
- Enjoy!

Beef Steak and Pepper Fajitas

Preparation Time-15 minutes | Cook Time-10 minutes | Servings-2 | Difficulty-Easy

Nutritional Facts- Calories-356 | Fats-8.7g | Carbohydrates-1.5g | Proteins-61.8g

Ingredients

- One pound of beef sirloin steak, cut into strips
- Two sliced shallots
- One sliced orange bell pepper
- One sliced red bell pepper
- Two minced cloves of garlic
- Two tablespoons of Cajun seasoning
- One tablespoon of paprika
- Salt and ground black pepper, to taste
- Four corn tortillas
- Half cup of shredded Cheddar cheese
- Cooking spray

Instructions

- Set the air fryer basket with cooking spray.
- Combine all the ingredients, except for the tortillas and cheese, in a large bowl. Toss to coat well.

- Pour the beef and vegetables in the basket and spritz with cooking spray.
- Slide the basket into the air fryer. Cook at the corresponding preset mode or Air Fry at 360F (182C) for 10 minutes.
- Stir the beef and vegetables halfway through the cooking time.
- When cooking is complete, the meat will be browned, and the vegetables will be soft and slightly wilted.
- Unfold the tortillas on a clean work surface and spread the cooked beef and vegetables on top. Scatter with cheese and fold to serve.

Beef Strips with Snow Peas and Mushrooms

Preparation Time-10 minutes | Cook Time-25 minutes | Servings-2 | Difficulty-Easy

Nutritional Facts- Calories-235 | Fats-9g | Carbohydrates-21.9g | Proteins-24g

Ingredients

- Salt and black pepper to the taste
- Eight ounces of white halved mushrooms
- Two tablespoons of soy sauce
- Two beef steaks, cut into strips
- Seven ounces of snow peas
- One yellow onion, cut into rings
- One teaspoon of olive oil

Instructions

- Whisk together the olive oil and soy sauce in a mixing dish, then toss in the beef strips.
- Mix onion, snow peas, and mushrooms with pepper, salt, and oil in a separate bowl, toss well and place in a pan that fits your air fryer. Cook for 16 minutes at 350 degrees F.
- Add the beef strips to the pan as well, and cook for another 6 minutes at 400 degrees F.
- Serve by dividing everything amongst plates.
- Enjoy!

Blackened Tilapia

Preparation Time-10 minutes | Cook Time-10 minutes | Servings-2 | Difficulty-Easy

Nutritional Facts- Calories-363 | Fats-12g | Carbohydrates-1g | Proteins-54g

Ingredients

- Two tilapia fillets
- Cooking spray
- One teaspoon of brown sugar
- One tablespoon of paprika
- A quarter teaspoon of cayenne pepper
- One teaspoon of garlic powder
- One teaspoon of dried oregano
- Half teaspoon of cumin
- Salt to taste

Instructions

- Spray fish fillets with oil.
- Mix the remaining ingredients in a bowl.
- Set both sides of fish with spice mixture.
- Add to the air fryer.
- Set it to air fry.
- Cook at 400 degrees F for 4 to 5 minutes per side.

Broccoli Beef

Preparation Time-10 minutes | Cook Time-12 minutes | Servings-2 | Difficulty-Easy

Nutritional Facts- Calories-302 | Fats-20g |Carbohydrates-7.8g |Proteins-24g

Ingredients

- Half lb. of round steak, cut into strips
- Half lb. of broccoli florets
- Two drops of liquid stevia
- One teaspoon of soy sauce
- 1/3 cup of sherry
- Two teaspoons of sesame oil
- 1/3 cup of oyster sauce
- One minced garlic clove
- One tablespoon of sliced ginger
- One teaspoon of arrowroot powder
- One tablespoon of olive oil

Instructions

- In a small bowl, merge together oyster sauce, stevia, soy sauce, sherry, arrowroot, and sesame oil.
- Add broccoli and meat to a large bowl.
- Pour oyster sauce mixture over meat and broccoli and toss well. Place in the fridge for 60 minutes.

- Add marinated meat broccoli to the air fryer basket. Drizzle with olive oil and sprinkle with ginger and garlic.
- Cook at 360 F for 12 minutes.
- Serve and enjoy.

Buffalo Chicken Wings

Preparation Time-5 minutes | Cook Time-30 minutes | Servings-2 to 4 | Difficulty-Easy

Nutritional Facts- Calories-402 | Fats-15.9g |Carbohydrates-4.8g |Proteins-31.8g

Ingredients

- One teaspoon of salt
- One tablespoon of brown sugar
- One tablespoon of Worcestershire sauce
- A quarter cup of vegan butter
- A quarter cup of cayenne pepper sauce
- Two pounds of chicken wings

Instructions

- Preparing the ingredients. Whisk salt, sugar, Worcester sauce, butter, and sauce together and set to the side.
- Dry wings and increase air fryer basket.
- Air Frying. Set temperature to 380°F, and set time to 25 minutes. Cook tossing halfway through.
- When timer sounds, shake wings, raise the temperature to 400 degrees and cook for another 5 minutes. Remove wings and place them into an enormous bowl. Add sauce and toss well. Serve alongside celery sticks!

Buttermilk Air fried chicken

Preparation Time-10 minutes | Cook Time-22 minutes | Servings-2 | Difficulty-Easy

Nutritional Facts- Calories-335 | Fats-12.9g |Carbohydrates-23.1g |Proteins-1g

Ingredients

- One cup of buttermilk
- One tablespoon of salt
- One tablespoon of sugar
- Half tablespoon of black pepper
- Two chicken legs
- Two chicken thighs
- One cup of flour

- Two eggs
- Two cups of flaked corn cereal, crushed
- One tablespoon of Emeril Essence seasoning

Instructions

- Pour buttermilk into a mixing bowl, then add salt, sugar, and pepper.
- Soak the chicken pieces in the buttermilk mixture.
- Add flour in a separate mixing bowl, beat eggs in a separate bowl and add cereal crumbs in a third bowl.
- Shake the chicken pieces for excess buttermilk and dip them in flour, then in eggs and in crumbs.
- Place the chicken pieces in the crisper tray. Slide the tray on position 2 of the Air Fryer.
- Select the air fry setting, then set the temperature at 375F for 40 minutes. Press the start button.
- When the cooking process is complete, the internal chicken temperature should be 160°F.

Cajun Cheese Shrimp

Preparation Time-10 minutes | Cook Time-5 minutes | Servings-2 | Difficulty-Easy

Nutritional Facts- Calories-175 | Fats-4.8g |Carbohydrates-1g|Proteins-27g

Ingredients

- One lb. of shrimp
- Half cup of almond flour
- One teaspoon of olive oil
- One tablespoon of Cajun seasoning
- Two tablespoons of parmesan cheese
- Two minced garlic cloves

Instructions

- Add all ingredients into the bowl and toss well.
- Spray air fryer basket with cooking spray.
- Transfer shrimp mixture into the air fryer basket and cook at 390 F for 5 minutes. Shake halfway through.
- Serve and enjoy.

Cheese Crust Salmon

Preparation Time-10 minutes | Cook Time-10 minutes | Servings-2 | Difficulty-Easy

Nutritional Facts- Calories-333 | Fats-18g |Carbohydrates-1.5g |Proteins-40g

Ingredients

- Two salmon fillets
- One teaspoon of Italian seasoning
- Two minced garlic cloves
- One cup of shredded parmesan cheese
- One teaspoon of paprika
- One tablespoon of olive oil
- A quarter cup of chopped fresh parsley
- Pepper
- Salt

Instructions

- Preheat the air fryer to 425 F.
- Add salmon, seasoning, and olive oil to the bowl and mix well.
- Place salmon fillet into the air fryer basket.
- In another bowl, mix together cheese, garlic, and parsley.
- Sprinkle cheese mixture on top of salmon and cook for 10 minutes.
- Serve and enjoy.

Cheese Ravioli and Marinara Sauce

Preparation Time-10 minutes | Cook Time- 11 minutes | Servings-2 | Difficulty-Easy

Nutritional Facts- Calories-270 | Fats-12g |Carbohydrates-6g |Proteins-15g

Ingredients

- Six ounces of cheese ravioli
- Three ounces of marinara sauce
- One tablespoon of olive oil
- Half cup of buttermilk
- One cup of bread crumbs
- A quarter cup of grated parmesan

Instructions

- Put the buttermilk in a bowl and breadcrumbs in another bowl.
- Dip ravioli in buttermilk, then in breadcrumbs and place them in your air fryer on a baking sheet.
- Drizzle olive oil over them, cook at 400 degrees F for 5 minutes, divide them among plates, sprinkle parmesan on top and serve for lunch

- Enjoy!

Cheesy Beef Empanadas

Preparation Time-15 minutes | Cook Time-Two hours | Servings-2 | Difficulty-Hard

Nutritional Facts- Calories-387 | Fats-9.9g |Carbohydrates-24g |Proteins-52g

Ingredients

- Half cup of cold butter, cut into cubes
- 3/4 cup of water
- One large egg
- One tablespoon of extra-virgin olive oil
- One yellow onion, chopped
- Two cloves minced garlic
- Two cups of all-purpose flour, plus more for surface
- One teaspoon of kosher salt
- One teaspoon of baking powder
- One lb. of ground beef
- One tablespoon of tomato paste
- One teaspoon of oregano
- One teaspoon of cumin
- Egg wash for brushing
- Freshly chopped cilantro for garnish
- Sour cream, for serving
- A half teaspoon of paprika
- Kosher salt
- Freshly ground black pepper
- Half cup of chopped tomatoes
- Half cup of chopped pickled jalapeños
- One cup of shredded Cheddar
- One cup of Shredded Monterey Jack

Instructions

- Whisk the flour, salt, and baking powder together in a big bowl. Use your hands or a pastry cutter to cut the butter into the flour until pea-sized. Add the water and egg and combine until it forms a dough. Turn the dough on a lightly floured surface and knead for around 5 minutes, until smooth.
- Wrap up and refrigerate for at least 1 hour in plastic wrap.
- Heat oil in a large skillet over medium heat. Add the onion & cook until soft, about 5 minutes, then add the garlic and cook for one more minute,

until fragrant. Add the ground beef and cook for 5 minutes, breaking the meat with a wooden spoon until it is no longer pink. Fat is to be drained.
- Return the pan to medium heat and stir in the beef with the tomato paste. Season with pepper and salt, and add oregano, cumin, and paprika. Add the tomatoes and jalapeños and cook for about 3 minutes, until hot. Remove from heat and allow it to cool slightly. On a lightly floured surface, put the dough and divide it in half. Cut out rounds using a 4.5" round cookie cutter." Repeat with the dough that remains.
- Lightly moisten the outer edge of a dough round with water and put around Two tablespoons of cheddar and Monterey filling in the middle and top. Fold dough in half over the filling. Crimp the edges together with a fork. Then brush them with egg wash. Repeat with the leftover filling and dough.
- Put empanadas in a parchment-lined Air Fryer basket to ensure they do not touch, and cook for 10 minutes in batches at 400 ° F.
- It is to be garnished with cilantro. Finally, serve with sour cream.

Chicken and Capers

Preparation Time-10 minutes | Cook Time-20 minutes | Servings-2 | Difficulty-Easy

Nutritional Facts- Calories-198 | Fats-9g |Carbohydrates-16.8g |Proteins-9.9g

Ingredients

- Four chicken thighs
- Three tablespoons of capers
- Four minced garlic cloves
- Three tablespoons of melted butter
- Salt and black pepper to the taste
- Half cup of chicken stock
- One sliced lemon
- Four chopped green onions

Instructions

- Brush the chicken with butter, season with salt & pepper to taste, and place in an air fryer-safe baking dish.
- Also, throw in the capers, chicken stock, garlic, and lemon slices to coat, then place in the

- air fryer and cook for 20 minutes, tossing halfway through.
- Serve with green onions sprinkled on top and divided among plates.
- Enjoy!

Chicken and Corn Casserole

Preparation Time-10 minutes | Cook Time- 30 minutes | Servings-2 | Difficulty-Easy

Nutritional Facts- Calories-332 | Fats-12g |Carbohydrates-30g |Proteins-43.8g

Ingredients

- One cup of clean chicken stock
- Two teaspoons of garlic powder
- Salt and black pepper to the taste
- Three ounces of canned coconut milk
- One and a half cups of green lentils
- One pound of skinless, boneless and cubed chicken breasts
- 1/3 cup of chopped cilantro
- One cup of corn
- One handful of spinach
- One chopped green onion

Instructions

- In a pan that fits your air fryer, mix stock with coconut milk, salt, pepper, garlic powder, chicken and lentils.
- Add corn, green onions, cilantro and spinach, stir well, introduce in your air fryer and cook at 350 degrees F for 30 minutes.
- Enjoy!

Chicken and Creamy Mushrooms

Preparation Time-10 minutes | Cook Time- 30 minutes | Servings-2 | Difficulty-Easy

Nutritional Facts- Calories-321 | Fats-9.9g |Carbohydrates-21.9g |Proteins-12g

Ingredients

- Two chicken thighs
- Salt and black pepper to the taste
- Two ounces of cremini halved mushrooms
- Three minced garlic cloves
- Three tablespoons of melted butter
- Half cup of chicken stock

- A quarter cup of heavy cream
- Half teaspoon of basil, dried
- Half teaspoon of dried thyme
- Half teaspoon of dried oregano
- One tablespoon of mustard
- A quarter cup of grated parmesan

Instructions

- Rub chicken pieces with two tablespoons of butter, season with salt and pepper, put in your air fryer's basket, cook at 370 degrees F for 5 minutes and leave aside in a bowl for now.
- Meanwhile, heat up a pan with the rest of the butter over medium-high heat, add mushrooms and garlic, stir and cook for 5 minutes.
- Add salt, pepper, stock, oregano, thyme and basil, stir well and transfer to a heat-proof dish that fits your air fryer.
- Add chicken, toss everything, put in your air fryer and cook at 370 degrees F for 20 minutes.
- Add mustard, parmesan and heavy cream, toss everything again, cook for 5 minutes more, divide among plates and serve.
- Enjoy!

Chicken and Green Onions Sauce

Preparation Time-10 minutes | Cook Time-20 minutes | Servings-2 | Difficulty-Easy

Nutritional Facts- Calories-321 | Fats-12g |Carbohydrates-21.9g |Proteins-20g

Ingredients

- Five roughly chopped green onions
- A chopped one-inch piece of ginger root
- Two minced garlic cloves
- One tablespoon of fish sauce
- Two tablespoons of soy sauce
- One teaspoon of Chinese five-spice
- Four chicken drumsticks
- One cup of coconut milk
- Salt and black pepper to the taste
- One teaspoon of melted butter
- A quarter cup of chopped cilantro
- One tablespoon of lime juice

Instructions

- In your food processor, mix green onions with

ginger, garlic, soy sauce, fish sauce, five-spice, salt, pepper, butter and coconut milk and pulse well.

- In a bowl, mix chicken with green onions mix, toss well, transfer everything to a pan that fits your air fryer and cook at 370 degrees F for 16 minutes, shaking the fryer once.
- Divide among plates, sprinkle cilantro on top, drizzle lime juice and serve with a side salad.
- Enjoy!

Chicken and Zucchini Lunch Mix

Preparation Time-10 minutes | Cook Time- 20 minutes | Servings-2 | Difficulty-Easy

Nutritional Facts- Calories-322 | Fats-9g |Carbohydrates-19g |Proteins-15.9g

Ingredients

- Two zucchinis, cut with a spiralizer
- Half pound of skinless, boneless and cubed chicken breasts
- Two minced cloves of garlic
- One teaspoon of olive oil
- Salt and black pepper to the taste
- One cup of halved cherry tomatoes
- A quarter cup of chopped almonds

For the pesto

- One cup of basil
- One cup of chopped kale
- One tablespoon of lemon juice
- One garlic clove
- 3/4 cup of pine nuts
- Half cup of olive oil
- A pinch of salt

Instructions

- In your food processor, mix basil with kale, lemon juice, garlic, pine nuts, oil and a pinch of salt, pulse really well and leave aside.
- Heat up a pan that fits your air fryer with the oil over medium heat, add garlic, stir and cook for 1 minute.
- Add chicken, salt, pepper, stir, almonds, zucchini noodles, garlic, cherry tomatoes and the pesto you've made at the beginning, stir gently, introduce in the preheated air fryer and cook at 360 degrees F for 17 minutes.

- Divide among plates and serve for lunch.
- Enjoy!

Chicken Fillets, Brie and Ham

Preparation Time-5 minutes | Cook Time-15 minutes | Servings-2 | Difficulty-Easy

Nutritional Facts- Calories-276 | Fats-12g |Carbohydrates-10.2g |Proteins-17g

Ingredients

- Two Large Chicken Fillets
- Freshly Ground Black Pepper
- Four Small Slices of Brie
- One tablespoon of Freshly Chopped Chives
- Four Slices Cured Ham

Instructions

- Preparing the Ingredients. Slice the fillets into four and make incisions as you'd for a hamburger roll. Leave a little "hinge" uncut at the rear. Season the INS and pop some brie and chives in there.
- Close them, and wrap them each in a slice of ham. Brush with oil and pop them into the basket.
- Air Frying. Heat your fryer to 350 F.
- Roast the small parcels until they appear tasty.

Chicken Kabobs

Preparation Time-10 minutes | Cook Time- 20 minutes | Servings-2 | Difficulty-Easy

Nutritional Facts- Calories-261 | Fats-9g |Carbohydrates-12.9g |Proteins-21g

Ingredients

- Three orange bell peppers, cut into squares
- A quarter cup of honey
- 1/3 cup of soy sauce
- Salt and black pepper to the taste
- Cooking spray
- Six halved mushrooms
- Two chicken breasts, skinless, boneless and roughly cubed

Instructions

- In a bowl, mix chicken with salt, pepper, honey, say sauce and some cooking spray and toss well.
- Thread chicken, bell peppers and mushrooms on skewers place them in your air fryer and cook at

338 degrees F for 20 minutes.

- Divide among plates and serve for lunch.
- Enjoy!

Chicken Pie

Preparation Time-10 minutes | Cook Time-16 minutes | Servings-2 | Difficulty-Easy

Nutritional Facts- Calories-257 | Fats-10.8g |Carbohydrates-19g |Proteins-23g

Ingredients

- Two boneless, skinless and cubed chicken thighs
- One chopped carrot
- One chopped yellow onion
- One chopped potato
- Two chopped mushrooms
- One teaspoon of soy sauce
- Salt and black pepper to the taste
- One teaspoon of Italian seasoning
- Half teaspoon of garlic powder
- One teaspoon of Worcestershire sauce
- One tablespoon of flour
- One tablespoon of milk
- Two puff pastry sheets
- One tablespoon of melted butter

Instructions

- Heat up a pan over medium-high heat, add potatoes, carrots and onion, stir and cook for 2 minutes.
- Add chicken and mushrooms, salt, soy sauce, pepper, Italian seasoning, garlic powder, Worcestershire sauce, flour and milk, stir really well and take off the heat.
- Place one puff pastry sheet on the bottom of your air fryer's pan and trim edge excess.
- Add chicken mix, top with the other puff pastry sheet, trim excess as well and brush pie with butter.
- Place in your air fryer and cook at 360 degrees F for 6 minutes.
- Leave the pie to cool down, slice and serve for breakfast.
- Enjoy!

Chicken, Beans, Corn and Quinoa Casserole

Preparation Time-10 minutes | Cook Time- 30 minutes | Servings-2 | Difficulty-Moderate

Nutritional Facts- Calories-365 | Fats-13.8g |Carbohydrates-27.9g |Proteins-26g

Ingredients

- Half cup of already cooked quinoa
- One cup of cooked and shredded chicken breast
- Four ounces of canned black beans
- Four ounces of corn
- Half cup of chopped cilantro
- Two chopped kale leaves
- Half cup of chopped green onions
- One cup of clean tomato sauce
- One cup of clean salsa
- Two teaspoons of chili powder
- Two teaspoons of ground cumin
- One cup of shredded mozzarella cheese
- One tablespoon of garlic powder
- Cooking spray
- One chopped jalapeno pepper

Instructions

- Spray a baking dish that fits your air fryer with cooking spray, add quinoa, chicken, black beans, corn, cilantro, kale, green onions, tomato sauce, salsa, chili powder, cumin, garlic powder, jalapenos and mozzarella, toss, introduce in your fryer and cook at 350 degrees F for 17 minutes.
- Slice and serve warm for lunch.
- Enjoy!

Chinese Pork Lunch Mix

Preparation Time-10 minutes | Cook Time- 15 minutes | Servings-2 | Difficulty-Easy

Nutritional Facts- Calories-321 | Fats-12.9g |Carbohydrates-15.9g |Proteins-27g

Ingredients

- One egg
- One pound pork, cut into medium cubes
- Half cup of cornstarch
- One teaspoon of sesame oil
- Salt and black pepper to the taste

- A pinch of Chinese five-spice
- One and a half tablespoons of canola oil
- Sweet tomato sauce for serving

Instructions

- In a bowl, mix five-spice with salt, pepper and cornstarch and stir.
- In another bowl, mix eggs with sesame oil and whisk well.
- Dredge pork cubes in cornstarch mix, then dip in eggs mix and place them in your air fryer, which you've greased with the canola oil.
- Cook at 340 degrees F for 12 minutes, shaking the fryer once.
- Serve pork for lunch with the sweet tomato sauce on the side.
- Enjoy!

Coconut and Chicken Casserole

Preparation Time-10 minutes | Cook Time- 25 minutes | Servings-2 | Difficulty-Easy

Nutritional Facts- Calories-176 | Fats-6g |Carbohydrates-12g |Proteins-16.8g

Ingredients

- Two torn lime leaves
- One cup of veggie stock
- One chopped lemongrass stalk
- One-inch grated piece of ginger
- Half a pound chicken breast, skinless, boneless, and cut into thin strips
- Four ounces of chopped mushrooms
- Two chopped Thai chilies
- Two tablespoons of fish sauce
- Three ounces of coconut milk
- A quarter cup of lime juice
- A quarter cup of chopped cilantro
- Salt and black pepper to the taste

Instructions

- Put the stock into a pan that fits your air fryer, bring to a simmer over medium heat, add lemongrass, ginger and lime leaves, stir and cook for 10 minutes.
- Strain soup, return to pan, add chicken, mushrooms, milk, chilies, fish sauce, lime juice, cilantro, salt and pepper, stir, introduce in your

air fryer and cook at 360 degrees F for 15 minutes.
Divide into bowls and serve.
Enjoy!

Cod and Vinaigrette

Preparation Time-10 minutes | Cook Time-15 minutes | Servings-2 | Difficulty-Easy

Nutritional Facts- Calories-291 | Fats-10.8g |Carbohydrates-20g |Proteins-9g

Ingredients

- Two skinless and boneless cod fillets
- Six halved cherry tomatoes
- Four pitted and roughly chopped black olives
- One tablespoon of lemon juice
- Salt and black pepper to the taste
- One tablespoon of olive oil
- Cooking spray
- One bunch of chopped basil

Instructions

- Season cod with salt and pepper to the taste, place in your air fryer's basket and cook at 360 degrees F for 10 minutes, flipping after 5 minutes.
- Meanwhile, heat up a pan with the oil over medium heat, add tomatoes, olives and lemon juice, stir, bring to a simmer, add basil, salt and pepper, stir well and take off the heat.
- Divide fish among plates and serve with the vinaigrette drizzled on top.
- Enjoy!

Cod Fillets and Peas

Preparation Time- 10 minutes | Cook Time- 10 minutes | Servings-2 | Difficulty-Easy

Nutritional Facts- Calories-261 | Fats-7.8g |Carbohydrates-20g |Proteins-21.9g

Ingredients

- Two boneless cod fillets
- Two tablespoons of chopped parsley
- One cup of peas
- Two tablespoons of wine
- Half teaspoon of dried oregano
- Half teaspoon of sweet paprika
- Two minced cloves of garlic

- Salt and pepper to the taste

Instructions

- In your food processor, mix garlic with parsley, salt, pepper, oregano, paprika and wine and blend well.
- Rub fish with half of this mix, place in your air fryer and cook at 360 degrees F for 10 minutes.
- Meanwhile, put peas in a pot, add water to cover, add salt, bring to a boil over medium-high heat, cook for 10 minutes, drain and divide among plates.
- Also, divide fish among plates, spread the rest of the herb dressing all over and serve.
- Enjoy!

Cod Fillets with Fennel and Grapes Salad

Preparation Time-10 minutes | Cook Time-15 minutes | Servings-2 | Difficulty-Easy

Nutritional Facts- Calories-301 | Fats-6g |Carbohydrates-31.8g |Proteins-25g

Ingredients

- Two boneless black cod fillets
- One tablespoon of olive oil
- Salt and black pepper to the taste
- One thinly sliced fennel bulb
- One cup of halved grapes
- Half cup of pecans

Instructions

- Drizzle half of the oil over fish fillets, season with salt and pepper, rub well, place fillets in your air fryer's basket, cook for 10 minutes at 400 degrees F and transfer to a plate.
- In a bowl, mix pecans with grapes, fennel, the rest of the oil, salt and pepper, toss to coat, add to a pan that fits your air fryer and cook at 400 degrees F for 5 minutes.
- Divide cod among plates, add fennel and grapes, mix on the side and serve.
- Enjoy!

Cod Steaks with Plum Sauce

Preparation Time-10 minutes | Cook Time-20 minutes | Servings-2 | Difficulty-Easy

Nutritional Facts- Calories-245 | Fats-6g |Carbohydrates-15g |Proteins-13.8g

Ingredients

- Two big cod steaks
- Salt and black pepper to the taste
- Half teaspoon of garlic powder
- Half teaspoon of ginger powder
- A quarter teaspoon of turmeric powder
- One tablespoon of plum sauce
- Cooking spray

Instructions

- Season cod steaks with salt and pepper, spray them with cooking oil, add garlic powder, ginger powder and turmeric powder and rub well.
- Place cod steaks in your air fryer and cook at 360 degrees F for 15 minutes, flipping them after 7 minutes.
- Heat up a pan over medium heat, add plum sauce, stir and cook for 2 minutes.
- Divide cod steaks among plates, drizzle the plum sauce all over and serve.

Coffee Flavored Steaks

Preparation Time-10 minutes | Cook Time-15 minutes | Servings-2 | Difficulty-Easy

Nutritional Facts- Calories-160 | Fats-9.9g |Carbohydrates-13.8g |Proteins-12g

Ingredients

- One and a half tablespoons of ground coffee
- Two rib-eye steaks
- Half tablespoon of sweet paprika
- One tablespoon of chili powder
- One teaspoon of garlic powder
- One teaspoon of onion powder
- A quarter teaspoon of ground ginger
- A quarter teaspoon of ground coriander
- A pinch of cayenne pepper
- Black pepper to the taste

Instructions

- In a bowl, mix coffee with paprika, chili powder, garlic powder, onion powder, ginger, coriander, cayenne and black pepper, stir, rub steaks with this mix, put in the preheated air fryer and cook at 360 degrees F for 15 minutes.

- Divide steaks among plates and serve with a side salad.
- Enjoy!

Collard Greens and Turkey Wings

Preparation Time-12 minutes | Cook Time- 22 minutes | Servings-2 | Difficulty-Easy

Nutritional Facts- Calories-231 | Fats-6g |Carbohydrates-20g |Proteins-18g

Ingredients

- Half chopped sweet onion
- Two smoked turkey wings
- Two tablespoons of olive oil
- Three minced garlic cloves
- Two pounds of chopped collard greens
- Salt and black pepper to the taste
- Half teaspoon of crushed red pepper
- Two tablespoons of apple cider vinegar
- One tablespoon of brown sugar

Instructions

- Heat the oil in an air fryer-compatible pan over medium-high heat, then add the onions, stir, and cook for 2 minutes.
- Add the garlic, pepper, vinegar, greens, salt, pepper, sugar, crushed red pepper, and smoked turkey to the air fryer and cook for 15 minutes at 350 degrees F.
- Serve the greens and turkey on separate plates.
- Enjoy!

Corn Casserole

Preparation Time-10 minutes | Cook Time-15minutes | Servings-2 | Difficulty-Easy

Nutritional Facts- Calories-281 | Fats-10.8g |Carbohydrates-34.8g |Proteins-1g

Ingredients

- One cup of corn
- Two tablespoons of flour
- One egg
- A quarter cup of milk
- Half cup of light cream
- Half cup of grated Swiss cheese
- Two tablespoons of butter
- Salt and black pepper to the taste

- Cooking spray

Instructions

- In a bowl, mix the corn with flour, egg, milk, light cream, cheese, salt, pepper and butter and stir well.
- Grease your air fryer's pan with cooking spray, pour the cream mix, spread and cook at 320 degrees F for 15 minutes.
- Serve warm for lunch.
- Enjoy!

Country Steak

Preparation Time-15 minutes | Cook Time-20 minutes | Servings-2 | Difficulty-Moderate

Nutritional Facts- Calories-325 | Fats-16.2g |Carbohydrates-0.8g |Proteins-41.4g

Ingredients

- A quarter cup of cornstarch
- Half cup of flour
- One teaspoon of paprika
- One teaspoon of onion powder
- One teaspoon of garlic powder
- Two rib-eye steaks
- Salt and pepper to taste
- One egg, beaten
- Cooking spray

Instructions

- Combine cornstarch, flour, paprika, onion powder and garlic powder in a bowl.
- Season steaks with salt and pepper.
- Coat steaks with egg.
- Dredge with cornstarch mixture.
- Spray with oil.
- Choose bake setting in the air fryer.
- Cook at 400 F for 8 to 10 minutes per side or until golden.

Crisp Pork Chops

Preparation Time-10 minutes | Cook Time-12 minutes | Servings-2 | Difficulty-Easy

Nutritional Facts- Calories-230 | Fats-10.8g |Carbohydrates-1.5g |Proteins-27g

Ingredients

- Half lbs. pork chops, boneless
- One teaspoon of paprika
- One teaspoon of creole seasoning
- One teaspoon of garlic powder
- A quarter cup of grated parmesan cheese
- 1/3 cup of almond flour

Instructions

- Preheat the air fryer to 360 F.
- Add all ingredients except pork chops in a zip-lock bag.
- Add pork chops to the bag. Seal bag and shake well to coat pork chops.
- Remove pork chops from the zip-lock bag and place them in the air fryer basket.
- Cook pork chops for 10-12 minutes.
- Serve and enjoy.

Crispy Chicken Breast

Preparation Time-5 minutes | Cook Time-22 minutes | Servings-2 | Difficulty-Easy

Nutritional Facts- Calories-188 | Fats-6g |Carbohydrates-4.8g |Proteins-23g

Ingredients

- Two chicken breasts, skinless and boneless
- Four eggs
- Two cups of buttermilk
- Two cups of all-purpose flour
- Two cups of yellow cornmeal
- One ounce of applewood smoked salt
- One ounce of old bay seasoning
- One tablespoon of ground black pepper
- Cooking spray

Instructions

- Merge the wet ingredients in a mixing bowl, and then combine the dry ingredients in a separate bowl.
- Place the pizza rack on position 2 in your Air Fryer.
- Dip each chicken breast in the wet mixture, then in the dry mixture. Spray the chicken with cooking spray and place them on the crisper tray.
- Place the crisper tray on a level higher than the pizza rack. Select the bake setting. Set the

temperature at 425F for 30 minutes. Press the start button.

- Check the meat when cooking is complete. The meat should at least have an internal temperature of 165F.
- Serve and enjoy.

Crispy Fish Fillet

Preparation Time-15 minutes | Cook Time-12 minutes | Servings-2 | Difficulty-Easy

Nutritional Facts- Calories-356 | Fats-9g |Carbohydrates-1.5g |Proteins-60g

Ingredients

- Two cod fillets
- One teaspoon of Old Bay seasoning
- Salt and pepper to taste
- Half cup of all-purpose flour
- One beaten egg
- One cup of breadcrumbs

Instructions

- Sprinkle both sides of cod with Old Bay seasoning, salt and pepper.
- Coat with flour, dip in egg and dredge with breadcrumbs.
- Add fish to the air fryer.
- Select air fry setting.
- Cook at 400 degrees F for 5 to 6 minutes per side.

Crispy Fish Sticks

Preparation Time-10 minutes | Cook Time-10 minutes | Servings-2 | Difficulty-Easy

Nutritional Facts- Calories-397 | Fats-1.6g |Carbohydrates-4g |Proteins-13.8g

Ingredients

- Half lb. of white fish, cut into pieces
- 3/4 teaspoon of Cajun seasoning
- Half cup of crushed pork rind
- Two tablespoons of water
- Two tablespoons of Dijon mustard
- A quarter cup of mayonnaise
- Pepper
- Salt

Instructions

- Using cooking spray, coat the air fryer basket.
- Combine water, mayonnaise, and mustard in a small mixing basin.
- Combine pork rind, Cajun seasoning, pepper, and salt in a small basin.
- Place the fish pieces in the air fryer basket after dipping them in the mayo mixture and coating them with the pork rind mixture.
- Cook for 5 minutes at 400 degrees Fahrenheit. Cook for another 5 minutes on the other side of the fish sticks.
- Serve and have fun.

Crispy Lamb

Preparation Time-10 minutes | Cook Time-30 minutes | Servings-2 | Difficulty-Easy

Nutritional Facts- Calories-230 | Fats-4g |Carbohydrates-12g |Proteins-13.8g

Ingredients

- One tablespoon of bread crumbs
- Two tablespoons of toasted and crushed macadamia nuts
- One tablespoon of olive oil
- One minced garlic clove
- Fourteen ounces rack of lamb
- Salt and black pepper to the taste
- One egg
- One tablespoon of chopped rosemary

Instructions

- In a bowl, mix oil with garlic and stir well.
- Season lamb with salt, pepper and brush with the oil.
- In another bowl, mix nuts with breadcrumbs and rosemary.
- Put the egg in a separate bowl and whisk well.
- Dip lamb in egg, then in macadamia mix, place them in your air fryer's basket, cook at 360 degrees F and cook for 25 minutes, increase heat to 400 degrees F and cook for 5 minutes more.
- Divide among plates and serve right away.
- Enjoy!

Crumbled Chicken Tenderloins

Preparation Time-15 minutes | Cook Time-30 minutes | Servings-2 | Difficulty-Moderate

Nutritional Facts- Calories-253 | Fats-10.8g |Carbohydrates-3g |Proteins-26g

Ingredients

- One egg
- Half cup of breadcrumbs
- Two tablespoons of vegetable oil
- Four chicken tenderloins

Instructions

- Whisk the egg in a mixing bowl.
- Mix bread crumbs and oil in a separate bowl until the mixture is crumbly.
- Dip each chicken tenderloin in egg, then in the crumb mixture until well coated.
- Lay the tenderloins on the crisper tray and place the tray on the pizza rack.
- Select air fry on Air Fryer and set the temperature at 350F for 12 minutes. Press start.
- The internal temperature should be 165F when the tenderloins are well cooked.
- Serve and enjoy immediately.

Delicious Beef Cubes

Preparation Time-10 minutes | Cook Time- 12 minutes | Servings-2 | Difficulty-Easy

Nutritional Facts- Calories-271 | Fats-7.8g |Carbohydrates-21g |Proteins-28.9g

Ingredients

- Half pound of cubed sirloin
- Eight ounces of jarred pasta sauce
- One and a half cups of bread crumbs
- Two tablespoons of olive oil
- White rice, already cooked for serving
- Half teaspoon of marjoram, dried

Instructions

- Toss beef chunks with pasta sauce in a mixing basin.
- Combine marjoram, bread crumbs, and oil in a separate bowl and toss well.
- Cook beef cubes in your air fryer at 360 degrees F for 12 minutes after dipping them in this

- mixture.
- Serve with white rice on the side and divide among plates.
- Enjoy!

Delicious White Fish

Preparation Time-10 minutes | Cook Time-10 minutes | Servings-2 | Difficulty-Easy

Nutritional Facts- Calories-358 | Fats-20g |Carbohydrates-1.2g |Proteins-41g

Ingredients

- Twelve ounces of white fish fillets
- Half teaspoon of onion powder
- Half teaspoon of lemon pepper seasoning
- Half teaspoon of garlic powder
- One tablespoon of olive oil
- Pepper
- Salt

Instructions

- Spray air fryer basket with cooking spray.
- Preheat the air fryer to 360 F.
- Set fish fillets with olive oil and season with onion powder, lemon pepper seasoning, garlic powder, pepper, and salt.
- Place fish fillets in an air fryer basket and cook for 10-12 minutes.
- Serve and enjoy.

Dijon Stuffed Chicken

Preparation Time-5 minutes | Cook Time-45 minutes | Servings-2 | Difficulty-Moderate

Nutritional Facts- Calories-340 | Fats-6g |Carbohydrates-34.8g |Proteins-19g

Ingredients

- Two chicken breasts
- One cubed potato
- One teaspoon of Dijon mustard
- Salt and pepper
- Two slices of provolone cheese
- Two teaspoons of olive oil
- Half an Apple
- Spinach

Instructions

- Preheat the Air Fryer Grill to 218C or 425F.
- Bake the potatoes for 10 minutes.
- Make two slits on the breasts and rub in some Dijon mustard.
- Put the apple slices and cheese slices in the slits and rub them with salt, pepper, and vegetable oil.
- Bake for a half-hour.

Duck and Plum Sauce

Preparation Time- 10 minutes | Cook Time-35 minutes | Servings-2 | Difficulty-Easy

Nutritional Facts- Calories-372 | Fats-25g |Carbohydrates-28.9g |Proteins-43.8g

Ingredients

- Two duck breasts
- One tablespoon of butter, melted
- One star anise
- One tablespoon of olive oil
- One chopped shallot
- Nine ounces red plumps, stoned, cut into small wedges
- Two tablespoons of sugar
- Two tablespoons of red wine
- One cup of beef stock

Instructions

- Heat up a pan with the olive oil over medium heat, add shallot, stir and cook for 5 minutes.
- Add sugar and plums, stir and cook until sugar dissolves.
- Add stock and wine, stir, cook for 15 minutes, take off the heat and keep warm for now.
- Score duck breasts, season with salt and pepper, rub with melted butter, transfer to a heat-proof dish that fits your air fryer, add star anise and plum sauce, introduce in your air fryer and cook at 360 degrees F for 12 minutes.
- Divide everything among plates and serve.
- Enjoy!

Duck Breast with Fig Sauce

Preparation Time-10 minutes | Cook Time- 20 minutes | Servings-2 | Difficulty-Easy

Nutritional Facts- Calories-246 | Fats-12g

|Carbohydrates-26g |Proteins-20g

Ingredients

- Two skin-on halved duck breasts
- One tablespoon of olive oil
- Half teaspoon of chopped thyme
- Half teaspoon of garlic powder
- A quarter teaspoon of sweet paprika
- Salt and black pepper to the taste
- One cup of beef stock
- Three tablespoons of melted butter
- One chopped shallot
- Half cup of port wine
- Four tablespoons of fig preserves
- One tablespoon of white flour

Instructions

- Season duck breasts with salt and pepper, drizzle half of the melted butter, rub well, put in your air fryer's basket and cook at 350 degrees F for 5 minutes on each side.
- Meanwhile, heat up a pan with the olive oil and the rest of the butter over medium-high heat, add shallot, stir and cook for 2 minutes.
- Add thyme, garlic powder, paprika, stock, salt, pepper, wine and figs, stir and cook for 7-8 minutes.
- Add flour, stir well, cook until sauce thickens a bit and take off the heat.
- Divide duck breasts among plates, drizzle figs sauce all over and serve.
- Enjoy!

Duck Breasts with Endives

Preparation Time- 10 minutes | Cook Time-25 minutes | Servings-2 | Difficulty-Easy

Nutritional Facts- Calories-400 | Fats-12g |Carbohydrates- 28.9g |Proteins-27.9g

Ingredients

- Two duck breasts
- Salt and black pepper to the taste
- One tablespoon of sugar
- One tablespoon of olive oil
- Four julienned endives
- Two tablespoons of cranberries
- Four ounces white wine

- One tablespoon of minced garlic
- Two tablespoons of heavy cream

Instructions

- Score duck breasts and season them with salt and pepper, put in the preheated air fryer and cook at 350 degrees F for 20 minutes, flipping them halfway.
- Meanwhile, heat up a pan with the oil over medium heat, add sugar and endives, stir and cook for 2 minutes.
- Add salt, pepper, wine, garlic, cream and cranberries, stir and cook for 3 minutes.
- Divide duck breasts among plates, drizzle the endives sauce all over and serve.
- Enjoy!

Easy Bacon Shrimp

Preparation Time-10 minutes | Cook Time-7 minutes | Servings-2 | Difficulty-Easy

Nutritional Facts- Calories-498 | Fats-1g |Carbohydrates-1g|Proteins-45g

Ingredients

- Eight shrimp, deveined
- A quarter teaspoon of pepper
- Eight bacon slices

Instructions

- Preheat the air fryer to 390 F.
- Spray air fryer basket with cooking spray.
- Wrap shrimp with bacon slice and place into the air fryer basket and cook for 5 minutes.
- Turn shrimp to another side and cook for 2 minutes more. Season shrimp with pepper.
- Serve and enjoy.

Easy Burger Patties

Preparation Time-10 minutes | Cook Time-45 minutes | Servings-2 | Difficulty-Moderate

Nutritional Facts- Calories-175 | Fats-6.9g |Carbohydrates-1.5g|Proteins-25g

Ingredients

- Five ounces of ground beef
- One teaspoon of dried basil
- One teaspoon of mustard

- One teaspoon of tomato paste
- A half-ounce of cheddar cheese
- One teaspoon of mixed herbs
- One teaspoon of garlic puree
- Pepper
- Salt

Instruction

- Set all ingredients into the large bowl and mix until combined.
- Spray air fryer basket with cooking spray.
- Make patties from the meat mixture and place them into the air fryer basket.
- Cook at 390 F for 25 minutes, then turn patties to another side and cook at 350 F for 20 minutes more.
- Serve and enjoy.

Easy Chicken Lunch

Preparation Time-10 minutes | Cook Time-20 minutes | Servings-2 | Difficulty-Easy

Nutritional Facts- Calories-180 | Fats-6.9g |Carbohydrates-12g |Proteins-10.8g

Ingredients

- Half chopped bunch of kale
- Salt and black pepper to the taste
- A quarter cup of chicken stock
- One cup of shredded chicken
- One chopped carrot
- One cup of roughly sliced shiitake mushrooms

Instructions

- In a blender, mix stock with kale, pulse a few times and pour into a pan that fits your air fryer.
- Add chicken, mushrooms, carrots, salt and pepper to the taste, toss, introduce in your air fryer and cook at 350 degrees F for 18 minutes.
- Enjoy!

Easy Chicken Thighs and Baby Potatoes

Preparation Time-10 minutes | Cook Time-30 minutes | Servings-2 | Difficulty-Easy

Nutritional Facts- Calories-363 | Fats-13.8g |Carbohydrates-21g |Proteins-34g

Ingredients

- Four chicken thighs
- One tablespoon of olive oil
- Half pound of halved baby potatoes
- One teaspoon of dried oregano
- One teaspoon of dried rosemary
- Half teaspoon of sweet paprika
- Salt and black pepper to the taste
- Two minced cloves of garlic
- One chopped red onion
- Two teaspoons of chopped thyme

Instructions

- In a bowl, mix chicken thighs with potatoes, salt, pepper, thyme, paprika, onion, rosemary, garlic, oregano and oil.
- Toss to coat, spread everything in a heat-proof dish that fits your air fryer and cook at 400 degrees F for 30 minutes, shaking halfway.
- Divide among plates and serve.
- Enjoy!

Easy Duck Breasts

Preparation Time-10 minutes | Cook Time- 40 minutes | Servings-2 | Difficulty-Moderate

Nutritional Facts- Calories-320 | Fats-27.9g |Carbohydrates-24g |Proteins-42g

Ingredients

- Two halved duck breasts
- Salt and black pepper to the taste
- One and a half tablespoons of flour
- Three tablespoons of melted butter
- Two cups of chicken stock
- Half cup of white wine
- A quarter cup of chopped parsley
- Two cups of chopped mushrooms

Instructions

- Season duck breasts with salt and pepper, place them in a bowl, add melted butter, toss and transfer to another bowl.
- Combine melted butter with flour, wine, salt, pepper and chicken stock and stir well.
- Arrange duck breasts in a baking dish that fits your air fryer, pour the sauce over them, add parsley and mushrooms, introduce them to your

air fryer and cook at 350 degrees F for 40 minutes.

- Divide among plates and serve.
- Enjoy!

Easy Hot Dogs

Preparation Time-10 minutes | Cook Time- 8 minutes | Servings-2 | Difficulty-Easy

Nutritional Facts- Calories-211 | Fats-7.8g | Carbohydrates-13.8g | Proteins-19g

Ingredients

- Two hot dog buns
- Two hot dogs
- One tablespoon of Dijon mustard
- Two tablespoons of grated cheddar cheese

Instructions

- Cook the hot dogs for 5 minutes at 390 degrees F in a preheated air fryer.
- Return everything to your air fryer and cook for another 2 minutes at 390 degrees F. Divide hot dogs between hot dog buns, put mustard and cheese on top, and cook for another 2 minutes at 390 degrees F.
- Serve at lunchtime.
- Enjoy!

Fast Chicken Sausage and Broccoli Casserole

Preparation Time-10 minutes | Cook Time-20 minutes | Servings-2 | Difficulty-Easy

Nutritional Facts- Calories-442 | Fats-19g | Carbohydrates-41g | Proteins-1.5g

Ingredients

- Four eggs
- One cup of shredded Cheddar cheese (divided)
- 1/3 cup of heavy whipping cream
- One (Twelve ounces) package cooked chicken sausage
- One cup of chopped broccoli
- Two minced garlic cloves
- Half tablespoon of salt
- A quarter tablespoon of ground black pepper
- Cooking spray

Instructions

- Spritz a baking pan with cooking spray.
- Whisk the eggs with Cheddar and cream in a large bowl to mix well.
- Combine the garlic, broccoli, cooked sausage, salt, and ground black pepper in a separate bowl. Stir to mix well.
- Pour the sausage mixture into the baking pan, and then spread the egg mixture over to cover.
- Place the pan on the bake position.
- Select Bake, set temperature to 400°F (205°C) and set time to 20 minutes.
- When cooking is complete, the egg should be set, and a toothpick inserted in the center should come out clean.
- Serve immediately.

Filet Mignon and Mushrooms Sauce

Preparation Time-10 minutes | Cook Time-25 minutes | Servings-2 | Difficulty-Easy

Nutritional Facts- Calories-340 | Fats-12g | Carbohydrates-15g | Proteins-23g

Ingredients

- Six sliced mushrooms
- One chopped shallot
- Two fillet mignons
- Two minced cloves of garlic
- Two tablespoons of olive oil
- A quarter cup of Dijon mustard
- A quarter cup of wine
- One cup of coconut cream
- Two tablespoons of chopped parsley
- Salt and black pepper to the taste

Instructions

- Heat up a pan with the oil over medium-high heat, add garlic and shallots, stir and cook for 3 minutes.
- Add mushrooms, stir and cook for 4 minutes more.
- Add wine, stir and cook until it evaporates.
- Add coconut cream, mustard, parsley, a pinch of salt and black pepper to the taste, stir, cook for 6 minutes more and take off the heat.
- Season fillets with salt and pepper, put them in your air fryer, and cook at 360 degrees F for 10

- minutes.
- Divide fillets among plates and serve with the mushroom sauce on top.
- Enjoy!

Fresh Chicken Mix

Preparation Time-10 minutes | Cook Time- 22 minutes | Servings-2 | Difficulty-Easy

Nutritional Facts- Calories-167 | Fats-6.9g |Carbohydrates-7.8g |Proteins-12g

Ingredients

- Two skinless, boneless and cubed chicken breasts
- Eight sliced button mushrooms
- One chopped red bell pepper
- One tablespoon of olive oil
- Half teaspoon of dried thyme
- Five ounces of alfredo sauce
- Four bread slices
- Two tablespoons of soft butter

Instructions

- Combine the chicken, bell pepper, mushrooms, and oil in your air fryer, stir to coat well, and cook for 15 minutes at 350 degrees mF.
- Return the chicken mixture to the air fryer, toss in the alfredo sauce and thyme, and cook for another 4 minutes at 350 degrees F.
- Spread butter on the bread slices, place them butter side up in the fryer and cook for another 4 minutes.
- Serve for lunch by arranging toasted bread slices on a dish and topping each with chicken mixture.
- Enjoy!

Fried Salmon

Preparation Time-10 minutes | Cook Time-15 minutes | Servings-2 | Difficulty-Easy

Nutritional Facts- Calories-215 | Fats-12.9g |Carbohydrates-1g |Proteins-18g

Ingredients

- Freshly ground black pepper
- Two teaspoons of extra-virgin olive oil
- Two tablespoons of whole grain mustard
- One tablespoon of brown sugar
- One clove minced garlic

- Two (6-oz.) salmon fillets
- Kosher salt
- A half teaspoon of thyme leaves

Instructions

- Season salmon with pepper and salt all over. Whisk the sugar, oil, mustard, garlic and thyme together in a small dish. Spread at the top of the salmon.
- Arrange salmon in a basket of the air fryer. Set the air fryer to 400 degrees F. Now cook for 10 minutes.

Garlic Butter Lobster Tails

Preparation Time-15 minutes | Cook Time-10 minutes | Servings-2 | Difficulty-Easy

Nutritional Facts- Calories-400 | Fats-30g |Carbohydrates-1.5g |Proteins-27.9g

Ingredients

- Two lobster tails
- Two minced cloves of garlic
- Two tablespoons of butter
- One teaspoon of lemon juice
- One teaspoon of chopped chives
- Salt to taste

Instructions

- Butterfly the lobster tails.
- Bring the meat on top of the shell.
- Mix the remaining ingredients in a bowl.
- Add lobster tails inside the air fryer.
- Set it to air fry.
- Spread garlic butter on the meat.
- Cook at 380 degrees F for 5 minutes.
- Spread more butter on top.
- Cook for another 2 to 3 minutes.

Garlic Butter Steak with Herbs

Preparation Time-15 minutes | Cook Time-15 minutes | Servings-2 | Difficulty-Easy

Nutritional Facts- Calories-233 | Fats-7.8g |Carbohydrates-3.18g |Proteins-35.4g

Ingredients

- Two minced cloves of garlic
- Four tablespoons of butter

- One teaspoon of chopped chives
- Two teaspoons of chopped parsley
- One teaspoon of chopped rosemary
- One teaspoon of chopped thyme
- Two rib-eye steaks
- Salt and pepper to taste

Instructions

- Combine the garlic, butter and herbs in a bowl.
- Refrigerate for 20 minutes.
- Roll the butter mixture into a log.
- Sprinkle both sides of steaks with salt and pepper.
- Set air fryer to grill.
- Air fry at 400 degrees F for 15 minutes, flipping once or twice.
- Slice the herb butter.
- Top the steaks with herb butter.

Garlic Herb Turkey Breast

Preparation Time-10 minutes | Cook Time-One hour | Servings-2 | Difficulty-Moderate

Nutritional Facts- Calories-270 | Fats-12.9g|Carbohydrates-7.8g|Proteins-30g

Ingredients

- One pound turkey breast, skin on
- Kosher salt
- Freshly ground black pepper
- One teaspoon of freshly chopped thyme
- Two tablespoons of melted butter
- Two minced garlic cloves
- One teaspoon of freshly chopped rosemary

Instructions

- Dry the turkey breast and season with pepper and salt on both sides.
- Combine the thyme, melted butter, garlic and rosemary in a shallow bowl. Brush the butter all over the breast of the turkey.
- Put in the air fryer basket, skin side up. Now cook for 40 minutes at 375 ° F or until the internal temperature exceeds 160 °F, turning halfway through.
- Allow 5 minutes to rest before slicing.

Garlic Pork Chops with Roasted Broccoli

Preparation Time-10 minutes | Cook Time-10 minutes | Servings-2 | Difficulty-Easy

Nutritional Facts- Calories-268 | Fats-17g |Carbohydrates-28.9g |Proteins-6g

Ingredients

- Two pork chops
- Two tablespoons of avocado oil, divided
- One teaspoon of garlic powder
- Half teaspoon of paprika
- Salt to taste
- Two cups of broccoli florets
- Two minced cloves of garlic

Instructions

- Warm your air fryer to 350 degrees F.
- Choose air fry setting.
- Drizzle pork chops with half of the avocado oil.
- Season with garlic powder, paprika and salt.
- Add to the air fryer.
- Cook for 5 minutes.
- Toss the broccoli in the remaining oil.
- Sprinkle with minced garlic and salt.
- Add broccoli to the air fryer.
- Cook for another 5 minutes.

Herbed Parmesan Shrimp

Preparation Time-10 minutes | Cook Time-10 minutes | Servings-2 | Difficulty-Easy

Nutritional Facts- Calories-233 | Fats-7.8g |Carbohydrates-3.18g |Proteins-34.8g

Ingredients

- One lb. of cooked shrimp, peeled and deveined
- Two tablespoons of olive oil
- Half teaspoon of onion powder
- One teaspoon of basil
- Half teaspoon of oregano
- 2/3 cup of grated parmesan cheese
- Two minced cloves of garlic
- A quarter teaspoon of pepper

Instructions

- In a large mixing bowl, merge together garlic, oil, onion powder, oregano, pepper, and cheese.

- Add shrimp in a bowl and toss until well coated.
- Spray air fryer basket with cooking spray.
- Add shrimp into the air fryer basket and cook at 350 F for 8-10 minutes.
- Serve and enjoy.

Herbed Pork Chops

Preparation Time-10 minutes | Cook Time-20 minutes | Servings-2 | Difficulty-Easy

Nutritional Facts- Calories-311 | Fats-15.9g|Carbohydrates-7.8g|Proteins-31.8g

Ingredients

- Two boneless pork chops
- One teaspoon of kosher salt
- One teaspoon of paprika
- One teaspoon of garlic powder
- One teaspoon of onion powder
- Two tablespoons of extra-virgin olive oil
- Half cup of freshly grated Parmesan
- A half teaspoon of freshly ground black pepper

Instructions

- Pat-dry pork chops with paper towels. Cover the two sides with oil. Combine the parmesan and spices in a medium bowl. Coat the pork chops with Parmesan paste on both sides.
- Place pork chops in an air-fryer basket and cook for 9 minutes at 375 ° F, flipping midway through.

Herbed Rotisserie Chicken

Preparation Time-10 minutes | Cook Time-One hour and 10 minutes | Servings-2 | Difficulty-Hard

Nutritional Facts- Calories-260 | Fats-13.8g |Carbohydrates-4g |Proteins-18g

Ingredients

- One pound of chicken
- Two tablespoons of dried oregano
- Two teaspoons of garlic powder
- Two teaspoons of onion powder
- One teaspoon of smoked paprika
- Kosher salt
- Freshly ground black pepper
- One tablespoon of dried thyme
- A quarter teaspoon of cayenne

Instructions

- Season the chicken pieces with pepper and salt all over. Whisk the herbs and spices together in a medium bowl and then brush the spice mix all over the chicken bits.
- Insert dark pieces of meat into the air fryer basket and cook 10 minutes at 350 ° F. Then flip and cook ten minutes more. Repeat for chicken breasts. However, reduce the time per side to eight minutes. To ensure the chicken is cooked through, using a meat thermometer, each piece should reach 165 ° F.

Herbed Steak

Preparation Time-10 minutes | Cook Time-45 minutes | Servings-2 | Difficulty-Moderate

Nutritional Facts- Calories-432 | Fats-18g |Carbohydrates-2.7g |Proteins-30g

Ingredients

- Two teaspoons of freshly chopped parsley
- Kosher salt
- Freshly ground black pepper
- One teaspoon of freshly chopped chives
- One teaspoon of freshly chopped thyme
- One teaspoon of freshly chopped rosemary
- Four tablespoons of butter softened
- Two cloves minced garlic
- One (two lb.) bone-in rib eye

Instructions

- Combine the butter and spices in a shallow bowl. Place it in the middle of the plastic piece middle and roll it into a log. Twist ends together. It should be refrigerated for twenty minutes till hardened.
- Season the steak with pepper and salt on both sides.
- Put the steak in the air fryer basket and cook at 400 ° F for twelve to fourteen minutes, for medium, based on steak thickness, flipping halfway through.
- Top steak with an herb butter slice.

Honey and Wine Chicken Breasts

Preparation Time-5 minutes | Cook Time-15 minutes | Servings-2 | Difficulty-Easy

Nutritional Facts- Calories-189 | Fats-13.8g

|Carbohydrates-1.5g |Proteins-10.8g

Ingredients

- Two chicken breasts, rinsed and halved
- One tablespoon of melted butter
- Half teaspoon of freshly ground pepper,
- 3/4 teaspoon of sea salt
- One teaspoon of paprika
- One teaspoon of dried rosemary
- Two tablespoons of dry white wine
- One tablespoon of honey

Instructions

- Preparing the Ingredients. Firstly, pat the chicken breasts dry. Lightly coat them with melted butter.
- Then, add the remaining ingredients.
- Air Frying. Transfer them to the air fryer basket; bake about a quarter-hour at 330 degrees F. Serve warm and enjoy!

Honey Glazed Salmon

Preparation Time-15 minutes | Cook Time-30 minutes | Servings-2 | Difficulty-Moderate

Nutritional Facts- Calories-388 | Fats-15g |Carbohydrates-3.18g |Proteins-55.8g

Ingredients

- Half cup of soy sauce
- One cup of honey
- Two tablespoons of lemon juice
- Two ounces of orange juice
- Two tablespoons of brown sugar
- Two teaspoons of olive oil
- Two tablespoons of red wine vinegar
- Two chopped scallions
- Two minced garlic cloves
- Salt and pepper to taste
- Two salmon fillets

Instructions

- Merge all the ingredients except salt, pepper and salmon.
- Place mixture in a pan over medium heat.
- Bring to a boil.
- Reduce heat.
- Simmer for 15 minutes.
- Turn off heat and transfer sauce to a bowl.

- Whisk salt and pepper on both sides of salmon.
- Add salmon to the air fryer.
- Select grill function.
- Cook at 320 degrees F for 6 minutes per side.
- Brush with the sauce.
- Cook for another 5 minutes per side.
- Serve with remaining sauce.

Japanese Chicken Mix

Preparation Time-10 minutes | Cook Time- 8 minutes | Servings-2 | Difficulty-Easy

Nutritional Facts- Calories-287 | Fats-12.9g |Carbohydrates-18g |Proteins-21g

Ingredients

- Two skinless and boneless chicken thighs
- Two chopped ginger slices
- Three minced garlic cloves
- A quarter cup of soy sauce
- A quarter cup of mirin
- 1/8 cup of sake
- Half teaspoon of sesame oil
- 1/8 cup of water
- Two tablespoons of sugar
- One tablespoon of cornstarch mixed with Two tablespoons of water
- Sesame seeds for serving

Instructions

- In a bowl, mix chicken thighs with ginger, garlic, soy sauce, mirin, sake, oil, water, sugar and cornstarch, toss well, transfer to preheated air fryer and cook at 360 degrees F for 8 minutes.
- Divide among plates, sprinkle sesame seeds on top and serve with a side salad for lunch.
- Enjoy!

Korean Chicken Wings

Preparation Time-5 minutes | Cook Time-22 minutes | Servings-2 | Difficulty-Easy

Nutritional Facts- Calories-356 | Fats-26g |Carbohydrates-9.9g |Proteins-23g

Ingredients

- One teaspoon of pepper
- One teaspoon of salt

- One pound of chicken wings

Sauce

- One packet of Splenda
- Half tablespoon of minced garlic
- Half tablespoon of minced ginger
- Half tablespoon of sesame oil
- One teaspoon of agave nectar
- One tablespoon of mayo
- One tablespoon of gochujang

Finishing

- A quarter cup of chopped green onions
- Two teaspoons of sesame seeds

Instructions

- Get the ingredients ready. Preheat the air fryer to 400 degrees Fahrenheit.
- Line a small pan with foil, place a rack on top, and place the pan in the air fryer.
- Season the wings with salt and pepper before placing them on the rack.
- Cook in the air fryer. Set the temperature to 160 degrees Fahrenheit and the timer to 20 minutes. Air fry for 20 minutes, flipping after 10 minutes.
- As the chicken air fries, combine all of the sauce ingredients.
- Remove the wings and set them in a bowl once the chicken has achieved 160 degrees on a thermometer.
- Pour half of the sauce mixture over the wings and toss to coat completely.
- Return the coated wings to the air fryer for another five minutes or until they reach 165°F. Remove and then add sesame seeds and green onions.

Lamb and Cabbage Mix

Preparation Time-5 minutes | Cook Time-30 minutes | Servings-2 | Difficulty-

Nutritional Facts- Calories- 250| Fats-13.8g |Carbohydrates-18g |Proteins-24g

Ingredients

- One lb. of lamb
- Two pressed garlic cloves
- Half cup of beef stock
- Two teaspoons of coriander

- Two teaspoons of nutmeg
- Half cabbage cut into wedges
- One bay leaf
- Two chopped carrots
- One turnip (cut into smaller pieces)
- Salt and black pepper to taste

Instructions

- Preheat the air fryer to 360 F.
- Put the beef in a pan, add the stock, coriander, nutmeg, salt, pepper, carrots, cabbage, bay leaves, garlic, turnip, stir, transfer to the air fryer, and cover. Cook for 20 minutes.
- Serve and enjoy.

Lamb and Creamy Brussels Sprouts

Preparation Time-5 minutes | Cook Time-One hour and 30 minutes | Servings-2 | Difficulty-

Nutritional Facts- Calories-420 | Fats-19g |Carbohydrates-6g |Proteins-37.8g

Ingredients

One lb. of scored lamb leg
- Half tablespoon of melted butter
- One tablespoon of olive oil
- Half cup of sour cream
- One tablespoon of thyme
- One lb. of trimmed Brussels sprouts
- One minced garlic clove
- One tablespoon of rosemary
- Salt and black pepper to taste

Instructions

- Preheat the air fryer to 375F.
- Season the lamb with salt, rosemary, thyme, and pepper. Brush with oil and transfer to the air fryer basket. Close the lid and cook for 1 hour, remove and set aside.
- In a pan that fits into the air fryer, mix Brussels sprouts with salt, pepper, garlic, sour cream. Transfer into the air fryer and cook for 10 minutes at 400F.
- Serve and enjoy!

Lamb and Green Pesto

Preparation Time- One hour | Cook Time- 45 minutes | Servings-2 | Difficulty-Easy

Nutritional Facts- Calories-200 | Fats-4g |Carbohydrates-15g |Proteins-12.9g

Ingredients

- One cup of parsley
- One cup of mint
- One small, roughly chopped yellow onion
- 1 /3 cup of chopped pistachios
- One teaspoon of grated lemon zest
- Five tablespoons of olive oil
- Salt and black pepper to the taste
- Two pounds lamb riblets
- Half chopped onion
- Five minced cloves of garlic
- Juice from one orange

Instructions

- In your food processor, mix parsley with mint, onion, pistachios, lemon zest, salt, pepper and oil and blend very well.
- Rub lamb with this mix, place in a bowl, cover and leave in the fridge for 1 hour.
- Transfer lamb to a baking dish that fits your air fryer, also add garlic, drizzle orange juice and cook in your air fryer at 300 degrees F for 45 minutes.
- Divide lamb among plates and serve.
- Enjoy!

Lamb and Lemon Sauce

Preparation Time-10 minutes | Cook Time-30 minutes | Servings-2 | Difficulty-Easy

Nutritional Facts- Calories-260 | Fats-6.9g |Carbohydrates-18g |Proteins-13.8g

Ingredients

- Two lamb shanks
- Salt and black pepper to the taste
- Two minced cloves of garlic
- Four tablespoons of olive oil
- Juice from half lemon
- Zest from half lemon
- Half teaspoon of dried oregano

Instructions

- Season lamb with salt, pepper, rub with garlic, put in your air fryer and cook at 350 degrees F for 30 minutes.
- Meanwhile, in a bowl, mix lemon juice with lemon zest, some salt and pepper, olive oil and oregano and whisk very well.
- Shred lamb, discard bone, divide among plates, drizzle the lemon dressing all over and serve.
- Enjoy!

Lamb and Snow Pea

Preparation Time-10 minutes | Cook Time-25 minutes | Servings-2 | Difficulty-Easy

Nutritional Facts- Calories-259 | Fats-6.9g |Carbohydrates-1.5g |Proteins-21g

Ingredients

- One lb. of sliced lean lamb back strap
- Seventeen ounces of trimmed snow pea
- One crushed garlic clove
- One chopped lemongrass stem
- 1/3 cup of rice wine
- One and a half teaspoons of peanut oil
- 1/3 cup of soy sauce
- One small sliced white onion
- Steamed jasmine rice to serve

Instructions

- Preheat the air fryer to 350F.
- In a bowl, mix peanut oil, soy sauce, and whisk. Toss in the lamb strip to coat. In another bowl, mix snow pea, onions, salt, lemongrass stem, rice wine, garlic, and pepper. Transfer to a pan and fit into the air fryer, set time to 16 minutes.
- Increase the air fryer's temperature to 400F, add the lamb strip, and cook for another 6 minutes.
- Serve and enjoy!

Lamb and Spinach Mix

Preparation Time-10 minutes | Cook Time- 35 minutes | Servings-2 | Difficulty-Easy

Nutritional Facts- Calories-172 | Fats-7.8g |Carbohydrates-20g |Proteins-20g

Ingredients

- Two tablespoons of grated ginger

- Two minced cloves of garlic
- Two teaspoons of ground cardamom
- One chopped red onion
- One pound of cubed lamb meat
- Two teaspoons of cumin powder
- One teaspoon of garam masala
- Half teaspoon of chili powder
- One teaspoon of turmeric
- Two teaspoons of ground coriander
- One pound of spinach
- Fourteen ounces of chopped canned tomatoes

Instructions

- Combine lamb, tomatoes, spinach, garlic, ginger, onion, cloves, cardamom, cumin, chilli, garam masala, turmeric, and coriander in a heatproof dish that fits your air fryer, stir, and cook at 360 degrees F for 35 minutes.
- Divide into bowls and serve.
- Enjoy!

Lamb Shanks and Carrots

Preparation Time-10 minutes | Cook Time-45 minutes | Servings-2 | Difficulty-Moderate

Nutritional Facts- Calories-423 | Fats-16.8g |Carbohydrates-25g |Proteins-43g

Ingredients

- Two lamb shanks
- Two tablespoons of olive oil
- One finely chopped yellow onion
- Three roughly chopped carrots
- Two minced cloves of garlic
- Two tablespoons of tomato paste
- One teaspoon of dried oregano
- One roughly chopped tomato
- Two tablespoons of water
- Four ounces of red wine
- Salt and black pepper to the taste

Instructions

- Season lamb with salt and pepper, rub with oil, put in your air fryer and cook at 360 degrees F for 10 minutes.
- In a pan that fits your air fryer, mix the onion with carrots, garlic, tomato paste, tomato, oregano, wine and water and toss.

- Add lamb, toss, introduce in your air fryer and cook at 370 degrees F for 35 minutes. Divide everything among plates and serve.
- Enjoy!

Lemon Butter Salmon

Preparation Time-10 minutes | Cook Time-15 minutes | Servings-2 | Difficulty-Easy

Nutritional Facts- Calories-379 | Fats-23g |Carbohydrates-1.5g |Proteins-34.8g

Ingredients

- Two salmon fillets
- Half teaspoon of olive oil
- Two teaspoons of minced garlic
- Two tablespoons of butter
- Two tablespoons of fresh lemon juice
- A quarter cup of white wine
- Pepper
- Salt

Instructions

- Preheat the air fryer to 350 F.
- Spray air fryer basket with cooking spray.
- Season salmon with pepper and salt and place into the air fryer basket, and cook for 6 minutes.
- Meanwhile, in a saucepan, add remaining ingredients and heat over low heat for 4-5 minutes.
- Place cooked salmon on the serving dish, then pour prepared sauce over salmon.
- Serve and enjoy.

Lemon Crab Patties

Preparation Time-15 minutes | Cook Time-15 minutes | Servings-2 | Difficulty-Easy

Nutritional Facts- Calories-184 | Fats-10.8g |Carbohydrates-4.8g |Proteins-12g

Ingredients

- One egg
- Six ounces of crabmeat
- Two chopped green onions
- A quarter cup of mayonnaise
- One cup of almond flour
- One teaspoon of old bay seasoning
- One teaspoon of red pepper flakes

- One tablespoon of fresh lemon juice

Instructions

- Preheat the air fryer to 400 F.
- Spray air fryer basket with cooking spray.
- Add 1/2 almond flour into the mixing bowl.
- Set remaining ingredients and mix until well combined.
- Make patties from mixture and coat with remaining almond flour and place into the air fryer basket.
- Cook patties for 5 minutes, then turn to another side and cook for 5 minutes more.
- Serve and enjoy.

Lemon Garlic Fish Fillet

Preparation Time-10 minutes | Cook Time-20 minutes | Servings-2 | Difficulty-Easy

Nutritional Facts- Calories-298 | Fats-12g |Carbohydrates-1g |Proteins-45.9g

Ingredients

- Two white fish fillets
- Cooking spray
- Half teaspoon of lemon pepper
- Half teaspoon of garlic powder
- Salt and pepper to taste
- Two teaspoons of lemon juice

Instructions

- Choose bake setting in your air fryer oven.
- Preheat it to 360 degrees F.
- Spray fish fillets with oil.
- Season fish fillets with lemon pepper, garlic powder, salt and pepper.
- Add to the air fryer.
- Cook at 360 F for 20 minutes.
- Drizzle with lemon juice.

Lemony Saba Fish

Preparation Time-10 minutes | Cook Time- 10 minutes | Servings-2 | Difficulty-Easy

Nutritional Facts- Calories-291 | Fats-4g |Carbohydrates-15g |Proteins-21g

Ingredients

- Four boneless Saba fish fillet

- Salt and black pepper to the taste
- Three chopped red chili peppers
- Two tablespoons of lemon juice
- Two tablespoons of olive oil
- Two tablespoons of minced garlic

Instructions

- Season fish fillets with salt and pepper and put them in a bowl.
- Add lemon juice, oil, chili and garlic toss to coat, transfer fish to your air fryer and cook at 360 degrees F for8 minutes, flipping halfway.
- Divide among plates and serve with some fries.
- Enjoy!

Lunch Egg Rolls

Preparation Time-10 minutes | Cook Time-15 minutes | Servings-2 | Difficulty-Easy

Nutritional Facts- Calories-172 | Fats-6g |Carbohydrates-7.8g |Proteins-6.9g

Ingredients

- Half cup of grated carrots
- Two chopped green onions
- Four egg roll wrappers
- One tablespoon of cornstarch
- Half cup of chopped mushrooms
- Half cup of grated zucchini
- Two tablespoons of soy sauce
- One whisked egg

Instructions

- Stir green onions, carrots, zucchini, mushrooms, and soy sauce together in a basin.
- Arrange egg roll wrappers on a work surface, divide the veggie mixture among them, and roll tightly.
- Mix cornstarch and egg in a bowl, whisk well, then brush this mixture over the eggs rolls.
- Seal the edges, then set all of the rolls in your warmed air fryer and cook for 15 minutes at 370 degrees F.
- Serve them for lunch by arranging them on a dish.
- Enjoy!

Lunch Fajitas

Preparation Time-10 minutes | Cook Time- 14 minutes | Servings-2 | Difficulty-Easy

Nutritional Facts- Calories-311 | Fats-7.8g |Carbohydrates-19g |Proteins-21g

Ingredients

- One teaspoon of garlic powder
- A quarter teaspoon of ground cumin
- Half teaspoon of chili powder
- Salt and black pepper to the taste
- A quarter teaspoon of ground coriander
- Half pound of chicken breasts, cut into strips
- Half sliced red bell pepper
- Half sliced green bell pepper
- Half chopped yellow onions
- One tablespoon of lime juice
- Cooking spray
- Two warmed up tortillas
- Salsa for serving
- Sour cream for serving
- One cup of lettuce leaves, torn for serving

Instructions

- In a bowl, mix chicken with garlic powder, cumin, chili, salt, pepper, coriander, lime juice, red bell pepper, green bell pepper and onion, toss, leave aside for 10 minutes, transfer to your air fryer and drizzle some cooking spray all over.
- Toss and cook at 400 degrees F for 10 minutes.
- Arrange tortillas on a working surface, divide chicken mix, also add salsa, sour cream and lettuce, wrap and serve for lunch.
- Enjoy!

Lunch Gnocchi

Preparation Time-10 minutes | Cook Time- 17 minutes | Servings-2 | Difficulty-Easy

Nutritional Facts- Calories-212 | Fats-4.8g |Carbohydrates-12.9g |Proteins-10.8g

Ingredients

- One chopped yellow onion
- One tablespoon of olive oil
- Two minced garlic cloves
- Eight ounces gnocchi

- A quarter cup of grated parmesan
- Four ounces of spinach pesto

Instructions

- Grease your air fryer's pan with olive oil, add gnocchi, onion and garlic, toss, put the pan in your air fryer and cook at 400 degrees F for 10 minutes.
- Add pesto, toss and cook for 7 minutes more at 350 degrees F.
- Divide among plates and serve for lunch.
- Enjoy!

Lunch Pizza

Preparation Time-10 minutes | Cook Time-15 minutes | Servings-2 | Difficulty-Easy

Nutritional Facts- Calories-283| Fats-15g|Carbohydrates-42g|Proteins-12g

Ingredients

- Two (eight ounces) packages of pizza dough
- One tablespoon of extra-virgin olive oil, divided
- Freshly ground black pepper
- Half (eight ounces) mozzarella ball, cut into Quarter" slices
- Basil leaves for serving
- One-third cup of crushed tomatoes
- One clove minced garlic
- A half teaspoon of oregano
- Kosher salt

Instructions

- Gently flatten the dough ball with your hands up to about 8" in diameter on a smooth, floured surface (or smaller than the basket of the air fryer). Repeat it with the second ball of dough. Brush both with olive oil and pass one to your air fryer's basket, oil side up.
- Stir to mix crushed tomatoes, garlic, then oregano, and season with pepper and salt in a medium bowl. On the middle of the rolled-out pizza dough, spoon half the tomato mixture, then spread into an even layer, leaving 1/2" bare outer crust.
- Apply half the slices of mozzarella to the pie. Air fry for 10 to 12 minutes at 400 ° F, or until the crust is golden and the cheese is melted.
- Using two sets of tongs, remove the first pizza

from the air fryer basket and garnish it with basil leaves. Prepare and cook the second pizza, garnish and serve.

Lunch Pork and Potatoes

Preparation Time-10 minutes | Cook Time-25 minutes | Servings-2 | Difficulty-Easy

Nutritional Facts- Calories-323 | Fats-15g |Carbohydrates-34g |Proteins-21g

Ingredients

- Two pounds pork loin
- Salt and black pepper to the taste
- Two red potatoes, cut into medium wedges
- Half teaspoon of garlic powder
- Half teaspoon of red pepper flakes
- One teaspoon of dried parsley
- A drizzle of balsamic vinegar

Instructions

- In your air fryer's pan, mix pork with potatoes, salt, pepper, garlic powder, pepper flakes, parsley and vinegar, toss and cook at 390 degrees F for 25 minutes.
- Slice pork, divide it and potatoes among plates and serve for lunch.
- Enjoy!

Lunch Shrimp Croquettes

Preparation Time-10 minutes | Cook Time-8 minutes | Servings-2 | Difficulty-Easy

Nutritional Facts- Calories-142 | Fats-6.9g |Carbohydrates-9g |Proteins-4.8g

Ingredients

- 2/3 pound of shrimp, cooked, peeled, deveined and chopped
- One and a half cups of bread crumbs
- One whisked egg
- Two tablespoons of lemon juice
- Two chopped green onions
- Half teaspoon of dried basil
- Salt and black pepper to the taste
- Two tablespoons of olive oil

Instructions

- In a bowl, mix half of the bread crumbs with egg

and lemon juice and stir well.
- Add green onions, basil, salt, pepper and shrimp and stir really well.
- In a separate bowl, mix the rest of the bread crumbs with the oil and toss well.
- Shape round balls out of shrimp mix, dredge them in bread crumbs, place them in the preheated air fryer and cook for 8 minutes at 400 degrees F.
- Serve them with a dip for lunch.
- Enjoy!

Lunch Special Pancake

Preparation Time-10 minutes | Cook Time- 10 minutes | Servings-2 | Difficulty-Easy

Nutritional Facts- Calories-189 | Fats-7.8g |Carbohydrates-12g |Proteins-6g

Ingredients

- One tablespoon of butter
- Three whisked eggs
- Half cup of flour
- Half cup of milk
- One cup of salsa
- One cup of peeled and deveined small shrimp

Instructions

- Preheat your air fryer at 400 degrees F, add fryer's pan, add one tablespoon of butter and melt it.
- In a bowl, mix eggs with flour and milk, whisk well and pour into the air fryer's pan; spread, cook at 350 degrees for 12 minutes and transfer to a plate.
- In a bowl, mix shrimp with salsa, stir and serve your pancake with this on the side.
- Enjoy!

Macaroni and Cheese

Preparation Time-10 minutes | Cook Time- 30 minutes | Servings-2 | Difficulty-Easy

Nutritional Facts- Calories-321 | Fats-10.8g |Carbohydrates-34g |Proteins-1.5g

Ingredients

- One and a half cups of favorite macaroni
- Cooking spray

- Half cup of heavy cream
- One cup of chicken stock
- 3/4 cup of shredded cheddar cheese
- Half cup of shredded mozzarella cheese
- A quarter cup of shredded parmesan
- Salt and black pepper to the taste

Instructions

- Spray a pan with cooking spray, then add macaroni, mozzarella, stock, heavy cream, cheddar cheese, and parmesan cheese, as well as salt and pepper, combine well, and cook for 30 minutes in an air fryer basket.
- Serve for lunch by dividing the mixture among plates.
- Enjoy!

Meatballs

Preparation Time-10 minutes | Cook Time-20 minutes | Servings-2 | Difficulty-Easy

Nutritional Facts- Calories-356 | Fats-25g |Carbohydrates-1g |Proteins-31.8g

Ingredients

- A quarter lb. of ground beef
- A quarter lb. of Italian sausage
- Half cup of cheddar cheese, shredded
- 1/3 teaspoon of pepper
- Half teaspoon of garlic powder
- One teaspoon of onion powder

Instructions

- Spray air fryer basket with cooking spray.
- Merge all ingredients into the large bowl and mix until combined.
- Set small balls from the meat mixture and place them in the air fryer basket.
- Cook at 370 F for 15 minutes. Turn to another side and cook for 5 minutes more.
- Serve and enjoy.

Meatballs with Tomato Sauce

Preparation Time-10 minutes | Cook Time-15 minutes | Servings-2 | Difficulty-Easy

Nutritional Facts- Calories-278 | Fats-8.58g |Carbohydrates-25g |Proteins-12.9g

Ingredients

- Half pound of lean ground beef
- Two chopped green onions
- Two minced cloves of garlic
- One egg yolk
- A quarter cup of bread crumbs
- Salt and black pepper to the taste
- One tablespoon of olive oil
- Eight ounces of tomato sauce
- One tablespoon of mustard

Instructions

- In a bowl, mix beef with onion, garlic, egg yolk, bread crumbs, salt and pepper, stir well and shape medium meatballs out of this mix.
- Grease meatballs with the oil, place them in your air fryer and cook them at 400 degrees F for 10 minutes.
- In a bowl, mix tomato sauce with mustard, whisk, add over meatballs, toss them and cook at 400 degrees F for 5 minutes more.
- Divide meatballs and sauce among plates and serve for lunch.
- Enjoy!

Meatloaf Sliders

Preparation Time-10 minutes | Cook Time-15 minutes | Servings-2 | Difficulty-Easy

Nutritional Facts- Calories-228 | Fats-15.9g |Carbohydrates-6g |Proteins-12.9g

Ingredients

- Half lb. of ground beef
- Half teaspoon of dried tarragon
- One teaspoon of Italian seasoning
- One tablespoon of Worcestershire sauce
- A quarter cup of ketchup
- A quarter cup of coconut flour
- Half cup of almond flour
- One minced clove of garlic
- A quarter cup of chopped onion
- Two lightly beaten eggs
- A quarter teaspoon of pepper
- Half teaspoon of sea salt

Instructions

- Set all ingredients into the mixing bowl and mix

until well combined.

- Make the equal shape of patties from the mixture and place them on a plate. Place in refrigerator for 10 minutes.
- Spray air fryer basket with cooking spray.
- Preheat the air fryer to 360 F.
- Place prepared patties in an air fryer basket and cook for 10 minutes.
- Serve and enjoy.

Parmesan Pork Chops

Preparation Time-10 minutes | Cook Time-15 minutes | Servings-2 | Difficulty-Easy

Nutritional Facts- Calories-329 | Fats-24g |Carbohydrates-1.5g |Proteins-23g

Ingredients

- Two boneless pork chops
- Two tablespoons of grated parmesan cheese
- One cup of pork rind
- Two lightly beaten eggs
- Half teaspoon of chili powder
- Half teaspoon of onion powder
- One teaspoon of paprika
- A quarter teaspoon of pepper
- Half teaspoon of salt

Instructions

- Preheat the air fryer to 400 F.
- Season pork chops with pepper and salt.
- Add pork rind in the food processor and process until crumbs form.
- Mix together pork rind crumbs and seasoning in a large bowl.
- Place egg in a separate bowl.
- Dip pork chops in egg mixture, then coat with pork crumb mixture and place in the air fryer basket.
- Cook pork chops for 12-15 minutes.
- Serve and enjoy.

Pastrami and Veggies Casserole

Preparation Time-10 minutes | Cook Time-10 minutes | Servings-2 | Difficulty-Easy

Nutritional Facts- Calories-218 | Fats-9g |Carbohydrates-12g |Proteins-21g

Ingredients

- One cup of sliced pastrami
- One chopped bell pepper
- A quarter cup of Greek yogurt
- Two chopped spring onions
- Half cup of grated cheddar cheese
- Two eggs
- A quarter teaspoon of ground black pepper
- Sea salt, to taste
- Cooking spray

Instructions

- Spritz a baking pan with cooking spray.
- Set together all the ingredients in a large bowl. Stir to mix well. Pour the mixture into the baking pan.
- Place the pan on the bake position.
- Select Bake, set temperature to 330F (166C) and set time to 8 minutes.
- When cooking is complete, the eggs should be set, and the casserole edges should be lightly browned.
- Remove the baking pan from the air fryer grill and allow it to cool for 10 minutes before serving.

Pecan Crusted Chicken

Preparation Time-10 minutes | Cook Time-25 minutes | Servings-2 | Difficulty-Easy

Nutritional Facts- Calories-259 | Fats-15.9g |Carbohydrates-9.9g |Proteins-21g

Ingredients

- Half cup of breadcrumbs
- Two eggs
- One lb. of chicken breast, skinless and boneless
- One tablespoon of honey
- One pinch of salt
- Half cup of pecan pieces
- Two tablespoons of Creole seasoning
- Half cup of olive oil
- Half cup of mayonnaise
- One tablespoon of Creole mustard
- One pinch of cayenne pepper

Instructions

- In a food processor, combine pecans, breadcrumbs and two teaspoons of

Creole seasoning. To combine, pulse for a minute. Fill a dish halfway with the mixture.

- Beat the eggs in a mixing dish, then add the oil and the remaining Creole.
- Shake off any excess after dipping the chicken breast in the egg mixture and then in the pecan mixture.
- Place the chicken on a baking sheet and bake it. Place the crisper tray on top of the pizza rack, followed by the baking pan.
- Set the temperature to 360°F for 15 minutes and select the air fry setting. Start by pressing the start button.
- Meanwhile, whisk together the honey, salt, mustard, and pepper.
- During the cooking process, season the chicken breasts with salt and pepper. Serve with the sauce and take pleasure in it.

Perfect Chicken Parmesan

Preparation Time-5 minutes | Cook Time-25 minutes | Servings-2 | Difficulty-Easy

Nutritional Facts- Calories-262 | Fats-17g |Carbohydrates-8.19g |Proteins-16.2g

Ingredients

- Two large white meat chicken breasts, approximately 5-6 ounces
- One cup of breadcrumbs
- Two medium-sized eggs
- Pinch of salt and pepper
- One tablespoon of dried oregano
- One cup of marinara sauce
- Two slices of provolone cheese
- One tablespoon of parmesan cheese

Instructions

- Prepare the Ingredients. Cover the basket of the power air fryer with a lining of tin foil, leaving the sides uncovered to permit air to circulate through the basket.
- Preheat the air fryer to 350 degrees.
- In a bowl, set the eggs until fluffy until the yolks and whites are thoroughly combined and put aside.
- In a separate bowl, combine the breadcrumbs, oregano, salt and pepper, and put aside.

- One by one, dip the raw chicken breasts into the bowl with dry ingredients, coating both sides; then submerge into the bowl with wet ingredients, then dip again into the dry ingredients. This double coating will ensure an additional crisp-and-delicious air-fry!
- Lay the coated chicken breasts on the foil covering the power air fryer basket in a single flat layer.
- Set the power air fryer timer for 10 minutes.
- After 10 minutes, the air fryer will switch off, and the chicken should be mid-way cooked and the breaded coating beginning to brown.
- Using tongs, turn each bit of chicken over to make sure a full all-over fry.
- Reset the air fryer to 320 degrees for an additional 10 minutes.
- While the chicken is cooking, pour half the marinara sauce into a 7-inch heat-safe pan.
- After a quarter-hour, when the air fryer shuts off, remove the fried chicken breasts using tongs and set them in the marinara-covered pan. Drizzle the remainder of the marinara sauce over the fried chicken, then place the slices of provolone cheese atop both of them and sprinkle the parmesan cheese over the whole pan.
- Reset the air fryer to 350 degrees for five minutes.
- After 5 minutes, when the air fryer shuts off, remove the dish from the air fryer using tongs or oven mitts. The chicken is going to be perfectly crisped and the cheese melted and lightly toasted. Serve while hot!

Pesto Fish

Preparation Time-15 minutes | Cook Time-10 minutes | Servings-2 | Difficulty-Easy

Nutritional Facts- Calories-342 | Fats-15.9g |Carbohydrates-1.5g |Proteins-45g

Ingredients

- One tablespoon of olive oil
- Two fish fillets
- Salt and pepper to taste
- One cup of olive oil
- Two cloves of garlic
- Half cup of fresh basil leaves
- Two tablespoons of grated Parmesan cheese
- Two tablespoons of pine nuts

Instructions

- Set olive oil over fish fillets and season with salt and pepper.
- Add remaining ingredients to a food processor.
- Pulse until smooth.
- Bring pesto to a bowl and set it aside.
- Add fish to the air fryer.
- Select grill setting.
- Cook at 320 degrees F for 5 minutes per side.
- Spread pesto on top of the fish before serving.

Philadelphia Chicken Lunch

Preparation Time-10 minutes | Cook Time- 30 minutes | Servings-2 | Difficulty-Easy

Nutritional Facts- Calories-301 | Fats-10.8g |Carbohydrates-36.9g |Proteins-12.9g

Ingredients

- One teaspoon of olive oil
- One sliced yellow onion
- Two skinless, boneless and sliced chicken breasts
- Salt and black pepper to the taste
- One tablespoon of Worcestershire sauce
- Fourteen ounces of pizza dough
- One and a half cups of grated cheddar cheese
- Half cup of jarred cheese sauce

Instructions

- Preheat your air fryer at 400 degrees F, add half of the oil and onions and fry them for 8 minutes, stirring once.
- Add chicken pieces, Worcestershire sauce, salt and pepper, toss, air fry for 8 minutes more, stirring once and transfer everything to a bowl.
- Roll pizza dough on a working surface and shape a rectangle.
- Spread half of the cheese all over, add chicken and onion mix and top with cheese sauce.
- Roll your dough and shape it into a U.
- Place your roll in your air fryer's basket, brush with the rest of the oil and cook at 370 degrees for 12 minutes, flipping the roll halfway.
- Slice your roll when it's warm and serve for lunch.
- Enjoy!

Pork with Mushrooms

Preparation Time-10 minutes | Cook Time-18 minutes | Servings-2 | Difficulty-Easy

Nutritional Facts- Calories-420 | Fats-2.1g |Carbohydrates-1g |Proteins-27g

Ingredients

- Half lb. of rinsed and pat dry pork chops
- Half teaspoon of garlic powder
- One teaspoon of soy sauce
- Two tablespoons of melted butter
- Four ounces of halved mushrooms
- Pepper
- Salt

Instructions

- Preheat the air fryer to 400 F.
- Cut pork chops into the 3/4-inch cubes and place them in a large mixing bowl.
- Add remaining ingredients into the bowl and toss well.
- Transfer pork and mushroom mixture into the air fryer basket and cook for 15-18 minutes. Shake basket halfway through.
- Serve and enjoy.

Quick and Easy Steak

Preparation Time-10 minutes | Cook Time-7 minutes | Servings-2 | Difficulty-Easy

Nutritional Facts- Calories-356 | Fats-8.7g |Carbohydrates-1.2g |Proteins-60g

Ingredients

- Twelve ounces of steaks
- Half tablespoon of unsweetened cocoa powder
- One tablespoon of Montreal steak seasoning
- One teaspoon of liquid smoke
- One tablespoon of soy sauce
- Pepper
- Salt

Instructions

- Add steak, liquid smoke, and soy sauce in a zip-lock bag and shake well.
- Season steak with seasonings and place in the refrigerator overnight.

- Place marinated steak in an air fryer basket and cook at 375 F for 5 minutes.
- Turn steak to another side and cook for 2 minutes more.
- Serve and enjoy.

Quick and Simple Bratwurst with Vegetables

Preparation Time-10 minutes | Cook Time-20 minutes | Servings-2 | Difficulty-Easy

Nutritional Facts- Calories-70 | Fats-4g | Carbohydrates-4g | Proteins-1.5g

Ingredients

- Half package of bratwurst sliced 1/2-inch rounds
- Half tablespoon of Cajun seasoning
- A quarter cup of diced onion
- One sliced bell pepper

Instructions

- Set all ingredients into the mixing bowl and toss well.
- Line air fryer basket with foil.
- Add vegetable and bratwurst mixture into the air fryer basket and cook at 390 F for 10 minutes.
- Toss well and cook for 10 minutes more.
- Serve and enjoy.

Quick and Tender Pork Chops

Preparation Time-5 minutes | Cook Time-15 minutes | Servings-2 | Difficulty-Easy

Nutritional Facts- Calories-285 | Fats-7.8g | Carbohydrates-1.5g | Proteins-21g

Ingredients

- Two pork chops, rinsed and pat dry
- A quarter teaspoon of smoked paprika
- Half teaspoon of garlic powder
- Two teaspoons of olive oil
- Pepper
- Salt

Instructions

- Set pork chops with olive oil and season with paprika, garlic powder, pepper, and salt.

- Place pork chops in the air fryer basket and cook at 380 F for 10-14 minutes. Turn halfway through.
- Serve and enjoy.

Quick Lunch Pizzas

Preparation Time-10 minutes | Cook Time-7 minutes | Servings-2 | Difficulty-Easy

Nutritional Facts- Calories-187 | Fats-4.8g | Carbohydrates-12g | Proteins-4g

Ingredients

- Two pitas
- One tablespoon of olive oil
- 3/4 cup of pizza sauce
- Two ounces sliced jarred mushrooms
- Half teaspoon of dried basil
- Two chopped green onions
- Two cups of grated mozzarella
- One cup of sliced grape tomatoes

Instructions

- Spread pizza sauce on each pita bread, sprinkle green onions and basil, divide mushrooms and top with cheese.
- Arrange pita pizzas in your air fryer and cook them at 400 degrees F for 7 minutes.
- Top each pizza with tomato slices, divide among plates and serve.
- Enjoy!

Rotisserie Chicken

Preparation Time-10 minutes | Cook Time-One hour | Servings-2 | Difficulty-Hard

Nutritional Facts- Calories-282 | Fats-13.8g | Carbohydrates-0g | Proteins-43.8g

Ingredients

- A quarter cup of Rustic rub
- Two lb. of whole chicken

Instructions

- Rub the chicken with the rustic rub.
- Fix the rotisserie spit on one side, then slide the chicken so the split can run through the chicken. Fix the fork and screws.

- Select the rotisserie setting in the Emeril Lagasse Air Fryer 360. Set the temperature at 350°F for 55 minutes. Press the start button.
- The chicken should have an internal temperature of 160°F when the cooking cycle is complete. Otherwise, add more minutes.
- Let the chicken rest for 15 minutes before serving.

Rutabaga and Cherry Tomatoes Mix

Preparation Time-10 minutes | Cook Time- 15 minutes | Servings-2 | Difficulty-Easy

Nutritional Facts- Calories-160 | Fats-1g|Carbohydrates-15g |Proteins-6.9g

Ingredients

- One minced garlic clove
- 3/4 cup of soaked for a couple of hours and drained cashews
- Two tablespoons of nutritional yeast
- Half cup of veggie stock
- Salt and black pepper to the taste
- Two teaspoons of lemon juice
One tablespoon of chopped shallot

For the pasta

- One cup of halved cherry tomatoes
- Five teaspoons of olive oil
- A quarter teaspoon of garlic powder
- Two peeled and cut into thick noodles rutabagas

Instructions

- Place tomatoes and rutabaga noodles into a pan that fits your air fryer, drizzle the oil over them, season with salt, black pepper and garlic powder, toss to coat and cook in your air fryer at 350 degrees F for 15 minutes.
- Meanwhile, in a food processor, mix garlic with shallots, cashews, veggie stock, nutritional yeast, lemon juice, a pinch of sea salt and black pepper to the taste and blend well.
- Divide rutabaga pasta among plates, top with tomatoes, drizzle the sauce over them and serve.
- Enjoy!

Salmon and Asparagus

Preparation Time-10 minutes | Cook Time- 23 minutes | Servings-2 | Difficulty-Easy

Nutritional Facts- Calories-121 | Fats-1g|Carbohydrates-4g |Proteins-24g

Ingredients

- Half pound of trimmed asparagus
- One tablespoon of olive oil
- A pinch of sweet paprika
- Salt and black pepper to the taste
- A pinch of garlic powder
- A pinch of cayenne pepper
- One halved red bell pepper
- Four ounces of smoked salmon

Instructions

- Put asparagus spears and bell pepper on a lined baking sheet that fits your air fryer, add salt, pepper, garlic
- powder, paprika, olive oil, cayenne pepper, toss to coat, introduce in the fryer, cook at 390 degrees F for 8 minutes, flip and cook for 8 minutes more.
- Add salmon, cook for 5 minutes, more, divide everything among plates and serve.
- Enjoy!

Scallops and Dill

Preparation Time-10 minutes | Cook Time- minutes | Servings-2 | Difficulty-Easy

Nutritional Facts- Calories-153 | Fats-4.8g |Carbohydrates-19g |Proteins-4.8g

Ingredients

- Half pound of debearded sea scallops
- Half tablespoon of lemon juice
- Half teaspoon of chopped dill
- One teaspoon of olive oil
- Salt and black pepper to the taste

Instructions

- In your air fryer, mix scallops with dill, oil, salt, pepper and lemon juice, cover and cook at 360 degrees F for 5 minutes.
- Discard unopened ones, divide scallops and dill sauce among plates and serve for lunch.

- Enjoy!

Seasoned Catfish Fillets

Preparation Time-10 minutes | Cook Time-20 minutes | Servings-2 | Difficulty-Easy

Nutritional Facts- Calories-245 | Fats-15g |Carbohydrates-1g |Proteins-24g

Ingredients

- Four catfish fillets
- Half tablespoon of olive oil
- A quarter cup of fish seasoning
- Half tablespoon of fresh chopped parsley

Instructions

- Preheat the air fryer to 400 F.
- Spray air fryer basket with cooking spray.
- Seasoned fish with seasoning and place into the air fryer basket.
- Drizzle fish fillets with oil and cook for 10 minutes.
- Turn fish to another side and cook for 10 minutes more.
- Garnish with parsley and serve.

Seasoned Cod

Preparation Time-10 minutes | Cook Time-30 minutes | Servings-2 | Difficulty-Moderate

Nutritional Facts- Calories-245 | Fats-15g |Carbohydrates-1g |Proteins-24g

Ingredients

- One lb. cod, cut into four strips
- One large egg, beaten
- Two cups of panko bread crumbs
- One teaspoon of Old Bay seasoning
- Lemon wedges, for serving
- Kosher salt
- Freshly ground black pepper
- Half cup of all-purpose flour
- Tartar sauce, for serving

Instructions

- Dry and season the fish with pepper and salt on both sides.
- Place in three shallow bowls the flour, egg, and panko. To mix, add Old Bay to panko & toss.

Acting one at a time, cover the fish with the flour, then with the egg, and then with the panko, and press to coat.
- Working in batches, put fish in the air fryer basket and cook for 10 to 12 minutes at 400 ° F, softly tossing halfway through or until the fish is golden and comfortably flakes with a fork.
- Serve with tartar sauce and lemon wedges.

Seasoned King Prawns

Preparation Time-10 minutes | Cook Time-8 minutes | Servings-2 | Difficulty-Easy

Nutritional Facts- Calories-130 | Fats-4.8g |Carbohydrates-4.8g |Proteins-15g

Ingredients

- Six king prawns
- Half tablespoon of vinegar
- Half tablespoon of ketchup
- One tablespoon of mayonnaise
- Half teaspoon of. pepper
- Half teaspoon of. chili powder
- Half teaspoon of. red chili flakes
- Half teaspoon of. sea salt

Instructions

- Preheat the air fryer to 350 F.
- Spray air fryer basket with cooking spray.
- Add prawns, chili flakes, chili powder, pepper, and salt to the bowl and toss well.
- Transfer shrimp to the air fryer basket and cook for 6 minutes.
- In a small bowl, mix together mayonnaise, ketchup, and vinegar.
- Serve with mayo mixture and enjoy.

Sesame Chicken Thighs

Preparation Time-10 minutes | Cook Time-55 minutes | Servings-2 | Difficulty-Hard

Nutritional Facts- Calories-484 | Fats-16.8g |Carbohydrates-26g |Proteins-40g

Ingredients

- One tablespoon of sesame oil
- One tablespoon of soy sauce
- Half tablespoon of honey
- Half tablespoon of sriracha sauce

- Half tablespoon of rice vinegar
- One lb. of chicken thighs
- One chopped green onion
- One tablespoon of toasted sesame seeds

Instructions

- Merge the first five ingredients in a mixing bowl. Add chicken to the bowl and stir until well coated.
- Seal and refrigerate for at least 30 minutes.
- Drain the marinade and place the chicken in the crisper tray. Place the crisp tray on the pizza rack of the Air Fryer.
- Select the air fry setting and set the temperature at 400F for 15 minutes. Press start.
- When you have cooked for 5 minutes, flip and cook for an additional 10 minutes.
- Let the chicken rest before serving.

Shrimp Bang

Preparation Time-10 minutes | Cook Time-4 minutes | Servings-2 | Difficulty-Easy

Nutritional Facts- Calories-304 | Fats-16.8g |Carbohydrates-15g |Proteins-21.9g

Ingredients

- One cup of cornstarch
- A quarter teaspoon of Sriracha powder
- One lb. of peeled and deveined shrimp
- A quarter cup of mayonnaise
- A quarter cup of sweet chili sauce

Instructions

- In a bowl, combine cornstarch and Sriracha powder.
- Dredge shrimp with this mixture.
- Place shrimp in the air fryer.
- Choose air fry setting.
- Cook at 400 F for 7 minutes per side.
- Mix the mayo and chili sauce.
- Serve shrimp with sauce.

Simple Air Fryer Salmon

Preparation Time-5 minutes | Cook Time-10 minutes | Servings-2 | Difficulty-Easy

Nutritional Facts- Calories-256 | Fats-13.2g |Carbohydrates-0g |Proteins-34g

Ingredients

- Two salmon fillets, skinless and boneless
- One teaspoon of olive oil
- Pepper
- Salt

Instructions

- Set salmon fillets with olive oil and season with pepper and salt.
- Place salmon fillets in the air fryer basket and cook at 360 F for 8-10 minutes.
- Serve and enjoy.

Simple Air Fryer Steak

Preparation Time-10 minutes | Cook Time-18 minutes | Servings-2 | Difficulty-Easy

Nutritional Facts- Calories-363 | Fats-10.8g |Carbohydrates-1g |Proteins-60g

Ingredients

- Twelve ounces of steaks, 3/4-inch thick
- One teaspoon of garlic powder
- One teaspoon of olive oil
- Pepper
- Salt

Instructions

- Coat steaks with oil and season with garlic powder, pepper, and salt.
- Preheat the air fryer to 400 F.
- Place steaks in an air fryer basket and cook for 15-18 minutes. Turn halfway through.
- Serve and enjoy.

Spiced Steak

Preparation Time-10 minutes | Cook Time-9 minutes | Servings-2 | Difficulty-Easy

Nutritional Facts- Calories-304 | Fats-6g |Carbohydrates-1.5g |Proteins-52.8g

Ingredients

- One lb. of rib-eye steak
- Half teaspoon of chipotle powder
- A quarter teaspoon of paprika
- A quarter teaspoon of onion powder
- Half teaspoon of garlic powder
- One teaspoon of chili powder

- A quarter teaspoon of black pepper
- One teaspoon of coffee powder
- 1/8 teaspoon of cocoa powder
- 1/8 teaspoon of coriander powder
- Half teaspoon of sea salt

Instructions

- In a small bowl, merge together all ingredients except steak.
- Rub spice mixture over the steak and let marinate the steak for 20 minutes.
- Spray air fryer basket with cooking spray.
- Preheat the air fryer to 390 F.
- Place marinated steak in the air fryer and cook for 9 minutes.
- Serve and enjoy.

Spicy Chicken Taquitos

Preparation Time-10 minutes | Cook Time-45 minutes | Servings-2 | Difficulty-Moderate

Nutritional Facts- Calories-216 | Fats-7.8g | Carbohydrates-18g | Proteins-11.1g

Ingredients

One teaspoon of cumin
- One teaspoon of chili powder
- Kosher salt
- Cooking spray
- Two cups of shredded cooked chicken
- One (eight ounces) block cream cheese, softened
- Freshly ground black pepper
- One chipotle in adobo sauce, chopped, plus one tablespoon of sauce
- Four small corn tortillas
- One and a half cups of shredded cheddar
- One and a half cups of shredded Pepper Jack
- Pico de Gallo, for serving
- One clove garlic
- Juice of lime
- Kosher salt
- Freshly ground black pepper
- Crumbled queso fresco for serving

For the avocado cream sauce

- One large avocado pitted
- Half cup of sour cream

- A quarter cup of packed cilantro leaves

Instructions

- Combine the chicken, cream cheese, chipotle, sauce, cumin, and chili powder in a large bowl with pepper and salt, season.
- Place the tortillas on a secure microwave plate and cover them with a wet paper towel. Microwave for 30 seconds or before more pliable and wet.
- Spread on one end of the tortilla about a quarter cup of filling, then scatter next to the filling a little cheddar and pepper jack. Tightly roll-up. Repeat with the filling and cheese.
- Place in the air fryer basket, seam side down, and cook for 7 minutes at 400 ° F.
- Serve with salsa, Pico de Gallo, and queso fresco with avocado cream.
- Mix the cilantro, avocado, sour cream, garlic and lime juice together in a food processor. With pepper and salt, season it. Pour into a bowl and press directly over the top with plastic wrap and refrigerate till ready to use.

Spicy Shrimp

Preparation Time-10 minutes | Cook Time-6 minutes | Servings-2 | Difficulty-Easy

Nutritional Facts- Calories-195 | Fats-9g | Carbohydrates-1.5g | Proteins-26g

Ingredients

- Half lb. of peeled and deveined shrimp
- Half teaspoon of old bay seasoning
- One teaspoon of cayenne pepper
- One tablespoon of olive oil
- A quarter teaspoon of paprika
- 1/8 teaspoon of salt

Instructions

- Preheat the air fryer to 390 F.
- Add all ingredients into the bowl and toss well.
- Transfer shrimp into the air fryer basket and cook for 6 minutes.
- Serve and enjoy.

Squash Fritters

Preparation Time-10 minutes | Cook Time-8 minutes | Servings-2 | Difficulty-Easy

Nutritional Facts- Calories-156 | Fats-4g |Carbohydrates-12g |Proteins-10.8g

Ingredients

- One and a half ounces of cream cheese
- One whisked egg
- Half teaspoon of dried oregano
- A pinch of salt and black pepper
- One grated yellow summer squash
- 1/3 cup of grated carrot
- 2/3 cup of bread crumbs
- Two tablespoons of olive oil

Instructions

- Combine cream cheese, pepper, salt, oregano, breadcrumbs, egg, carrots, and squash in a mixing dish and whisk well.
- Form medium patties from the mixture and brush with the oil.
- Cook the squash patties in your air fryer for 7 minutes at 400 degrees F.
- You can eat them for lunch.
- Enjoy!

Steak Bites with Mushrooms

Preparation Time-10 minutes | Cook Time-18 minutes | Servings-2 | Difficulty-Easy

Nutritional Facts- Calories-388 | Fats-5g |Carbohydrates-3.18g |Proteins-55.8g

Ingredients

- One lb. of steaks, cut into 1/2-inch cubes
- Half teaspoon of garlic powder
- One teaspoon of Worcestershire sauce
- Two tablespoons of melted butter
- Eight ounces of sliced mushroom
- Pepper
- Salt

Instructions

- Set all ingredients into the large mixing bowl and toss well.
- Set air fryer basket with cooking spray.
- Preheat the air fryer to 400 F.

- Add steak mushroom mixture into the air fryer basket and cook at 400 F for 15-18 minutes. Shake basket twice.
- Serve and enjoy.

Steak Fajitas

Preparation Time-10 minutes | Cook Time-15 minutes | Servings-2 | Difficulty-Easy

Nutritional Facts- Calories-301 | Fats-16.8g |Carbohydrates-12.9g |Proteins-21.9g

Ingredients

- Half lb. of sliced steak
- One tablespoon of olive oil
- One tablespoon of fajita seasoning, gluten-free
- Half cup of sliced onion
- Two sliced bell peppers

Instructions

- Line air fryer basket with aluminum foil.
- Add all ingredients large bowl and toss until well coated.
- Transfer fajita mixture into the air fryer basket and cook at 390 F for 5 minutes.
- Toss well and cook for 5-10 minutes more.
- Serve and enjoy.

Steaks and Cabbage

Preparation Time-10 minutes | Cook Time-15 minutes | Servings-2 | Difficulty-Easy

Nutritional Facts- Calories-282 | Fats-9g |Carbohydrates-26g |Proteins-30g

Ingredients

- Half pound sirloin steak, cut into strips
- Two teaspoons of cornstarch
- One tablespoon of peanut oil
- One cup of chopped green cabbage
- One chopped yellow bell pepper
- One chopped green onion
- Two minced cloves of garlic
- Salt and black pepper to the taste

Instructions

- In a bowl, mix cabbage with salt, pepper and peanut oil, toss, transfer to air fryer's basket, cook

at 370 degrees F for 4 minutes and transfer to a bowl.
- Add steak strips to your air fryer, also add green onions, bell pepper, garlic, salt and pepper, toss and cook for 5 minutes.
- Add over cabbage, toss, divide among plates and serve for lunch.
- Enjoy!

Stuffed Meatballs

Preparation Time-10 minutes | Cook Time- 15 minutes | Servings-2 | Difficulty-Easy

Nutritional Facts- Calories-201 | Fats-12g |Carbohydrates-9g |Proteins-21g

Ingredients

- 1/3 cup of bread crumbs
- Two tablespoons of milk
- One tablespoon of ketchup
- One egg
- Half teaspoon of dried marjoram
- Salt and black pepper to the taste
- Half pound of lean ground beef
- Ten cheddar cheese cubes
- One tablespoon of olive oil

Instructions

- In a bowl, mix bread crumbs with ketchup, milk, marjoram, salt, pepper and egg and whisk well.
- Add beef, stir and shape 20 meatballs out of this mix.
- Shape each meatball around a cheese cube, drizzle the oil over them and rub.
- Place all meatballs in your preheated air fryer and cook at 390 degrees F for 10 minutes.
- Serve them for lunch with a side salad.
- Enjoy!

Stuffed Mushrooms

Preparation Time-10 minutes | Cook Time-20 minutes | Servings-2 | Difficulty-Easy

Nutritional Facts- Calories-152 | Fats-1g|Carbohydrates-6.9g |Proteins-1.5g

Ingredients

- Two big Portobello mushroom caps
- One tablespoon of olive oil
- A quarter cup of ricotta cheese
- Three tablespoons of grated parmesan
- One cup of torn spinach, torn
- 1/3 cup of bread crumbs
- A quarter teaspoon of chopped rosemary

Instructions

- Rub mushrooms caps with the oil, place them in your air fryer's basket and cook them at 350 degrees F for 2 minutes.
- Meanwhile, in a bowl, mix half of the parmesan with ricotta, spinach, rosemary and bread crumbs and stir well.
- Stuff mushrooms with this mix, sprinkle the rest of the parmesan on top, place them in your air fryer's basket again and cook at 350 degrees F for 10 minutes.
- Divide them among plates and serve with a side salad for lunch.
- Enjoy!

Succulent Lunch Turkey Breast

Preparation Time-10 minutes | Cook Time-50 minutes | Servings-2 | Difficulty-Moderate

Nutritional Facts- Calories-280 | Fats-10.8g |Carbohydrates-23g |Proteins-13.8g

Ingredients

One turkey breast
- Two teaspoons of olive oil
- Half teaspoon of smoked paprika
- One teaspoon of dried thyme
- Half teaspoon of dried sage
- Salt and black pepper to the taste
- Two tablespoons of mustard
- A quarter cup of maple syrup
- One tablespoon of softened butter

Instructions

- Brush turkey breast with olive oil, season with salt, pepper, thyme, paprika and sage, rub, place in your air fryer's basket and fry at 350 degrees F for 25 minutes.
- Flip turkey, cook for 10 minutes more, flip one more time and cook for another 10 minutes.
- Meanwhile, heat up a pan with the butter over medium heat, add mustard and maple syrup, stir

well, cook for a couple of minutes and take off the heat.

- Slice turkey breast, divide among plates and serve with the maple glaze drizzled on top.
- Enjoy!

Sumptuous Chicken and Vegetable Casserole

Preparation Time-5 minutes | Cook Time-15 minutes | Servings-2 | Difficulty-Easy

Nutritional Facts- Calories-245 | Fats-13.8g |Carbohydrates-1g |Proteins-24g

Ingredients

- Two boneless and skinless chicken breasts, cut into cubes
- Two sliced carrots
- One yellow bell pepper
- One red bell pepper
- Eight ounces of broccoli florets
- One cup of snow peas
- One diced scallion
- Cooking spray

Sauce

- One teaspoon of Sriracha
- Three tablespoons of soy sauce
- Two tablespoons of oyster sauce
- One tablespoon of rice wine vinegar
- One teaspoon of cornstarch
- One tablespoon of grated ginger
- Two minced cloves of garlic
- One teaspoon of sesame oil
- One tablespoon of brown sugar

Instructions

- Spritz a baking pan with cooking spray.
- Combine the chicken, bell peppers, and carrot in a large bowl. Stir to mix well.
- Merge the ingredients for the sauce in a separate bowl. Stir to mix well.
- Pour the chicken mixture into the baking pan, and then pour the sauce over. Stir to coat well.
- Place the pan on the bake position.
- Select Bake, set temperature to 370F (188C) and set time to 13 minutes. Add the broccoli and snow peas to the pan halfway through.

- When cooking is complete, the vegetables should be tender.
- Remove the pan from the air fryer grill and sprinkle with sliced scallion before serving.

Sweet and Sour Chicken

Preparation Time-5 minutes | Cook Time-22 minutes | Servings-2 | Difficulty-Easy

Nutritional Facts- Calories-188 | Fats-6g |Carbohydrates-4.8g |Proteins-16.8g

Ingredients

- Two cubed chicken breasts
- Half cup of Flour
- Half cup of Cornstarch
- Two sliced red peppers
- One chopped onion
- Two julienned carrots
- 3/4 Cup of Sugar
- Two tablespoons of Cornstarch
- 1/3 Cup of Vinegar
- 2/3 Cup of Water
- A quarter cup of Soy sauce
- One tablespoon of Ketchup

Instructions

- Preheat the power air fryer to 375 degrees.
- Combine the flour, cornstarch and chicken in an airtight container and shake to mix. Remove chicken from the container and shake off any excess flour.
- Add chicken to the Air Fryer tray and cook for 20 minutes.
- In a saucepan, whisk together sugar, water, vinegar, soy and ketchup. Bring to a boil medium heat, reduce the warmth, then simmer for two minutes
- After cooking the chicken for 20 minutes, add the vegetables and sauce mixture to the power air fryer and cook for an additional 5 minutes. Serve over hot rice.

Sweet and Sour Sausage Mix

Preparation Time-10 minutes | Cook Time-10 minutes | Servings-2 | Difficulty-Easy

Nutritional Facts- Calories-162 | Fats-6g |Carbohydrates-13.8g |Proteins-9.9g

Ingredients

- Half pound of sliced sausages
- One chopped red bell pepper
- Half cup of chopped yellow onion
- Two tablespoons of brown sugar
- 1/3 cup of ketchup
- One tablespoon of mustard
- One tablespoon of apple cider vinegar
- Half cup of chicken stock

Instructions

- In a bowl, mix sugar with ketchup, mustard, stock and vinegar and whisk well.
- In your air fryer's pan, mix sausage slices with bell pepper, onion and sweet and sour mix, toss and cook at 350 degrees F for 10 minutes.
- Divide into bowls and serve for lunch.
- Enjoy!

Sweet Potato Lunch Casserole

Preparation Time-10 minutes | Cook Time- 50 minutes | Servings-2 | Difficulty-Moderate

Nutritional Facts- Calories-220 | Fats-4.8g |Carbohydrates-21g |Proteins-6g

Ingredients

- Two big sweet potatoes, pricked with a fork
- One cup of chicken stock or water
- Salt and black pepper to the taste
- A pinch of cayenne pepper
- A quarter teaspoon of ground nutmeg
- 1/3 cup of coconut cream

Instructions

- Place sweet potatoes in your air fryer, cook them at 350 degrees F for 40 minutes, cool them down, peel, roughly chop and transfer to a pan that fits your air fryer.
- Add stock, salt, pepper, cayenne and coconut cream, toss, introduce in your air fryer and cook at 360 degrees F for 10 minutes more.
- Divide casserole into bowls and serve.
- Enjoy!

Tasty and Cheesy Pork Chops

Preparation Time-10 minutes | Cook Time-10 minutes | Servings-2 | Difficulty-Easy

Nutritional Facts- Calories-332 | Fats-9g |Carbohydrates-1.5g |Proteins-17g

Ingredients

- Two pork chops, boneless
- One teaspoon of onion powder
- One teaspoon of smoked paprika
- Half cup of grated parmesan cheese
- Two tablespoons of olive oil
- Half teaspoon of pepper
- One teaspoon of kosher salt

Instructions

- Brush pork chops with olive oil.
- In a bowl, merge together parmesan cheese and spices.
- Spray air fryer basket with cooking spray.
- Coat pork chops with parmesan cheese mixture and place in the air fryer basket.
- Cook pork chops at 375 F for 9 minutes. Turn halfway through.
- Serve and enjoy.

Tasty Chicken Tenders

Preparation Time-10 minutes | Cook Time-One hour | Servings-2 | Difficulty-Hard

Nutritional Facts- Calories-188 | Fats-6g |Carbohydrates-4.8g |Proteins-23g

Ingredients

- One lb. of chicken tenders
- Kosher salt
- A quarter teaspoon of hot sauce (optional)
- Pinch of kosher salt
- Freshly ground black pepper
- Freshly ground black pepper
- One cup of all-purpose flour
- Two cups of panko bread crumbs
- One large egg
- A quarter cup of buttermilk
- Cooking spray
- 1/3 cup of mayonnaise
- Three tablespoons of honey

- One tablespoon of Dijon mustard

Instructions

- Chicken tenders are seasoned with pepper and salt on both sides. In two separate small pans, put flour and bread crumbs. Whisk the eggs and buttermilk together in a third bowl. Dip the chicken in the flour, then the mixture of the eggs, and finally in the bread crumbs, pressing to coat.
- Working in batches, put chicken tenders in the air fryer basket, making sure not to overcrowd them. Spray the chicken tops with cooking spray and roast for 5 minutes at 400 ° F. Flip over the chicken, coat the tops with some more cooking spray, and cook for five more minutes. Repeat for the remaining chicken tenders.
- Make the sauce: Whisk together Dijon, mayonnaise, honey and hot sauce, if used, in a small bowl. And use a pinch of salt and a few black pepper cracks to season.
- Serve with honey mustard the chicken tenders.

Tender and Juicy Chicken

Preparation Time-10 minutes | Cook Time-40 minutes | Servings-2 | Difficulty-Moderate

Nutritional Facts- Calories-336 | Fats-15.9g |Carbohydrates-1.5g |Proteins-43.8g

Ingredients

- One lb. of skinless and boneless chicken thighs
- Four sliced cloves of garlic
- Two tablespoons of olive oil
- One tablespoon of fresh chopped parsley
- One fresh lemon juice
- Pepper
- Salt

Instructions

- Place chicken on a baking dish and season with pepper and salt.
- Sprinkle parsley and garlic over the chicken and drizzle oil and lemon juice on top of the chicken.
- Place the inner pot in the grill air fryer combo base.
- Place the baking dish in the inner pot.
- Cover the inner pot with an air frying lid.
- Select bake mode then set the temperature to 450 F and time for 40 minutes. Press start.

- When the timer reaches 0, then press the cancel button.
- Serve and enjoy.

Tuna and Zucchini Tortillas

Preparation Time-10 minutes | Cook Time- 10 minutes | Servings-2 | Difficulty-Easy

Nutritional Facts- Calories-176 | Fats-6g |Carbohydrates-9.9g |Proteins-15.9g

Ingredients

- Two corn tortillas
- Two tablespoons of softened butter
- Three ounces of drained canned tuna
- Half cup of shredded zucchini
- 1/3 cup of mayonnaise
- Two tablespoons of mustard
- One cup of grated cheddar cheese

Instructions

- Spread butter on tortillas, place them in your air fryer's basket and cook them at 400 degrees F for 3 minutes.
- Meanwhile, in a bowl, mix tuna with zucchini, mayo and mustard and stir.
- Divide this mix on each tortilla, top with cheese, roll tortillas, place them in your air fryer's basket again and cook them at 400 degrees F for 4 minutes more.
- Serve for lunch.
- Enjoy!

Tuna Patties

Preparation Time-10 minutes | Cook Time-10 minutes | Servings-2 | Difficulty-Easy

Nutritional Facts- Calories-414 | Fats-15.9g |Carbohydrates-5.4g |Proteins-45g

Ingredients

- Two cans of tuna
- Juice of half lemon
- Half teaspoon of onion powder
- One teaspoon of garlic powder
- Half teaspoon of dried dill
- One and a half tablespoons of mayonnaise
- One and a half tablespoons of almond flour
- A quarter teaspoon of pepper

- A quarter teaspoon of salt

Instructions

- Preheat the air fryer to 400 F.
- Set all ingredients in a mixing bowl and mix until well combined.
- Spray air fryer basket with cooking spray.
- Make four patties from the mixture and place them in the air fryer basket.
- Cook patties for 10 minutes at 400 F. If you want crispier patties, then cook for 3 minutes more.
- Serve and enjoy.

Turkey Cakes

Preparation Time-10 minutes | Cook Time- 10 minutes | Servings-2 | Difficulty-Easy

Nutritional Facts- Calories-202 | Fats-6.9g |Carbohydrates-21g |Proteins-12g

Ingredients

- Three chopped mushrooms
- One teaspoon of garlic powder
- One teaspoon of onion powder
- Salt and black pepper to the taste
- One and a quarter pounds turkey meat, ground
- Cooking spray
- Tomato sauce for serving

Instructions

- In your blender, mix mushrooms with salt and pepper, pulse well and transfer to a bowl.
- Add turkey, onion powder, garlic powder, salt and pepper, stir and shape cakes out of this mix.
- Spray them with cooking spray, transfer them to your air fryer and cook at 320 degrees F for 10 minutes.
- Serve them with tomato sauce on the side and a tasty side salad.
- Enjoy!

Turkey Meatloaf

Preparation Time-5 minutes | Cook Time-One hour and 15 minutes | Servings-2 | Difficulty-Hard

Nutritional Facts- Calories-193 | Fats-10.8g |Carbohydrates-1g|Proteins-23g

Ingredients

- 2/3 cup of chopped yellow onion
- Half cup of dry unseasoned breadcrumbs
- One beaten egg
- One tablespoon of minced garlic
- Half tablespoon of salt
- One tablespoon of hot sauce
- One lb. of ground turkey
- Half cup of chopped green bell pepper
- 1/3 cup of chopped celery
- Half cup of ketchup
- One tablespoon of Emeril original Essence
- Half tablespoon of ground black pepper

Instructions

- In a mixing bowl, place the turkey. Combine the green bell pepper, yellow onion, breadcrumbs, egg, celery, one tablespoon ketchup, salt, essence, garlic, and black pepper in a mixing bowl.
- Mix until everything is well blended. Transfer the batter to a loaf pan and shape it into a dome.
- In a small mixing dish, combine the remaining ketchup with the spicy sauce. Spread the mixture over top of the meatloaf with the back of a spoon.
- Select bake and place the loaf pan on the Air Fryer rack. Preheat the oven to 375°F and bake for 50 minutes. Start by pressing the start button.
- The meatloaf should be golden brown on the outside and 165 degrees on the inside.
- Allow for a 5-minute rest period before serving. Enjoy.

Turkish Koftas

Preparation Time-10 minutes | Cook Time- 15 minutes | Servings-2 | Difficulty-Easy

Nutritional Facts- Calories-271 | Fats-16.8g |Carbohydrates-25g |Proteins-30g

Ingredients

- One chopped leek
- Two tablespoons of crumbled feta cheese
- Half pound lean minced beef
- One tablespoon of ground cumin
- One tablespoon of chopped mint
- One tablespoon of chopped parsley
- One teaspoon of minced garlic

- Salt and black pepper to the taste

Instructions

- In a bowl, mix beef with leek, cheese, cumin, mint, parsley, garlic, salt and pepper, stir well, shape your koftas and place them on sticks.
- Add koftas to your preheated air fryer at 360 degrees F and cook them for 15 minutes.
- Serve them with a side salad for lunch.
- Enjoy!

Veggie Toast

Preparation Time-10 minutes | Cook Time-15 minutes | Servings-2 | Difficulty-Easy

Nutritional Facts- Calories-152 | Fats-1g|Carbohydrates-6.9g |Proteins-1.5g

Ingredients

- One red bell pepper, cut into thin strips
- One cup of sliced cremini mushrooms
- One chopped yellow squash
- Two sliced green onions
- One tablespoon of olive oil
- Four bread slices
- Two tablespoons of soft butter
- Half cup of crumbled goat cheese

Instructions

- In a bowl, mix red bell pepper with mushrooms, squash, green onions and oil, toss, transfer to your air fryer, cook them at 350 degrees F for 10 minutes, shaking the fryer once and transfer them to a bowl.
- Spread butter on bread slices, place them in the air fryer and cook them at 350 degrees F for 5 minutes.
- Divide veggie mix on each bread slice, top with crumbled cheese and serve for lunch.
- Enjoy!

Yummy Kabab

Preparation Time-10 minutes | Cook Time-10 minutes | Servings-2 | Difficulty-Easy

Nutritional Facts- Calories-246 | Fats-10.8g |Carbohydrates-1g |Proteins-34.8g

Ingredients

- One lb. of ground beef
- A quarter cup of chopped fresh parsley
- One tablespoon of olive oil
- Two tablespoons of kabab spice mix
- One tablespoon of minced garlic
- One teaspoon of salt

Instructions

- Set all ingredients into the bowl and merge until combined. Place in the fridge for 60 minutes.
- Divide the meat mixture into four sections and wrap around four soaked wooden skewers.
- Spray air fryer basket with cooking spray.
- Place kabab into the air fryer and cook at 370 F for 10 minutes.
- Serve and enjoy.

Zingy and Nutty Chicken Wings

Preparation Time-5 minutes | Cook Time-18 minutes | Servings-2 | Difficulty-Easy

Nutritional Facts- Calories-253 | Fats-10.8g |Carbohydrates-13g |Proteins-26g

Ingredients

- One tablespoon of fresh lemon juice
- Six chicken middle wings, cut into half
- A quarter cup of crushed unsalted cashews
- One tablespoon of fish sauce
- One teaspoon of sugar
- Two fresh and finely chopped lemongrass stalks

Instructions

- Combine the fish sauce, juice, and sugar in a mixing bowl.
- Add the wings and liberally coat them in the mixture. Preheat the air fryer to 355 degrees F and marinate for around 1-2 hours.
- Place lemongrass stems in the air fryer pan. Cook for about a minute and a half. Transfer the cashew mixture from the Air fryer to a mixing basin. Preheat the air fryer to 390 degrees Fahrenheit.
- In an air fryer pan, place the chicken wings. Cook for another 13-15 minutes. Place the wings among plates to serve. Serve with a cashew mixture on top.

Zucchini Casserole

Preparation Time-10 minutes | Cook Time-16 minutes | Servings-2 | Difficulty-Easy

Nutritional Facts- Calories-133 | Fats-1g | Carbohydrates-13.8g | Proteins-4.8g

Ingredients

- One cup of veggie stock
- Two tablespoons of olive oil
- One sweet potato, peeled and cut into medium wedges
- Four zucchinis, cut into medium wedges
- Two chopped yellow onions
- One cup of coconut milk
- Salt and black pepper to the taste
- One tablespoon of soy sauce
- A quarter teaspoon of dried thyme
- A quarter teaspoon of dried rosemary
- Two tablespoons of chopped dill
- Half teaspoon of chopped basil

Instructions

- Heat up a pan that fits your air fryer with the oil over medium heat, add onion, stir and cook for 2 minutes.
- Add zucchinis, rosemary, thyme, basil, salt, potato, pepper, milk, stock, soy sauce and dill, stir, introduce in your air fryer, cook at 360 degrees F for 14 minutes, divide among plates and serve right away.

Chapter 3-Air Fried Dinner Recipes

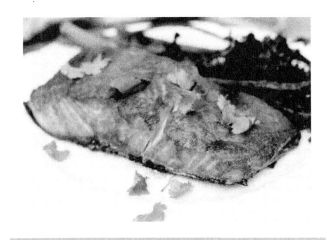

Asian Salmon

Preparation Time- One hour | Cook Time-15 minutes | Servings-2 | Difficulty-Hard

Nutritional Facts- Calories-305 | Fats-12g |Carbohydrates-21g |Proteins-30g

Ingredients

- Two medium salmon fillets
- Six tablespoons of light soy sauce
- Three teaspoons of mirin
- One teaspoon of water
- Six tablespoons of honey

Instructions

- In a bowl, mix soy sauce with honey, water and mirin, whisk well, add salmon, rub well and leave aside in the fridge for 1 hour.
- Transfer salmon to your air fryer and cook at 360 degrees F for 15 minutes, flipping them after 7 minutes.
- Meanwhile, put the soy marinade in a pan, heat up over medium heat, whisk well, cook for 2 minutes and take off the heat.
- Divide salmon among plates, drizzle marinade all over and serve.
- Enjoy!

Asian Steamed Tuna

Preparation Time-10 minutes | Cook Time-15 minutes | Servings-2 | Difficulty-Easy

Nutritional Facts- Calories-292 | Fats-13.8g |Carbohydrates-1.5g |Proteins-37.8g

Ingredients

- Four small tuna steaks
- Two tablespoons of low-sodium soy sauce
- Two teaspoons of sesame oil
- Two teaspoons of rice wine vinegar
- One teaspoon of grated fresh ginger
- 1/8 teaspoon of pepper
- One half-bent stalk of lemongrass
- Three tablespoons of lemon juice

Instructions

- Place the tuna steaks on a plate.
- In a small bowl, merge the soy sauce, sesame oil, rice wine vinegar, and ginger, and mix well. Pour this mixture over the tuna and marinate for 10 minutes. Rub the soy sauce mixture gently into both sides of the tuna. Sprinkle with pepper.
- Place the lemongrass on the air fryer basket and top with the steaks. Put the lemon juice and One tablespoon of water in the pan below the basket.
- Steam the fish until the tuna registers at least 145°F. Discard the lemongrass and serve the tuna.

Baja Cod Tacos with Mango Salsa

Preparation Time-15 minutes | Cook Time-20 minutes | Servings-2 | Difficulty-

Nutritional Facts- Calories-155 | Fats-1.5g |Carbohydrates-6g |Proteins-25g

Ingredients

- One egg
- Five ounces of Mexican beer
- 1/3 cup of all-purpose flour
- 1/3 cup of cornstarch
- A quarter teaspoon of chili powder
- Half teaspoon of ground cumin
- Half pound of cod, cut into large pieces
- Six corn tortillas
- Cooking spray

Salsa

- One peeled and diced mango
- A quarter diced red bell pepper
- Half diced small jalapeño
- A quarter minced red onion
- Juice of half a lime

- Pinch chopped fresh cilantro
- A quarter teaspoon of salt

A quarter teaspoon of ground black pepper

Instructions

- Set the air fryer basket with cooking spray.
- Whisk the egg with a beer in a bowl. Combine the flour, cornstarch, chili powder, and cumin in a separate bowl.
- Dredge the cod in the egg mixture first, then in the flour mixture to coat well. Shake the excess off.
- Arrange the cod in the air fryer basket and spritz with cooking spray.
- Slide the basket into the air fryer. Cook at the corresponding preset mode or Air Fry at 380F (193C) for 17 minutes.
- Flip the cod halfway through the cooking time.
- When cooked, the cod should be golden brown and crunchy.
- Meanwhile, merge the ingredients for the salsa in a small bowl. Stir to mix well.
- Unfold the tortillas on a clean work surface, then divide the fish on the tortillas and spread the salsa on top. Fold to serve.

Beef and Green Onions Marinade

Preparation Time-10 minutes | Cook Time-20 minutes | Servings-2 | Difficulty-

Nutritional Facts- Calories-329 | Fats-7.8g |Carbohydrates-37.8g |Proteins-21.9g

Ingredients

- One cup of chopped green onion
- One cup of soy sauce
- Half cup of water
- A quarter cup of brown sugar
- A quarter cup of sesame seeds
- Five minced garlic cloves
- One teaspoon of black pepper
- One pound of lean beef

Instructions

- In a bowl, mix onion with soy sauce, water, sugar, garlic, sesame seeds and pepper, whisk, add meat, toss and leave aside for 10 minutes.
- Drain beef, transfer to your preheated air fryer and cook at 390 degrees F for 20

- minutes.
- Slice, divide among plates and serve with a side salad.
- Enjoy!

Beef and Mushroom Stroganoff

Preparation Time-15 minutes | Cook Time-15 minutes | Servings-2 to 4 | Difficulty-Easy

Nutritional Facts- Calories-361 | Fats-16.8g |Carbohydrates-1.5g |Proteins-42g

Ingredient

- One pound of thinly sliced beef steak
- Eight ounces of sliced mushrooms
- One chopped whole onion
- Two cups of beef broth
- One cup of sour cream
- Four tablespoons of melted butter
- Two cups of cooked egg noodles

Instructions

- In a mixing bowl, combine the onion, mushrooms, sour cream, beef broth, and butter until well combined. Place the meat steak in a separate bowl.
- Allow 10 minutes for the mushroom mixture to marinade on the steak.
- In a baking pan, whisk the marinated steak.
- Bake, Super Convection is the option to choose. Preheat the oven to 400 degrees Fahrenheit (205 degrees Celsius) Set the timer to 14 minutes. To begin preheating, press Start/Stop.
- Place the pan in the bake position once it has been preheated. Halfway through the cooking period, turn the steak.
- When the steak is done, the vegetables should be soft and the meat should be browned.
- With the fried egg noodles, serve immediately.

Beef Jerky

Preparation Time-15 minutes | Cook Time-Three hours | Servings-2 | Difficulty-Hard

Nutritional Facts- Calories-372 | Fats-10.8g |Carbohydrates-12g |Proteins-54g

Ingredients

- One and a half pounds of trimmed beef round

- Half cup of Worcestershire sauce
- Half cup of low-sodium soy sauce
- Two teaspoons of honey
- One teaspoon of liquid smoke
- Two teaspoons of onion powder
- Half teaspoon of red pepper flakes
- Ground black pepper, as required

Instructions

- In a zip-top bag, place the beef and freeze for 1-2 hours to firm up.
- Bring the meat onto a cutting board and cut against the grain into 1/8-¼-inch strips.
- In a big bowl, add the remaining ingredients and mix until well combined.
- Add the steak slices and coat with the mixture.
- Refrigerate for around five to six hours to marinate.
- Remove the beef slices from the bowl, and with paper towels, pat dry them.
- Divide the steak strips onto the cooking trays and arrange them in an even layer.
- Select "Dehydrate" and then adjust the temperature to 160 degrees F.
- Set the timer for 3 hours and press the "Start".
- When the display shows "Add Food," inserts one tray in the top position and another in the center position.
- After 11/2 hours, switch the position of cooking trays.
- Meanwhile, in a small pan, add the remaining ingredients over medium heat and cook for about 10 minutes, stirring occasionally.
- When cooking time is complete, remove the trays from the air fryer.

Beef Stuffed Squash

Preparation Time-10 minutes | Cook Time-40 minutes | Servings-2 | Difficulty-Hard

Nutritional Facts- Calories-262 | Fats-7.8g |Carbohydrates-15.9g |Proteins-13.8g

Ingredients

- One pricked spaghetti squash, pricked
- One pound ground beef
- Salt and black pepper to the taste
- Three minced garlic cloves

- One chopped yellow onion
- One sliced Portobello mushroom
- Twenty-eight ounces of chopped canned tomatoes
- One teaspoon of dried oregano
- A quarter teaspoon of cayenne pepper
- Half teaspoon of dried thyme
- One chopped green bell pepper

Instructions

- Cook spaghetti squash in an air fryer for 20 minutes at 350 degrees F, then move to a chopping board and cut it into half, discarding seeds.
- Heat a pan over medium-high heat, then add the meat, onion, garlic, and mushroom, constantly stirring until the meat is browned.
- Season with salt, thyme, pepper, oregano, tomatoes, cayenne, and green pepper, then simmer for 10 minutes, stirring occasionally.
- Stuff squash with the meat mixture, place in the fryer and cook for 10 minutes at 360 degrees F.
- Divide among plates and serve.

Breaded Coconut Shrimp

Preparation Time-5 minutes | Cook Time-15 minutes | Servings-2 | Difficulty-Easy

Nutritional Facts- Calories-285 | Fats-13g |Carbohydrates-4g |Proteins-36.9g

Ingredients

- One lb. of Shrimp
- One cup of Panko breadcrumbs
- One cup of shredded coconut
- Two Eggs
- 1/3 cup of all-purpose flour

Instructions

- Fix the temperature of the Air Fryer at 360° Fahrenheit.
- Peel and devein the shrimp.
- Whisk the seasonings with the flour as desired. In another dish, whisk the eggs, and in the third container, combine the breadcrumbs and coconut.
- Dip the cleaned shrimp into the flour, egg wash, and finish it off with the coconut mixture.

- Lightly spray the basket of the fryer and set the timer for 10-15 minutes.
- Air-fry until it's a golden brown before serving.

Breaded Cod Sticks

Preparation Time-5 minutes | Cook Time-20 minutes | Servings-2 | Difficulty-Easy

Nutritional Facts- Calories-254 | Fats-14.1g |Carbohydrates-5.7g |Proteins-39g

Ingredients

Two large eggs
Three tablespoons of Milk
Two cups of Breadcrumbs
One cup of Almond flour
One lb. of Cod

Instructions

- Heat the Air Fryer at 350° Fahrenheit.
- Prepare three bowls; one with the milk and eggs, one with the breadcrumbs (salt and pepper if desired), and another with almond flour.
- Dip the sticks in the flour, egg mixture, and breadcrumbs.
- Place in the basket and set the timer for 12 minutes. Toss the basket halfway through the cooking process.
- Serve with your favorite sauce.

Buffalo Cauliflower

Preparation Time-10 minutes | Cook Time-15 minutes | Servings-2 | Difficulty-Easy

Nutritional Facts- Calories-145 | Fats-1g|Carbohydrates-12g |Proteins-4g

Ingredients

- Two teaspoons of avocado oil
- A quarter teaspoon of sea salt
- Two to Three tablespoons of Frank's Red-Hot Sauce
- One and a half teaspoons of maple syrup
- Two to three tablespoons of nutritional yeast
- One medium head cauliflower, chopped into 1 1/2" florets
- One tablespoon of cornstarch or arrowroot starch

Instructions

- Set the air fryer to 360 degrees F. To a large

mixing bowl, add all the ingredients except the cauliflower. Whisk thoroughly to mix. To cover uniformly, apply the cauliflower and flip.
- Apply part of the cauliflower to the fryer (no need to oil the basket). Cook for twelve to fourteen minutes, shaking halfway through, or until the perfect consistency is reached. Repeat with the remaining cauliflower, except for 9-10 minutes of shortened cooking time. Cauliflower must be kept securely packed for up to 4 days in the refrigerator. To reheat, add 1-2 minutes to the air fryer until hot and slightly crispy.

Buttered Shrimp Skewers

Preparation Time-10 minutes | Cook Time-8 minutes | Servings-2 | Difficulty-Easy

Nutritional Facts- Calories-155 | Fats-4g |Carbohydrates-15.9g |Proteins-7.8g

Ingredients

Eight deveined and peeled shrimps
Four minced garlic cloves
Eight green bell pepper slices
Salt and black pepper to the taste
One tablespoon of chopped rosemary
One tablespoon of melted butter

Instructions

- Toss shrimp with butter, garlic, salt, rosemary, pepper, and bell pepper slices in a mixing basin to coat, then set aside for 10 minutes.
- On a skewer, arrange two bell pepper slices and two shrimps, then repeat with the remaining bell pepper and shrimp slices.
- Place them all in the basket of your air fryer and cook for 6 minutes at 360 degrees F.
- Serve immediately after dividing among plates.
- Enjoy!

Caesar Chicken

Preparation Time-10 minutes | Cook Time-Six hours | Servings-2 | Difficulty-Hard

Nutritional Facts- Calories-378 | Fats-20g |Carbohydrates-13g |Proteins-41g

Ingredients

- Two skinless and boneless chicken breasts
- A quarter cup of creamy Caesar dressing
- A quarter teaspoon of dried parsley

- Two tablespoons of fresh chopped basil
- 1/8 teaspoon of black pepper
- 1/8 teaspoon of salt

Instructions

- Place the inner pot in the grill air fryer combo base.
- Add all ingredients into the inner pot and stir well.
- Cover the inner pot with a glass lid.
- Select slow cook mode, then press the temperature button and set the time for 6 hours. Press start.
- When the timer reaches 0, then press the cancel button.
- Shred the chicken using a fork and serve.

Cajun Shrimp

Preparation Time-5 minutes | Cook Time-5 minutes | Servings-2 | Difficulty-Easy

Nutritional Facts- Calories-356 | Fats-18g |Carbohydrates-6.9g |Proteins-34g

Ingredients

- Twenty Tiger shrimp
- One tablespoon of Olive oil
- Half teaspoon of Old Bay seasoning
- A quarter teaspoon of Smoked paprika
- A quarter teaspoon of Cayenne pepper

Instructions

- Set the Air Fryer at 390° Fahrenheit.
- Cover the shrimp using the oil and spices.
- Set them into the Air Fryer basket and set the timer for five minutes.
- Serve with your favorite side dish.

Caraway Crusted Beef Steaks

Preparation Time-5 minutes | Cook Time-10 minutes | Servings-2 | Difficulty-Easy

Nutritional Facts- Calories-327 | Fats-18g |Carbohydrates-15.9g |Proteins-34g

Ingredient

- Four beef steaks
- Two teaspoons of caraway seeds
- Two teaspoons of garlic powder

- Sea salt and cayenne pepper, to taste
- One tablespoon of melted butter
- 1/3 cup of almond flour
- Two beaten eggs

Instructions

- Attach the beef steaks to a large bowl and toss with the caraway seeds, garlic powder, and salt and pepper until well coated.
- Merge together the melted butter and almond flour in a bowl. Pour the eggs into a different bowl.
- Set the seasoned steaks in the eggs, then dip in the almond and butter mixture.
- Arrange the coated steaks in the air fry basket.
- Select Air Fry, Super Convection. Set temperature to 355F (179C) and set time to 10 minutes. Press Start/Stop to begin preheating.
- Once preheated, place the basket in the air fry position. Set the steaks once halfway through to ensure even cooking.
- When cooking is processed, the internal temperature of the beef steaks should reach at least 145F (63C) on a meat thermometer.
- Set the steaks to plates. Let cool and serve hot.

Cheese Herb Pork Chops

Preparation Time-5 minutes | Cook Time-10 minutes | Servings-2 | Difficulty-Easy

Nutritional Facts- Calories-340 | Fats-26g |Carbohydrates-4g |Proteins-25g

Ingredients

- Two boneless pork chops
- One teaspoon of herb de Provence
- One teaspoon of paprika
- Four tablespoons of grated parmesan cheese
- 1/3 cup of almond flour
- Half teaspoon of Cajun seasoning

Instructions

- Preheat the air fryer to 350 F.
- Mix together almond flour, Cajun seasoning, herb de Provence, paprika, and cheese.
- Spray pork chops with cooking spray and coat pork chops with almond flour mixture, and place into the air fryer basket.
- Cook for 9 minutes.

- Serve and enjoy.

Cheesy Spinach Stuffed Chicken Breasts

- Preparation Time-20 minutes | Cook Time-25 minutes | Servings-2 | Difficulty-Moderate
- Nutritional Facts- Calories-648 | Fats-37.8g |Carbohydrates-4.8g |Proteins-65g

Ingredients

- One (ten-ounce) package of thawed and drained frozen spinach
- One cup of crumbled feta cheese
- Four boneless chicken breasts
- Salt and ground black pepper, to taste
- Four to eight soaked toothpicks

Instructions

- Preheat the air fryer to 380F (193C). Set the air fryer basket with cooking spray.
- Make the filling: Chop the spinach and put it in a large bowl, then add the feta cheese and half a teaspoon of ground black pepper. Stir to mix well.
- On a clean work surface, using a knife, cut a 1-inch incision into the thicker side of each chicken breast horizontally. Make a 3-inch-long pocket from the incision and keep the sides and bottom intact.
- Stuff the chicken pockets with the filling and secure with 1 or 2 toothpicks.
- Arrange the stuffed chicken breasts in the preheated air fryer. Sprinkle with salt and black pepper and spritz with cooking spray. You may need to work in batches to avoid overcrowding.
- Cook for 12 minutes or until the internal temperature of the chicken reads at least 165F (74C). Set the chicken halfway through the cooking time.
- Remove the chicken from the air fryer basket. Discard the toothpicks and allow them to cool for 10 minutes before slicing to serve.

Chicken and Cabbage Egg Rolls

Preparation Time-10 minutes | Cook Time-25 minutes | Servings-2 to4 | Difficulty-Easy

Nutritional Facts- Calories-491 | Fats-27.9g |Carbohydrates-28.9g |Proteins-30g

Ingredients

- One pound of ground chicken
- Two teaspoons of olive oil
- Two minced cloves of garlic
- One teaspoon of grated fresh ginger
- Two cups of shredded white cabbage
- One chopped onion
- A quarter cup of soy sauce
- Eight egg roll wrappers
- One beaten egg
- Cooking spray

Instructions

- Set the air fryer basket with cooking spray.
- Warm olive oil in a saucepan over medium heat. Sauté the garlic and ginger in the olive oil for 1 minute, or until fragrant. Add the ground chicken to the saucepan. Sauté for 5 minutes or until the chicken is cooked through. Add the cabbage, onion and soy sauce and sauté for 5 to 6 minutes, or until the vegetables become soft. Remove the saucepan from the heat.
- On a clean work area, unfold the egg roll wrappers. Brush the edges of the wrappers with the beaten egg and divide the chicken mixture among them. Roll the egg rolls tightly to close the filling. Place the rolls in the basket and arrange them in a pleasing manner.
- Slide the basket into the air fryer. Cook at the corresponding preset mode or Air Fry at 370F (188C) for 12 minutes.
- Set the rolls halfway through the cooking time.
- When cooked, the rolls will be crispy and golden brown.
- Transfer to a platter and let cool for 5 minutes before serving.

Chicken and Garlic Sauce

Preparation Time-10 minutes | Cook Time-20 minutes | Servings-2 | Difficulty-Easy

Nutritional Facts- Calories-227 | Fats-9.9g |Carbohydrates-21.9g |Proteins-12g

Ingredients

- One tablespoon of melted butter
- Four skin-on and bone-in chicken breasts
- One tablespoon of olive oil

- Salt and black pepper to the taste
- Forty peeled and chopped garlic cloves
- Two thyme springs
- A quarter cup of chicken stock
- Two tablespoons of chopped parsley
- A quarter cup of dry white wine

Instructions

- Season chicken breasts with salt and pepper, rub with the oil, place in your air fryer, cook at 360 degrees F for 4 minutes on each side and transfer to a heat-proof dish that fits your air fryer.
- Add melted butter, garlic, thyme, stock, wine and parsley, toss, introduce in your air fryer and cook at 350 degrees F for 15 minutes more.
- Divide everything among plates and serve.

Chicken and Zucchini

Preparation Time-30 minutes | Cook Time-20 minutes | Servings-2 | Difficulty-Moderate

Nutritional Facts- Calories-283 | Fats-19g |Carbohydrates-3.5g |Proteins-21.8g

Ingredients

- A quarter cup of olive oil
- One tablespoon of lemon juice
- Two tablespoons of red wine vinegar
- One teaspoon of oregano
- One tablespoon of garlic, chopped
- Two cube-sliced chicken breast fillets
- One sliced zucchini
- One sliced red onion
- One cup of sliced cherry tomatoes,
- Salt and pepper to taste

Instructions

- In a bowl, merge the olive oil, lemon juice, vinegar, oregano and garlic.
- Pour half of the mixture into another bowl.
- Toss chicken in half of the mixture.
- Cover and marinate for 15 minutes.
- Toss the veggies in the remaining mixture.
- Season both chicken and veggies with salt and pepper.
- Add chicken to the air fryer basket.
- Spread veggies on top.

- Select the air fry function. Seal and cook at 380 degrees F for 15 to 20 minutes.

Chicken Cacciatore

Preparation Time-10 minutes | Cook Time-20 minutes | Servings-2 | Difficulty-Easy

Nutritional Facts- Calories-301 | Fats-12.9g |Carbohydrates-20g |Proteins-24g

Ingredients

- Eight bone-in chicken drumsticks
- One teaspoon of garlic powder
- Twenty-eight ounces of crushed canned tomatoes and juice
- Half cup of pitted and sliced black olives
- Salt and black pepper to the taste
- One bay leaf
- One chopped yellow onion
One teaspoon of dried oregano

Instructions

- Combine the chicken, pepper, salt, garlic powder, onion, bay leaf, oregano, tomatoes and juice, and olives in a heat-proof dish that fits your air fryer, toss, and cook at 365 degrees F for 20 minutes.
- Serve by dividing the mixture among plates.
- Enjoy!

Chicken Empanadas with Salsa Verde

Preparation Time-25 minutes | Cook Time-12 minutes | Servings-2 | Difficulty-Easy

Nutritional Facts- Calories-334 | Fats-9.9g |Carbohydrates-7.8g |Proteins-31.8g

Ingredients

- One cup of finely chopped boneless, skinless rotisserie chicken breast meat
- A quarter cup of salsa Verde
- 2/3 cup of shredded Cheddar cheese
- One teaspoon of ground cumin
- One teaspoon of ground black pepper
- Two purchased refrigerated pie crusts, from a minimum 14.1-ounce box
- One large egg
- Two tablespoons of water
- Cooking spray

Instructions

- Set the air fryer basket with cooking spray. Set aside.
- Combine the chicken meat, salsa Verde, cheddar, cumin, and black pepper in a large bowl. Stir to mix well. Set aside.
- Unfold the pie crusts on a clean work surface, and then use a large cookie cutter to cut out 31/2-inch circles as much as possible.
- Roll the remaining crusts to a ball and flatten them into a circle that has the same thickness as the original crust. Cut out more 31/2-inch circles until you have 12 circles in total.
- Make the empanadas: Divide the chicken mixture in the middle of each circle, about 1 and1/2 tablespoons of each. Set the edges of the circle with water. Fold the circle in half over the filling to shape like a half-moon and press to seal, or you can press with a fork.
- Whisk the egg with water in a small bowl.
- Arrange the empanadas in the basket and spritz with cooking spray. Brush with whisked egg.
- Slide the basket into the air fryer. Cook at the corresponding preset mode or Air Fry at 356 degrees F for 12 minutes.
- Set the empanadas halfway through the cooking time.
- When cooking is complete, the empanadas will be golden and crispy.
- Serve immediately.

Chicken Milanese

Preparation Time-10 minutes | Cook Time-30 minutes | Servings-2 | Difficulty-Moderate

Nutritional Facts- Calories-548 | Fats-20g |Carbohydrates-45g |Proteins-17g

Ingredients

- Two tablespoons of Extra Virgin Olive Oil
- One teaspoon of White wine vinegar
- Two cups of panko breadcrumbs
- A quarter cup of parmesan
- Half teaspoon of Garlic powder
- Two eggs
- Four chicken cutlets
- Three cups of arugula
- One beefsteak tomato

- Juice from half lemon
- Salt and Pepper
- Shaved parmesan

Instructions

- Combine panko breadcrumbs, Parmesan cheese, and garlic in a bowl.
- Drizzle the chicken cutlets with salt and pepper.
- Dip the cutlets in the egg.
- Top cutlets with panko mixture.
- Place the cutlets on the vegetable trays.
- Place the trays in the electric fryer. Press the Steaks/Chops button (350F) and decrease the cooking time to 15 minutes to start the cook cycle.
- While cooking the chicken, also prepare the salad.
- In a bowl, pour together the vinegar, lemon juice, olive oil and a pinch of salt and pepper.
- Add the arugula to the bowl and top with the dressing.
- Top chicken with diced tomatoes and arugula salad.
- Garnish with grated Parmesan.

Chicken Quesadilla

Preparation Time-20 minutes | Cook Time-30 minutes | Servings-2 | Difficulty-Moderate

Nutritional Facts- Calories-184 | Fats-14g |Carbohydrates-7.5g |Proteins-5.7g

Ingredients

- Four tortillas
- Cooking spray
- Half cup of sour cream
- Half cup of salsa
- Hot sauce
- Twelve ounces of chopped and grilled chicken breast fillet
- Three diced jalapeño peppers
- Two cups of shredded cheddar cheese
- Chopped scallions

Instructions

- Add grill grate to the Air fryer.
- Close the hood.
- Choose grill setting.
- Preheat for 5 minutes.

- While waiting, spray tortillas with oil.
- In a bowl, mix sour cream, salsa and hot sauce. Set aside.
- Add tortilla to the grate.
- Grill for 1 minute.
- Repeat with the other tortillas.
- Spread the toasted tortilla with the salsa mixture, chicken, jalapeño peppers, cheese and scallions.
- Place a tortilla on top. Press.
- Repeat these steps with the remaining two tortillas.
- Take the grill out of the pot.
- Choose a roast setting.
- Cook the Quesadillas at 350F for 25 minutes.

Chicken Tenders

Preparation Time-10 minutes | Cook Time-30 minutes | Servings-2 | Difficulty-Easy

Nutritional Facts- Calories-256 | Fats-6g |Carbohydrates-6.9g |Proteins-19g

Ingredients

- A half-cup of crushed potato sticks
- A quarter cup of melted butter
- A half-cup of crushed cheese crackers
- Two cooked and crumbled bacon strips
- Additional sour cream and chives
- A half-cup of panko bread crumbs
- Two teaspoons of minced fresh chives
- One tablespoon of sour cream
- A quarter cup of grated Parmesan cheese
- One pound of chicken tenderloins

Instructions

- Preheat the air fryer to 400 degrees Fahrenheit. Mix the ingredients in a shallow
- bowl. In another shallow bowl, whisk together the butter as well as sour cream. Dip the chicken in the butter mixture and then in the crumb mixture, patting it down to ensure the coating sticks.
- Then the chicken is to be arranged in a single layer on a greased tray in the air-fryer basket in batches; spritz with cooking spray. Cook for 7-8 minutes on each side, or until the coating turns golden brown well as the chicken is no longer

pink. Serve with a dollop of sour cream and a sprinkling of chives.

Chicken, Mushroom, And Pepper Kabobs

Preparation Time-One hour and 5 minutes | Cook Time-20 minutes | Servings-2 | Difficulty-Hard

Nutritional Facts- Calories-380 | Fats-15.9g |Carbohydrates-26g |Proteins-34g

Ingredients

- 1/3 cup of raw honey
- Two tablespoons of sesame seeds
- Two cube-cut boneless chicken breasts
- Six halved white mushrooms
- Three diced green or red bell peppers
- 1/3 cup of soy sauce
- Salt and ground black pepper, to taste
- Four soaked wooden skewers

Instructions

- Combine the honey, soy sauce, sesame seeds, salt, and black pepper in a large bowl. Stir to mix well.
- Dunk the chicken cubes in this bowl, then wrap the bowl in plastic and refrigerate to marinate for at least an hour.
- Preheat the air fryer to 390F (199C). Set the air fryer basket with cooking spray.
- Remove the chicken cubes from the marinade, and then run the skewers through the chicken cubes, mushrooms, and bell peppers alternatively.
- Baste the chicken, mushrooms, and bell peppers with the marinade, and then arrange them in the preheated air fryer.
- Spritz them with cooking spray and cook for 15 to 20 minutes or until the mushrooms and bell peppers are tender and the chicken cubes are well browned. Flip them halfway through the cooking time.
- Transfer the skewers to a large plate and serve hot.

Chili Garlic Shrimp

Preparation Time-10 minutes | Cook Time-8 minutes | Servings-2 | Difficulty-Easy

Nutritional Facts- Calories-170 | Fats-4.8g |Carbohydrates-1g|Proteins-25g

Ingredients

- One lb. of peeled and deveined shrimp
- One tablespoon of olive oil
- One sliced lemon
- One sliced red chili pepper
- Half teaspoon of garlic powder
- Pepper
- Salt

Instructions

- Preheat the air fryer to 400 F.
- Spray air fryer basket with cooking spray.
- Add all ingredients into the bowl and toss well.
- Add shrimp into the air fryer basket and cook for 5 minutes. Shake basket twice.
- Serve and enjoy.

Cinnamon-Beef Kofta

Preparation Time-10 minutes | Cook Time-15 minutes | Servings-2 | Difficulty-Easy

Nutritional Facts- Calories-342 | Fats-12g |Carbohydrates-6g |Proteins-42g

Ingredient

- One and a half pounds of lean ground beef
- One teaspoon of onion powder
- 1/3 teaspoon of ground cinnamon
- 1/3 teaspoon of ground dried turmeric
- One teaspoon of ground cumin
- 1/3 teaspoon of salt
- A quarter teaspoon of cayenne
- Twelve three-inch-long cinnamon sticks
- Cooking spray

Instructions

- Spritz the air fry basket with cooking spray.
- Merge all the ingredients, except for the cinnamon sticks, in a large bowl. Toss to mix well.
- Divide and shape the mixture into 12 balls, then wrap each ball around each cinnamon stick and leave a quarter of the length uncovered.

- Arrange the beef cinnamon sticks in the prepared basket and spritz with cooking spray.
- Select Air Fry, Super Convection. Set temperature to 375F (190C) and set time to 13 minutes. Press Start/Stop to begin preheating.
- Once preheated, place the basket in the air fry position. Flip the sticks halfway through the cooking.
- When cooking is processed, the beef should be browned.
- Serve immediately.

Coconut Shrimp

Preparation Time-15 minutes | Cook Time-10 minutes | Servings-2 | Difficulty-Easy

Nutritional Facts- Calories-524 | Fats-13.8g |Carbohydrates-45g |Proteins-23g

Ingredients

- One (Eight-ounce) can of crushed pineapple
- Half cup of sour cream
- A quarter cup of pineapple preserves
- Two egg whites
- 2/3 cup of cornstarch
- 2/3 cup of sweetened coconut
- One cup of panko bread crumbs
- One pound of deveined and shelled large uncooked shrimp, thawed if frozen
- Olive oil for misting

Instructions

- Rinse the crushed pineapple well, reserving the juice.
- In a small bowl, combine the pineapple, sour cream, and preserves, and merge well. Set aside.
- In a shallow bowl, set the egg whites with two tablespoons of the reserved pineapple liquid. Place the cornstarch on a plate. Merge the coconut and bread crumbs on another plate.
- Dip the shrimp into the cornstarch, shake it off, then dip into the egg white mixture and finally into the coconut mixture.
- Place the shrimp in the air fryer basket and mist with oil. Air-fry for 5 to 7 minutes or until the shrimp are crisp and golden brown.

Crab Ratatouille

Preparation Time-15 minutes | Cook Time-15 minutes | Servings-2 | Difficulty-Easy

Nutritional Facts- Calories-147 | Fats-4.8g |Carbohydrates-10.8g |Proteins-15.9g

Ingredients

- One and a half cups of peeled and cubed eggplant
- One chopped onion
- One chopped red bell pepper
- Two chopped large tomatoes
- One tablespoon of olive oil
- Half teaspoon of dried thyme
- Half teaspoon of dried basil
- Pinch salt
- Freshly ground black pepper
- One and a half cups of cooked crabmeat

Instructions

- Combine the eggplant, onion, bell pepper, tomatoes, olive oil, thyme, and basil in a 6-inch metal bowl. Sprinkle with salt and pepper.
- Roast for 9 minutes, then remove the bowl from the air fryer and stir.
- Add the crabmeat and roast for 2 to 5 minutes or until the ratatouille is bubbling and the vegetables are tender. Serve immediately.

Creamy Coconut Chicken

Preparation Time-Two hours | Cook Time-25 minutes | Servings-2 | Difficulty-Hard

Nutritional Facts- Calories-298 | Fats-4.8g |Carbohydrates-24g |Proteins-20g

Ingredients

- Two to four big chicken legs
- Five teaspoons of turmeric powder
- Two tablespoons of grated ginger
- Salt and black pepper to the taste
- Four tablespoons of coconut cream

Instructions

- In a bowl, mix cream with turmeric, ginger, salt and pepper, whisk, add chicken pieces, toss them well and leave aside for 2 hours.

- Transfer chicken to your preheated air fryer, cook at 370 degrees F for 25 minutes, divide among plates and serve with a side salad.

Creamy Salmon

Preparation Time-5 minutes | Cook Time-20 minutes | Servings-2 | Difficulty-Easy

Nutritional Facts- Calories-340 | Fats-15.9g |Carbohydrates-1g |Proteins-30g

Ingredients

- One tablespoon of chopped dill
- One tablespoon of olive oil
- Three tablespoons of sour cream
- Two ounces of Plain yogurt
- Six pieces of salmon

Instructions

- Heat the Air Fryer and wait for it to reach 285° Fahrenheit.
- Shake the salt over the salmon and add them to the fryer basket with the olive oil to air-fry for 10 minutes.
- Whisk the yogurt, salt, and dill.
- Serve the salmon with the sauce with your favorite sides.

Creamy Shrimp

Preparation Time-10 minutes | Cook Time-10 minutes | Servings-2 | Difficulty-Easy

Nutritional Facts- Calories-185 | Fats-4.8g |Carbohydrates-7.8g |Proteins-25g

Ingredients

- One lb. of peeled shrimp
- One tablespoon of minced garlic
- One tablespoon of tomato ketchup
- Three tablespoons of mayonnaise
- Half teaspoon of paprika
- One teaspoon of sriracha
- Half teaspoon of salt

Instructions

- In a bowl, mix together mayonnaise, paprika, sriracha, garlic, ketchup, and salt. Add shrimp and stir well.
- Add shrimp mixture into the air fryer baking dish

and place in the air fryer.

- Cook at 325 F for 8 minutes. Stir halfway through.
- Serve and enjoy.

Creole Pork Chops

Preparation Time-10 minutes | Cook Time-12 minutes | Servings-2 | Difficulty-Easy

Nutritional Facts- Calories-400 | Fats-30g | Carbohydrates-1.5g | Proteins-27.9g

Ingredients

- One and a half lbs. of boneless pork chops
- One teaspoon of garlic powder
- Five tablespoons of grated parmesan cheese
- 1/3 cup of almond flour
- One and a half teaspoons of paprika
- One teaspoon of Creole seasoning

Instructions

- Preheat the air fryer to 360 F.
- Add all ingredients except pork chops into the zip-lock bag. Mix well.
- Add pork chops into the bag. Seal bag and shake until well coated.
- Spray air fryer basket with cooking spray.
- Place pork chops into the air fryer basket and cook for 12 minutes.
- Serve and enjoy.

Crispy Herbed Salmon

Preparation Time-5 minutes | Cook Time-15 minutes | Servings-2 | Difficulty-Easy

Nutritional Facts- Calories-373 | Fats-21g | Carbohydrates-12.9g | Proteins-34g

Ingredients

- Four (six-ounce) skinless salmon fillets
- Three tablespoons of honey mustard
- Half teaspoon of dried thyme
- Half teaspoon of dried basil
- A quarter cup of panko bread crumbs
- 1/3 cup of crushed potato chips
- Two tablespoons of olive oil

Instructions

- Place the salmon on a plate. In a small bowl, merge the mustard, thyme, and basil, and spread evenly over the salmon.
- In another small bowl, merge the bread crumbs and potato chips and mix well. Set in the olive oil and mix until combined.
- Place the salmon in the air fryer basket and gently but firmly press the bread crumb mixture onto the top of each fillet.
- Bake until the salmon reaches at least 145°F on a meat thermometer and the topping is browned and crisp.

Cumin Lamb

Preparation Time-10 minutes | Cook Time-10 minutes | Servings-2 | Difficulty-Easy

Nutritional Facts- Calories-285 | Fats-15.9g | Carbohydrates-1.5g | Proteins-1g

Ingredients

- One lb. of chopped lamb
- A quarter teaspoon of liquid stevia
- Two tablespoons of olive oil
- Half teaspoon of cayenne
- Two tablespoons of ground cumin
- Two chopped red chili peppers
- One tablespoon of minced garlic
- One tablespoon of soy sauce
- One teaspoon of salt

Instructions

- In a small bowl, mix together cumin and cayenne.
- Rub meat with cumin mixture and place in a large bowl.
- Add oil, soy sauce, garlic, chili peppers, stevia, and salt over the meat. Coat well and place in the refrigerator overnight.
- Add marinated meat to the air fryer and cook at 360 F for 10 minutes.
- Serve and enjoy.

Duck Breasts with Raspberry Sauce

Preparation Time-10 minutes | Cook Time-15 minutes | Servings-2 | Difficulty-Easy

Nutritional Facts- Calories-456 | Fats-21.9g | Carbohydrates-18g | Proteins-45g

Ingredients

- Two skin-on and scored duck breasts
- Salt and black pepper to the taste
- Cooking spray
- Half teaspoon of cinnamon powder
- Half cup of raspberries
- One tablespoon of sugar
- One teaspoon of red wine vinegar
- Half cup of water

Instructions

- Season duck breasts with salt and pepper, spray them with cooking spray, put in preheated air fryer skin side down and cook at 350 degrees F for 10 minutes.
- Heat up a pan with the water over medium heat, add raspberries, cinnamon, sugar and wine, stir, bring to a simmer, transfer to your blender, puree and return to pan.
- Add air fryer duck breasts to the pan as well, toss to coat, divide among plates and serve right away.

Easy Beef Broccoli

Preparation Time-10 minutes | Cook Time-10 minutes | Servings-2 | Difficulty-Easy

Nutritional Facts- Calories-230 | Fats-4.8g |Carbohydrates-6.9g |Proteins-39g

Ingredients

- One lb. of round beef cubes
- Half medium diced onion
- One tablespoon of Worcestershire sauce
- Half lb. of steamed broccoli floret
- One teaspoon of olive oil
- One teaspoon of onion powder
- One teaspoon of garlic powder
- Pepper
- Salt

Instructions

- Spray air fryer basket with cooking spray.
- Add all ingredients except broccoli into the large bowl and toss well.
- Add bowl mixture into the air fryer basket and cook at 360 F for 10 minutes.
- Serve with broccoli and enjoy.

Fish and Chips

Preparation Time-10 minutes | Cook Time-20 minutes | Servings-2 | Difficulty-Easy

Nutritional Facts- Calories-374 | Fats-15.9g |Carbohydrates-37.8g |Proteins-30g

Ingredients

- Four (four-ounce) fish fillets
- Pinch salt
- Freshly ground black pepper
- Half teaspoon of dried thyme
- One egg white
- 1/3 cup of crushed potato chips
- Two tablespoons of olive oil, divided
- Two peeled russet potatoes

Instructions

- Set the fish fillets dry and sprinkle with salt, pepper, and thyme. Set aside.
- In a shallow bowl, beat the egg white until foamy. In another bowl, combine the potato chips and one tablespoon of olive oil and mix until combined.
- Set the fish fillets into the egg white, then into the crushed potato chip mixture to coat.
- Toss the fresh potato strips with the remaining One tablespoon of olive oil.
- Use your separator to divide the air fryer basket in half, and then fry the chips and fish. The chips will take about 20 minutes; the fish will take about 10 to 12 minutes to cook.

Fish Tacos with Slaw and Mango Salsa

Preparation Time-15 minutes | Cook Time-6 minutes | Servings-2 | Difficulty-Easy

Nutritional Facts- Calories-323 | Fats-12g |Carbohydrates-30g |Proteins-24g

Ingredients

- Four Tortillas
- One pound of Cod
- Three tablespoons of melted butter
- Half teaspoon of Paprika
- A quarter teaspoon of Garlic Onion
- One teaspoon of Thyme
- Half teaspoon of Onion Powder
- Half teaspoon of Cayenne Pepper

- One teaspoon of Brown Sugar
- One cup of prepared (or store-bought) Slaw
- Salt and Pepper, to taste

Mango Salsa

- A quarter cup of diced Red Onions
- Juice of one Lime
- One diced Mango
- One deseeded and minced Jalapeno Pepper
- One tablespoon of chopped Parsley or Cilantro

Instructions

- Preheat your Air fryer grill to medium.
- Brush the butter over the cod and sprinkle with the spices.
- When ready, open the grill, and arrange the cod fillets onto the bottom plate.
- Close the lid and cook for about 4-5 minutes in total.
- Transfer to a plate and cut into chunks.
- Place all of the mango salsa ingredients in a bowl and mix to combine.
- Assemble the tacos by adding slaw, topped with grilled cod, and adding a tablespoon of or so of the mango salsa.
- Enjoy!

Fried Chicken

Preparation Time-20 minutes | Cook Time-40 minutes | Servings-2 | Difficulty-Moderate

Nutritional Facts- Calories-200 | Fats-9.9g | Carbohydrates-4.8g | Proteins-9g

Ingredients

- Two cups of buttermilk
- Three teaspoons of kosher salt, divided
- A quarter teaspoon of cayenne pepper
- One teaspoon of garlic powder
- A half teaspoon of Oregano
- Two pounds bone-in skin-on chicken pieces (mix of cuts)
- Half cup of hot sauce
- A half teaspoon of freshly ground black pepper
- Two cups of all-purpose flour
- One teaspoon of onion powder

Instructions

- Trim the chicken with the extra fat and put it in a large bowl. Combine the buttermilk, hot sauce, and Two tablespoons of salt in a medium bowl.
- Pour the paste over the chicken, ensuring that all parts are coated. For at least sixty minutes and up to overnight, cover and refrigerate.
- Combine the flour, the remaining one teaspoon of salt and seasonings in a shallow bowl or pie dish. Remove the chicken from the buttermilk and shake off the extra buttermilk, working one at a time. Place in the mixture of flour and turn to coat.
- Place coated chicken in the air fryer basket, running in batches as required to prevent overcrowding the basket. Cook at 400 ° F until the chicken is golden and the internal temperature hits 165 ° F, turning midway through for 20 to 25 minutes.
- Repeat for leftover chicken.

Fried Pork Shoulder

Preparation Time-30 minutes | Cook Time-One hour and 20 minutes | Servings-2 | Difficulty-Hard

Nutritional Facts- Calories-221 | Fats-6g | Carbohydrates-7.8g | Proteins-15g

Ingredients

- Three tablespoons of minced garlic
- Three tablespoons of olive oil
- Four pounds of pork shoulder
- Salt and black pepper to the taste

Instructions

- In a bowl, mix olive oil with salt, pepper and oil, whisk well and brush pork shoulder with this mix.
- Place in the preheated air fryer and cook at 390 degrees F for 1 0 minutes.
- Reduce heat to 300 degrees F and roast pork for 1 hour and 10 minutes.
- Slice pork shoulder, divide among plates and serve with a side salad.

Garlic and Bell Pepper Beef

Preparation Time-30 minutes | Cook Time-30 minutes | Servings-2 | Difficulty-Hard

Nutritional Facts- Calories-343 | Fats-6.9g |Carbohydrates-26g |Proteins-37.8g

Ingredients

- Eleven ounces of sliced steak fillets
- Four minced garlic cloves
- Two tablespoons of olive oil
- One chopped red bell pepper
- Black pepper to the taste
- One tablespoon of sugar
- Two tablespoons of fish sauce
- Two teaspoons of cornflour
- Half cup of beef stock
- Four sliced green onions

Instructions

- In a pan that fits your air fryer, mix beef with oil, garlic, black pepper and bell pepper, stir, cover and keep in the fridge for 30 minutes.
- Put the pan in your preheated air fryer and cook at 360 degrees F for 14 minutes.
- In a bowl, mix sugar with fish sauce, stir well, pour over beef and cook at 360 degrees F for 7 minutes more.
- Add stock mixed with cornflour and green onions, toss and cook at 370 degrees F for 7 minutes more.
- Divide everything among plates and serve.

Garlic Lamb Chops

Preparation Time-10 minutes | Cook Time-10 minutes | Servings-2 | Difficulty-Easy

Nutritional Facts- Calories-231 | Fats-6.9g |Carbohydrates-15g |Proteins-23g

Ingredients

- Three tablespoons of olive oil
- Four lamb chops
- Salt and black pepper to the taste
- Four minced garlic cloves
- One tablespoon of chopped oregano
- One tablespoon of chopped coriander

Instructions

- In a bowl, mix oregano with salt, pepper, oil, garlic and lamb chops and toss to coat.
- Transfer lamb chops to your air fryer and cooks at 400 degrees F for 10 minutes.
- Divide lamb chops among plates and serve with a side salad.

Garlic Parmesan Chicken

Preparation Time-10 minutes | Cook Time-33 minutes | Servings-2 | Difficulty-Moderate

Nutritional Facts- Calories-246 | Fats-10.8g |Carbohydrates-16.8g |Proteins-30g

Ingredients

- Two large eggs
- Freshly ground black pepper
- One teaspoon of garlic powder
- One teaspoon of Italian seasoning
- 2/3 cup of freshly grated Parmesan
- Kosher salt
- One cup of Panko breadcrumbs
- Four bone-in, skin-on chicken thighs

Instructions

- With pepper and salt, season the chicken. Whisk together the parmesan, panko, garlic powder and Italian seasoning in a shallow bowl. Beat the eggs in yet another shallow bowl.
- Dip the chicken thighs in the egg and then roll until thoroughly covered in the Panko mix.
- Cook at 360 F for about 30 minutes or until golden.

Garlic Pork Chops

Preparation Time-5 minutes | Cook Time-20 minutes | Servings-2 | Difficulty-Easy

Nutritional Facts- Calories-545 | Fats-27g |Carbohydrates-4g |Proteins-40g

Ingredients

- Two lbs. of pork chops
- Two tablespoons of minced garlic
- One tablespoon of fresh parsley
- Two tablespoons of olive oil
- Two tablespoons of fresh lemon juice
- Pepper

- Salt

Instructions

- In a small bowl, merge together garlic, parsley, oil, and lemon juice.
- Season pork chops with pepper and salt.
- Rub garlic mixture over the pork chops and allow to marinate for 30 minutes.
- Add marinated pork chops into the air fryer and cook at 400 F for 10 minutes.
- Turn pork chops to another side and cook for 10 minutes more.
- Serve and enjoy.

Garlic-Herb Fried Patty Pan Squash

Preparation Time-15 minutes | Cook Time-25 minutes | Servings-2 | Difficulty-Easy

Nutritional Facts- Calories-163 | Fats-1g | Carbohydrates-21.9g | Proteins-7.8g

Ingredients

- A half teaspoon of salt
- A quarter teaspoon of dried thyme
- Two minced garlic cloves
- One tablespoon of minced fresh parsley
- One tablespoon of olive oil
- Five cups of halved small pattypan squash
- A one-fourth teaspoon of dried oregano
- A one-fourth teaspoon of pepper

Instructions

- Preheat the air fryer to 375 degrees F. Squash should be placed in a big mixing bowl. Drizzle squash with salt, oil, garlic, thyme, oregano, and pepper. Toss in order to coat evenly. In an air-fryer basket, place the squash on a greased tray.
- Then cook, occasionally stirring until the vegetable is tender for about 13-15 minutes. Serve after sprinkling with parsley.

Ground Beef with Zucchini

Preparation Time-5 minutes | Cook Time-15 minutes | Servings-2 | Difficulty-Easy

Nutritional Facts- Calories-311 | Fats-20g | Carbohydrates-4g | Proteins-39g

Ingredient

- One and a half pounds of ground beef
- One pound of chopped zucchini
- Two tablespoons of extra-virgin olive oil
- One teaspoon of dried oregano
- One teaspoon of dried basil
- One teaspoon of dried rosemary
- Two tablespoons of chopped fresh chives

Instructions

- In a large bowl, merge all the ingredients, except for the chives, until well blended.
- Place the beef and zucchini mixture in the baking pan.
- Select Bake, Super Convection, set the temperature to 400°F (205°C) and set the time to 12 minutes. Press Start/Stop to begin preheating.
- Once preheated, place the pan in the bake position.
- When cooking is processed, the beef should be browned, and the zucchini should be tender.
- Divide the beef and zucchini mixture among four serving dishes. Top with fresh chives and serve hot.

Herbed Cornish Hens

Preparation Time-Two hours and 15 minutes | Cook Time-30 minutes | Servings-2 | Difficulty-Hard

Nutritional Facts- Calories-245 | Fats-15g | Carbohydrates-1.5g | Proteins-24g

Ingredients

- Two (One and a quarter pound) of giblets removed, split lengthwise Cornish hens
- Two cups of white wine, divided
- Two minced cloves of garlic
- One small minced onion
- Half teaspoon of celery seeds
- Half teaspoon of poultry seasoning
- Half teaspoon of paprika
- Half teaspoon of dried oregano
- A quarter teaspoon of freshly ground black pepper

Instructions

- Place the hens, cavity side up, on a rack in a

baking pan. Pour 1Half cup of the wine over the hens; set aside.

- In a shallow bowl, combine the onion, garlic, paprika, oregano, celery seeds, poultry seasoning, and pepper. Sprinkle half of the combined seasonings over the cavity of each split half. Cover and refrigerate. Allow the hens to marinate for 2 hours.
- Place the basket on the bake position.
- Transfer the hens in the air fry basket. Select Bake, set temperature to 356 degrees F and set time to 90 minutes.
- Remove the pan basket from the air fryer grill halfway through the baking, turn the breast side up, and remove the skin. Pour the remaining half cup of wine over the top, and sprinkle with the remaining seasonings.
- When cooking is complete, the inner temperature of the hens should be at least 165F (74C). Bring the hens to a serving platter and serve hot.

Honey Mustard Chicken

Preparation Time-10 minutes | Cook Time-Four hours | Servings-2 | Difficulty-Hard

Nutritional Facts- Calories-599 | Fats-16.5g |Carbohydrates-57.9g |Proteins-52.8g

Ingredients

- One lb. of skinless, boneless and cut into pieces chicken breast
- Two tablespoons of soy sauce
- A quarter cup of orange juice
- Half cup of ground mustard
- A quarter cup of honey
- Two tablespoons of water
- Two tablespoons of cornstarch

Instructions

- Place the inner pot in the grill air fryer combo base.
- Add chicken into the inner pot.
- In a small bowl, combine together soy sauce, orange juice, ground mustard, and honey.
- Pour bowl mixture over the chicken.
- Cover the inner pot with a glass lid.

- Select slow cook mode, then press the temperature button and set the time for 4 hours. Press start.
- When the timer reaches 0, then press the cancel button.
- Mix together water and cornstarch and pour over the chicken mixture and stir well.
- Serve and enjoy.

Jerk Pork

Preparation Time-10 minutes | Cook Time-20 minutes | Servings-2 | Difficulty-Easy

Nutritional Facts- Calories-325 | Fats-12g |Carbohydrates-1g |Proteins-51g

Ingredients

- One and a half lbs. of chopped pork butt
- Three tablespoons of jerk paste

Instructions

- Add meat and jerk paste into the bowl and coat well. Place in the fridge overnight.
- Spray air fryer basket with cooking spray.
- Preheat the air fryer to 390 F.
- Add marinated meat into the air fryer and cook for 20 minutes. Turn halfway through.
- Serve and enjoy.

Jersey Hot Fried Chicken

Preparation Time-20 minutes | Cook Time-30 minutes | Servings-2 | Difficulty-Moderate

Nutritional Facts- Calories-626 | Fats-30g |Carbohydrates-9.9g |Proteins-69g

Ingredients

- Two chicken thighs
- Two cups of flour
- Two chicken legs
- Two tablespoons of Tomato paste
- One teaspoon of sugar
- One tablespoon of Garlic powder
- One teaspoon of cumin
- Five tablespoons of smoked or sweet paprika
- Two teaspoons of ground cumin
- Two tablespoons of cayenne pepper
- One teaspoon of Garlic powder
- Four cups of olive oil

- Two chicken breasts
- One teaspoon of onion powder
- One cup of buttermilk
- One tablespoon of salt
- One tablespoon of olive oil
- One tablespoon of freshly ground black pepper
- Two chicken wings
- One tablespoon of Paprika
- One teaspoon of turmeric

Instructions

- Set the chicken parts in a bowl with the buttermilk for a minimum of 1 hour, if possible, overnight.
- Bring together the seasoning ingredients in another bowl.
- Dredge the chicken in the flour; place in the buttermilk and back again in the flour.
- Drop the chicken on 2 Air Flow racks. Sprinkle the chicken with olive oil spray. Place the racks on the bottom and middle shelves of the Air Fryer.
- Set the power button and increase the cooking temperature to 390F and the cooking time to 35 minutes. Turn racks halfway through cook time (17 1/2 minutes).
- Bring together ground cumin, paprika, turmeric, cayenne pepper, garlic powder, tomato paste, salt and sugar in a skillet.
- Cook the spices over medium-low heat for a few minutes, being careful not to burn the sugars.
- Whisk four cups of olive oil into the sauce and cook for about 5 minutes over medium heat.
- Drizzle sauce over chicken.

Juicy and Tender Steak

Preparation Time-10 minutes | Cook Time-12 minutes | Servings-2 | Difficulty-Easy

Nutritional Facts- Calories-490 | Fats-21g |Carbohydrates-4g |Proteins-28.9g

Ingredients

- Two rib-eye steak
- Three tablespoons of fresh chopped parsley
- One stick of softened butter
- One and a half teaspoons of Worcestershire sauce
- Three minced garlic cloves
- Pepper

- Salt

Instructions

- In a bowl, merge together butter, Worcestershire sauce, garlic, parsley, and salt and place in the refrigerator.
- Preheat the air fryer to 400 F.
- Season steak with pepper and salt.
- Place seasoned steak in the air fryer and cook for 12 minutes. Turn halfway through.
- Remove steak from the air fryer and top with butter mixture.
- Serve and enjoy.

Lahmacun (Turkish Pizza)

Preparation Time-20 minutes | Cook Time-10 minutes | Servings-2 | Difficulty-Easy

Nutritional Facts- Calories-313 | Fats-27g |Carbohydrates-1g|Proteins-30g

Ingredient

Two (6-inch) flour tortillas

For the Meat Topping

- Two ounces of ground lamb or 85% lean ground beef
- A quarter cup of chopped green bell pepper
- A quarter cup of chopped fresh parsley
- One small deseeded and chopped plum tomato
- Two tablespoons of chopped yellow onion
- One minced garlic clove
- Two teaspoons of tomato paste
- A quarter teaspoon of sweet paprika
- A quarter teaspoon of ground cumin
- A quarter teaspoon of red pepper flakes
- 1/8 teaspoon of ground allspice
- 1/8 teaspoon of kosher salt
- 1/8 teaspoon of black pepper

For Serving

- A quarter cup of chopped fresh mint
- One teaspoon of extra-virgin olive oil
- One lemon, cut into wedges

Instructions

- Combine all the ingredients for the meat topping in a medium bowl until well mixed.

- Lay the tortillas on a clean work surface. Spoon the meat mixture on the tortillas and spread it all over.
- Place the tortillas in the air fry basket.
- Select Air Fry, Super Convection. Set temperature to 400°F (205°C) and set time to 10 minutes. Press Start/Stop to begin preheating.
- Once preheated, place the basket in the air fry position.
- When cooking is complete, the edge of the tortilla should be golden, and the meat should be lightly browned.
- Transfer them to a serving dish. Top with chopped fresh mint and drizzle with olive oil. Squeeze the lemon wedges on top and serve.

Lamb Loin Chops with Horseradish Cream Sauce

Preparation Time-15 minutes | Cook Time-14 minutes | Servings-2 to 4 | Difficulty-Easy

Nutritional Facts- Calories-230 | Fats-21.9g | Carbohydrates-9.9g | Proteins-4.8g

Ingredients

For the Lamb

- Four lamb loin chops
- Two tablespoons of vegetable oil
- One minced clove of garlic
- Half teaspoon of kosher salt
- Half teaspoon of black pepper

For the Horseradish Cream Sauce

- One and a half tablespoons of prepared horseradish
- One tablespoon of Dijon mustard
- Half cup of mayonnaise
- Two teaspoons of sugar
- Cooking spray

Instructions

- Spritz the airflow racks with frying spray.
- Position the lamb chops on a plate; after rubbing with oil, season with salt, garlic, and black pepper. Allow 30 minutes at room temperature to marinate.

- Combine the mayonnaise, mustard, horseradish, and sugar in a mixing basin. Set aside half of the sauce until you're ready to serve it.
- Place the marinated lamb in the airflow racks.
- Close the door and place the racks in the air fryer oven. Turn on and off the Power Button. Preheat oven to 325°F and bake for 10 minutes.
- Flip the lamb chops halfway through the cooking time.
- During the cooking process, the lamb should be browned.
- Move the chops from the air fryer to the bowl with the horseradish sauce. To coat completely, roll it out.
- Replace the coated chops in the airflow racks of the air fryer oven. Turn on and off the Power Button. Preheat the oven to 400 degrees Fahrenheit with a 3-minute timer.
- During the cooking process, the internal temperature should reach 145 degrees F on a meat thermometer. Flip the lamb halfway through.
- Serve hot with prepared sauce.

Lamb Rack with Pistachio

Preparation Time-15 minutes | Cook Time-20 minutes | Servings-2 | Difficulty-Easy

Nutritional Facts- Calories-300 | Fats-12g | Carbohydrates-1g | Proteins-45.9g

Ingredients

- One teaspoon of fresh rosemary
- Two teaspoons of chopped fresh oregano
- Black pepper and salt as per taste
- One tablespoon of Dijon mustard
- Half cup of pistachios
- Three tablespoons of panko breadcrumbs
- One tablespoon of olive oil
- One lamb rack

Instructions

- Combine the rosemary, pistachios, breadcrumbs, olive oil, oregano, salt, and black pepper in a food processor. Pulse until smooth to blend.
- Season the lamb rack with black pepper and salt on a clean work surface before placing it on the airflow racks.

- Close the door and place the racks in the air fryer oven. Turn on and off the Power Button. Preheat oven to 380°F and bake for 12 minutes.
- Flip the lamb midway through.
- During the cooking process, the lamb should be nicely browned.
- Rub the fat side of the lamb rack with Dijon mustard, then equally coat the lamb rack with the pistachios mixture.
- Return the lamb rack to the air fryer oven and cook for an additional eight minutes, or until the internal temperature reaches 145°F.
- Remove the lamb rack from the air fryer with tongs and lay aside for 5 minutes to cool before slicing to serve.

Lamb Roast and Potatoes

Preparation Time-10 minutes | Cook Time-45 minutes | Servings-2 | Difficulty-Moderate

Nutritional Facts- Calories-273 | Fats-4.8g |Carbohydrates-25g |Proteins-27.9g

Ingredients

- Two pounds of lamb roast
- One spring of rosemary
- Three minced garlic cloves
- Four halved potatoes
- Half cup of lamb stock
- Two bay leaves
- Salt and black pepper to the taste

Instructions

- Put potatoes in a dish that fits your air fryer, add lamb, garlic, rosemary spring, salt, pepper, bay leaves and stock, toss, introduce in your air fryer and cook at 360 degrees F for 45 minutes.
- Slice lamb, divide among plates and serve with potatoes and cooking juices.
- Enjoy!

Lamb Shanks

Preparation Time-10 minutes | Cook Time-45 | Servings-2 | Difficulty-Moderate

Nutritional Facts- Calories-283 | Fats-4.8g |Carbohydrates-16.8g |Proteins-26g

Ingredients

- Four lamb shanks
- One chopped yellow onion
- One tablespoon of olive oil
- Four teaspoons of crushed coriander seeds
- Two tablespoons of white flour
- Four bay leaves
- Two teaspoons of honey
- Five ounces of dry sherry
- Two and a half cups of chicken stock
- Salt and pepper to the taste

Instructions

- Season lamb shanks with salt and pepper, rub with half of the oil, put in your air fryer and cook at 360 degrees F for 10 minutes.
- Heat up a pan that fits your air fryer with the rest of the oil over medium-high heat, add onion and coriander, stir and cook for 5 minutes.
- Add flour, sherry, stock, honey and bay leaves, salt and pepper, stir, bring to a simmer, add lamb, introduce everything in your air fryer and cook at 360 degrees F for 30 minutes.
- Divide everything among plates and serve.
- Enjoy!

Lemon and Honey Glazed Game Hen

Preparation Time-10 minutes | Cook Time-20 minutes | Servings-2 | Difficulty-Easy

Nutritional Facts- Calories-623 | Fats-19g |Carbohydrates-30g |Proteins-55.8g

Ingredients

- One (Two pounds) halved Cornish game hen
- A quarter teaspoon of dried thyme
- Juice and zest of one lemon
- A quarter cup of honey
- One and a half teaspoons of chopped fresh thyme leaves
- One tablespoon of olive oil
- Salt and ground black pepper, to taste
- Half teaspoon of soy sauce

Instructions

- Preheat the air fryer to 390F (199C). Set the air fryer basket with cooking spray.
- On a clean work surface, brush the game hen

halves with olive oil, then sprinkle with dried thyme, salt, and black pepper to season.

- Cook the hen in the preheated air fryer for 15 minutes or until the hen is lightly browned. Flip the hen halfway through.
- Meanwhile, mix the lemon juice and zest, honey, thyme leaves, soy sauce, and black pepper in a bowl.
- Baste the game hen with the honey glaze, then cook for an additional 4 minutes or until the hen is well glazed and a meat thermometer inserted in the hen reads at least 165°F (74°C).
- Remove the game hen from the air fryer basket. Set to cool for a few minutes and slice to serve.

Lemon flavored Pork Loin Chop Schnitzel

Preparation Time-17 minutes | Cook Time-15 minutes | Servings-2 | Difficulty-Easy

Nutritional Facts- Calories-384 | Fats-23g |Carbohydrates-10.8g |Proteins-34g

Ingredients

- Two tablespoons of lemon juice
- A quarter teaspoon of marjoram
- One cup of panko breadcrumbs
- Lemon wedges
- Four thin boneless pork loin chops
- Half cup of flour
- One teaspoon of salt
- Two eggs
- Cooking spray

Instructions

- Lemon juice should be applied on both sides of the pork chops.
- Combine the marjoram, flour, and salt in a small dish. Place the breadcrumbs in a separate shallow dish. Whisk the eggs together in a large mixing dish.
- Coat the pork chops in flour, then dip them in beaten eggs to coat them completely. Remove any excess breadcrumbs and roll in them. Before putting the pork chops in the airflow racks, spray them with cooking spray.
- Close the door and place the racks in the air fryer oven. Turn on and off the Power Button. Preheat oven to 400 degrees F and bake for 15 minutes.

- After 7 minutes, extract the air fryer from the oven. On the other side, cook the pork. Bring to the air fryer oven for a couple more minutes of cooking.
- When the pork is done, it should be crunchy and golden.
- Serve with lemon wedges squeezed over the fried chops right away.

Lobster Tails

Preparation Time-10 minutes | Cook Time-7 minutes | Servings-2 | Difficulty-Easy

Nutritional Facts- Calories-255 | Fats-10.8g |Carbohydrates-1.5g |Proteins-34g

Ingredients

- Four thawed lobster tails
- One teaspoon of pepper
- Two tablespoons of melted butter
- Half teaspoon of salt

Instructions

- Melt the butter.
- With kitchen scissors, cut lobster right through the tail part.
- Then break the shell and pull backward with your fingers.
- Rub the lobster tail with butter and add salt and pepper.
- Place it in the air fryer and cook at 380 degrees F for 4 minutes.
- Add melted butter and cook for another 3 minutes.
- Serve with more butter.

Marinated Lamb and Veggies

Preparation Time-5 minutes | Cook Time-40 minutes | Servings-2 | Difficulty-Moderate

Nutritional Facts- Calories-265 | Fats-1g |Carbohydrates-18g |Proteins-21.9g

Ingredients

- Four ounces of sliced lamb loin
- One sliced onion
- One chopped carrot
- Three ounces of beans sprouts
- Half tablespoon of olive oil

Marinade

- Half grated apple
- One tablespoon of sugar
- One minced garlic clove
- Five tablespoons of soy sauce
- One tablespoon of grated ginger
- Two tablespoons of orange juice
- One grated onion
- Salt and pepper to taste

Instructions

- Preheat the air fryer to 350F.
- In a bowl, attach all the marinade ingredients, whisk and set aside. In a pan that fits into the air fryer, heat oil, add onions and beans sprout. Cook for 3 minutes; add the lamb and the marinade.
- Transfer into the air fryer, close the lid and cook for 25 minutes.
- Serve and enjoy!

Marinated Lamb and Veggies

Preparation Time-10 minutes | Cook Time-30 minutes | Servings-2 | Difficulty-Moderate

Nutritional Facts- Calories-274 | Fats-4g |Carbohydrates-18g |Proteins-24g

Ingredients

- One chopped carrot
- One sliced onion
- Half tablespoon of olive oil
- Three ounces of bean sprouts
- Eight ounces of sliced lamb loin

For the marinade

- One minced garlic clove
- Half grated apple
- Salt and black pepper to the taste
- One small grated yellow onion
- One tablespoon of grated ginger
- Five tablespoons of soy sauce
- One tablespoon of sugar
- Two tablespoons of orange juice

Instructions

- In a bowl, mix one grated onion with the apple, garlic, One tablespoon of ginger, soy sauce, orange juice, sugar and black pepper, whisk well, add lamb and leave aside for 10 minutes.
- Heat up a pan that fits your air fryer with the olive oil over medium-high heat, add one sliced onion, carrot and bean sprouts, stir and cook for 3 minutes.
- Add lamb and the marinade, transfer pan to your preheated air fryer and cook at 360 degrees F for 25 minutes.
- Divide everything into bowls and serve.

Meat and Rice Stuffed Bell Peppers

Preparation Time-20 minutes | Cook Time-18 minutes | Servings-2 | Difficulty-Easy

Nutritional Facts- Calories-177 | Fats-4g |Carbohydrates-10.8g |Proteins-26g

Ingredients

- Four ounces of lean ground pork
- One (Fifteen ounces) can of crushed tomatoes
- One teaspoon of barbecue seasoning
- Half teaspoon of dried basil
- Half teaspoon of garlic powder
- Half teaspoon of salt
- Cooking spray
- 1/3 pound of lean ground beef
- A quarter cup of minced onion
- One teaspoon of Worcestershire sauce
- One teaspoon of honey
- Half cup of cooked brown rice
- Half teaspoon of oregano
- Two small deseeded and halved bell peppers

Instructions

- Using cooking spray, coat a baking pan.
- In a baking pan, arrange the beef, pork, and onion.
- Place the pan in the air fryer and turn it on. Toggle the Power Button on and off. Cook for 8 minutes at 360°F (182°C).
- Halfway through the cooking time, break the ground beef into bits.
- The ground meat should be lightly browned after the cooking is finished.
- In a separate pot, add the tomatoes, barbecue seasoning, Worcestershire sauce, honey, and basil. Stir everything together thoroughly.

- Add the cooked rice, oregano, garlic powder, salt, and ¼ cup of tomato sauce to a large mixing bowl with the cooked meat mixture. Stir everything together thoroughly.
- Fill the pepper halves halfway with the mixture, then place them in the airflow racks.
- Place the pan in the air fryer and cook for another 10 minutes.
- When the peppers are done, they should be faintly browned.
- Serve with the remaining tomato sauce on top of the stuffed peppers.

Montreal Steak

Preparation Time-5 minutes | Cook Time-10 minutes | Servings-2 | Difficulty-Easy

Nutritional Facts- Calories-345 | Fats-9g |Carbohydrates-1g|Proteins-57.9g

Ingredients

- Twelve ounces of steak
- Half teaspoon of. liquid smoke
- One tablespoon of soy sauce
- Half tablespoon of cocoa powder
- One tablespoon of Montreal steak seasoning
- Pepper
- Salt

Instructions

- Add steak, liquid smoke, soy sauce, and steak seasonings into the large zip-lock bag. Coat well and place in the refrigerator overnight.
- Spray air fryer basket with cooking spray.
- Place marinated steaks into the air fryer
- Cook at 375 degrees F for 7 minutes. Turn after 5 minutes to another side.
- Serve and enjoy.

Mushroom in Bacon-Wrapped fillets Mignons

Preparation Time-10 minutes | Cook Time-13 minutes | Servings-2 | Difficulty-Easy

Nutritional Facts- Calories-352 | Fats-21g |Carbohydrates-6g |Proteins-52.8g

Ingredient

- One ounce of dried porcini mushrooms

- Half teaspoon of granulated white sugar
- Half teaspoon of salt
- Half teaspoon of ground white pepper
- Eight (Four ounces) fillets mignons or beef tenderloin steaks
- Eight thin-cut bacon strips

Instructions

- Put the mushrooms, sugar, salt, and white pepper in a spice grinder and grind to combine.
- On a clean work surface, rub the fillets mignons with the mushroom mixture, then wrap each filet with a bacon strip. Secure with toothpicks if necessary.
- Arrange the bacon-wrapped fillets mignons in the air fry basket, seam side down.
- Select Air Fry, Super Convection. Set temperature to 400°F (205°C) and set time to 13 minutes. Press Start/Stop to begin preheating.
- Once preheated, place the basket in the air fry position. Flip the fillets halfway through.
- When cooking is complete, the fillets should be medium-rare.
- Serve immediately.

New York Strip with Honey-Mustard Butter

Preparation Time-10 minutes | Cook Time-15 minutes | Servings-2 | Difficulty-Easy

Nutritional Facts- Calories-160 | Fats-1.5g |Carbohydrates-6g |Proteins-25g

Ingredients

- Two pounds of New York Strip
- One teaspoon of cayenne pepper
- One tablespoon of honey
- One tablespoon of Dijon mustard
- Half stick softened butter
- Sea salt and ground black pepper, to taste
- Cooking spray

Instructions

- Spritz the airflow racks with cooking spray.
- Sprinkle the New York Strip with cayenne pepper, salt, and black pepper on a clean work surface.
- Arrange the New York Strip in the prepared racks

and spritz with cooking spray.

- Slide the racks into the air fryer oven. Press the Power Button. Cook at 400F (205C) for 14 minutes.
- Flip the New York Strip halfway through.
- When cooking is processed, the strips should be browned.
- Meanwhile, combine the honey, mustard, and butter in a small bowl. Stir to mix well.
- Transfer the air-fried New York Strip onto a plate and bastes with the honey-mustard butter before serving.

Nutty Crusted Pork Rack

Preparation Time-5 minutes | Cook Time-35 minutes | Servings-2 | Difficulty-Easy

Nutritional Facts- Calories-323 | Fats-12g |Carbohydrates-30g |Proteins-24g

Ingredients

- Two tablespoons of olive oil
- One cup of chopped macadamia nuts
- One tablespoon of chopped rosemary
- Salt and ground black pepper, to taste
- One minced clove of garlic
- One pound of the rack of pork
- One tablespoon of breadcrumbs
- One egg

Instructions

- Combine the olive oil and garlic in a small bowl. Everything should be well mixed together.
- Place the pork rack on a clean work surface with the garlic oil and season both sides with salt and black pepper.
- Combine the breadcrumbs, macadamia nuts, and rosemary in a small dish. Whisk the egg in a large mixing bowl.
- Put the pork in the egg, then coat it completely in the macadamia nut mixture. By shaking off any surplus, you may get rid of it.
- Place the pork in the racks so that air may circulate freely.
- Close the door and place the racks in the air fryer oven. Turn on and off the Power Button. Preheat oven to 356 degrees Fahrenheit and bake for 30 minutes.

- After 30 minutes, take the air fryer out of the oven. Overturn the pork rack. Preheat the air fryer oven to 390 degrees F (199 degrees C) for 5 minutes. Cooking should be continued.
- Before cooking the pork, it should be browned.
- Serve immediately.

Panko Salmon and Carrot Croquettes

Preparation Time-15 minutes | Cook Time-10 minutes | Servings-2 | Difficulty-Easy

Nutritional Facts- Calories-172 | Fats-4.8g |Carbohydrates-7.8g |Proteins-25g

Ingredients

- Two egg whites
- One cup of almond flour
- One cup of panko bread crumbs
- One pound of chopped salmon fillet
- 2/3 cup of grated carrots
- Two tablespoons of minced garlic cloves
- Half cup of chopped onion
- Two tablespoons of chopped chives
Cooking spray

Instructions

- Spritz the air fry basket with cooking spray.
- Whisk the egg whites in a bowl. Put the flour in a second bowl. Pour the bread crumbs into a third bowl. Set aside.
- Combine the salmon, garlic, onion, carrots, and chives in a large bowl. Stir to mix well.
- Form the mixture into balls with your hands. Dredge the balls into the flour, then egg, and then bread crumbs to coat well.
- Arrange the salmon balls in the air fry basket and spritz with cooking spray.
- Place the basket on the air fry position.
- Select Air Fry, set temperature to 356 degrees Fahrenheit and set time to 10 minutes. Flip the salmon balls halfway through cooking.
- When cooking is complete, the salmon balls will be crispy and browned. Remove the basket from the air fryer grill.
- Serve immediately.

Paprika Pork Chops with Corn

Preparation Time-10 minutes | Cook Time-20 minutes | Servings-2 | Difficulty-Easy

Nutritional Facts- Calories-418 | Fats-23g |Carbohydrates-21g |Proteins-34.8g

Ingredients

- Two boneless pork chops
- One tablespoon of olive oil
- One teaspoon of paprika
- Half teaspoon of onion powder
- Salt and pepper to taste
- Two grilled ears of corn

Instructions

- Garnish both sides of pork chops with oil.
- Season with paprika, onion powder, salt and pepper.
- Add pork chops to the air fryer.
- Set it to the grill.
- Cook at 375 degrees F for 5 to 7 minutes per side.
- Serve with grilled corn.

Parmesan "Fried" Tortellini

Preparation Time-10 minutes | Cook Time-25 minutes | Servings-2 | Difficulty-Easy

Nutritional Facts- Calories-166 | Fats-12g |Carbohydrates-21g |Proteins-6g

Ingredients

- One teaspoon of dried oregano
- A half teaspoon of crushed red pepper flakes
- Freshly ground black pepper
- Two large eggs
- One cup of Panko breadcrumbs
- One-third cup of freshly grated Parmesan
- A half teaspoon of garlic powder
- Kosher salt
- One cup of all-purpose flour
- One (nine ounces) package cheese tortellini
- Marinara, for serving

Instructions

- Cook tortellini in a big pot of boiling salted water. Then drain.
- Mix together the garlic powder, Panko, Parmesan, oregano and red pepper flakes in a shallow bowl. With pepper and salt, season. Beat the eggs in another shallow bowl and add the flour to the third shallow bowl.
- Cover the tortellini in flour, then dredge them in eggs, then mix them in Panko. Continue until they are all covered with tortellini.
- Place in an air fryer and fry for 10 minutes at 370 °F until crispy.
- Serve with marinara as well.

Pork and Tri-colour Vegetables Kebabs

Preparation Time-1 hour and 20 minutes | Cook Time-10 minutes | Servings-2 | Difficulty-Hard

Nutritional Facts- Calories-233 | Fats-7.8g |Carbohydrates-3.18g |Proteins-35.4g

Ingredients

For the Pork

- One pound of pork steak, cut into cubes
- One tablespoon of white wine vinegar
- Three tablespoons of steak sauce
- A quarter cup of soy sauce
- One teaspoon of powdered chili
- One teaspoon of red chili flakes
- Two teaspoons of smoked paprika
- One teaspoon of garlic salt

For the Vegetable

- One deseeded and cube-cut green squash
- One deseeded and cube-cut yellow squash
- One cube-cut red pepper
- One cube-cut green pepper
- Salt and ground black pepper, to taste
- Cooking spray
- Four bamboo skewers, soaked in water for half an hour

Instructions

- Combine the ingredients for the pork in a large bowl. Press the pork to dunk in the marinade. Wrap the bowl in plastic and refrigerate for at least an hour.
- Spritz the airflow racks with cooking spray.
- Remove the pork from the marinade and run the skewers through the pork and vegetables

- alternatively. Sprinkle with salt and pepper to taste.
- Arrange the skewers in the racks and spritz with cooking spray.
- Slide the racks into the air fryer oven. Press the Power Button. Cook at 380F (193C) for 8 minutes.
- After 4 minutes, detach from the air fryer oven. Flip the skewers. Bring to the air fryer oven and continue cooking.
- When cooking is processed, the pork should be browned, and the vegetables should be lightly charred and tender.
- Serve immediately.

Pork Butt with Garlicky Coriander-Parsley Sauce

Preparation Time-One hour and 15 minutes | Cook Time-30 minutes | Servings-2 | Difficulty-Hard

Nutritional Facts- Calories-187 | Fats-4.8g |Carbohydrates-6.9g |Proteins-25g

Ingredients

- One teaspoon of golden flaxseeds meal
- One well-whisked egg white
- One tablespoon of soy sauce
- One teaspoon of freshly squeezed lemon juice
- One tablespoon of olive oil
- One pound of pork butt, cut into pieces
- Salt and ground black pepper, to taste

Coriander- Garlic-Parsley Sauce

- Three minced garlic cloves
- 1/3 cup of fresh coriander leaves
- 1/3 cup of fresh parsley leaves
- One teaspoon of lemon juice
- 1/Two tablespoons of salt
- 1/3 cup of extra-virgin olive oil

Instructions

- In a large mixing bowl, combine the egg white, flaxseed meal, soy sauce, salt, lemon juice, black pepper, and olive oil. Submerge the pork strips by dipping them in and pressing them down.
- Cover the bowl with plastic wrap and place it in the refrigerator for at least an hour to marinate.

- In the airflow racks, arrange the marinated pork strips.
- Place the racks in the air fryer oven and close the door. Toggle the Power Button on and off. Cook for 30 minutes at 380°F (193°C).
- Remove the air fryer oven after 15 minutes. Cook the pork on the other side. Return to the air fryer oven and cook for a few more minutes.
- When the pork is cooked, it should be thoroughly browned.
- In a small mixing dish, combine the sauce ingredients. Stir everything together thoroughly. Place the bowl in the fridge to chill until ready to use.
- Serve the cold sauce beside the air-fried pork slices.

Pork Chops and Mushrooms Mix

Preparation Time-10 minutes | Cook Time-40 minutes | Servings-2 | Difficulty-Moderate

Nutritional Facts- Calories-456 | Fats-9.9g |Carbohydrates-9g |Proteins-30g

Ingredients

- Eight ounces of sliced mushrooms
- One teaspoon of garlic powder
- One chopped yellow onion
- One cup of mayonnaise
- Three boneless pork chops
- One teaspoon of nutmeg
- One tablespoon of balsamic vinegar
- Half cup of olive oil

Instructions

- Heat up a pan that fits your air fryer with the oil over medium heat, add mushrooms and onions, stir and cook for 4 minutes.
- Add pork chops, nutmeg and garlic powder and brown on both sides.
- Introduce pan your air fryer at 330 degrees F and cook for 30 minutes.
- Add vinegar and mayo, stir, divide everything among plates and serve.
- Enjoy.

Pork Chops with Creamy Dip

Preparation Time-10 minutes | Cook Time-30 minutes | Servings-2 | Difficulty-Moderate

Nutritional Facts- Calories-398 | Fats-18g |Carbohydrates-4g |Proteins-13.8g

Ingredients

Sauce

- Three tablespoons of mayonnaise
- One teaspoon of apple cider vinegar
- One tablespoon of honey
- One tablespoon of mustard
- A quarter teaspoon of paprika
- Salt and pepper to taste

Pork

- Four pork chops
- Salt and pepper to taste
- A quarter cup of all-purpose flour
- Two eggs
- 1/3 cup of breadcrumbs

Instructions

- In a bowl, mix the ingredients for the sauce.
- Refrigerate until serving time.
- Season pork chops with salt and pepper.
- Coat with flour.
- Dip in eggs and dredge with breadcrumbs.
- Press air fry setting.
- Cook at 360 F for 30 minutes, flipping once.
- Serve pork chops with dip.

Pork Fried Rice with Scrambled Egg

Preparation Time-10 minutes | Cook Time-15 minutes | Servings-2 | Difficulty-Easy

Nutritional Facts- Calories-157 | Fats-4.8g |Carbohydrates-13.8g |Proteins-15.9g

Ingredients

- Three diced scallions
- Half cup of diced bell peppers
- Two teaspoons of sesame oil
- Half pound of diced pork tenderloin
- Half cup of frozen peas, thawed
- Half cup of roasted mushrooms
- Half cup of soy sauce
- Two cups of cooked rice
- One beaten egg

Instructions

- Place the scallions and red pepper on a baking pan. Set with the sesame oil and toss the vegetables to coat them in the oil.
- Bring the pan into the air fryer oven. Press the Power Button. Cook at 375F (190C) for 12 minutes.
- While the vegetables are cooking, place the pork in a large bowl. Add the peas, mushrooms, soy sauce, and rice and toss to coat the ingredients with the sauce.
- After about 4 minutes, remove from the air fryer oven. Place the pork mixture on the pan and stir the scallions and peppers into the pork and rice. Bring to the air fryer oven and continue cooking.
- After another 6 minutes, remove from the air fryer oven. Move the rice mixture to the sides to create an empty circle in the middle of the pan. Pour the egg into the circle. Bring to the air fryer oven and continue cooking.
- When cooking is processed, remove it from the air fryer oven and stir the egg to scramble it. Stir the egg into the fried rice mixture. Serve immediately.

Pork Leg Roast with Candy Onions

Preparation Time-10 minutes | Cook Time-One hour | Servings-2 | Difficulty-Hard

Nutritional Facts- Calories-290 | Fats-9.9g |Carbohydrates-4g |Proteins-37.8g

Ingredients

- Two teaspoons of sesame oil
- One teaspoon of dried sage, crushed
- One teaspoon of cayenne pepper
- One chopped rosemary spring
- One chopped thyme spring
- Sea salt and black pepper, to taste
- Two pounds of scored pork leg roast
- Half pound of sliced candy onions
- Four finely chopped cloves of garlic
- Two minced chili peppers

Instructions

- In a mixing bowl, combine the sesame oil, sage,

cayenne pepper, rosemary, thyme, salt and black pepper until well mixed. In another bowl, place the pork leg and brush with the seasoning mixture.

- Place the seasoned pork leg in a baking pan. Bring the pan into the air fryer oven. Press the Power Button. Cook at 400F (205C) for 40 minutes.

- After 20 minutes, detach from the air fryer oven. Flip the pork leg. Bring to the air fryer oven and continue cooking.

- After another 20 minutes, add the candy onions, garlic, and chili peppers to the pan and cook for another 12 minutes.

- When cooking is complete, the pork leg should be browned.

- Transfer the pork leg to a plate. Let cool for 5 minutes and slice. Spread the juices left in the pan over the pork and serve warm with the candy onions.

Pork with Couscous

Preparation Time-10 minutes | Cook Time-35 minutes | Servings-2 | Difficulty-Moderate

Nutritional Facts- Calories-310 | Fats-7.8g |Carbohydrates-31.8g |Proteins-28.9g

Ingredients

- Two pounds of boneless and trimmed pork loin
- 3/4 cup of chicken stock
- Two tablespoons of olive oil
- Half tablespoon of sweet paprika
- Two teaspoons of dried sage
- Half tablespoon of garlic powder
- A quarter teaspoon of dried rosemary
- A quarter teaspoon of dried marjoram
- One teaspoon of dried basil
- One teaspoon of dried oregano
- Salt and black pepper to the taste
- Two cups of cooked couscous

Instructions

- In a bowl, mix oil with stock, paprika, garlic powder, sage, rosemary, thyme, marjoram, oregano, salt and pepper to the taste, whisk well, add pork loin, toss well and leave aside for 1 hour.

- Transfer everything to a pan that fits your air fryer and cook at 370 degrees F for 35 minutes.

- Divide among plates and serve with couscous on the side.

Pretzel-Crusted Catfish

Preparation Time-10 minutes | Cook Time-15 minutes | Servings-2 | Difficulty-Easy

Nutritional Facts- Calories-431 | Fats-15.9g |Carbohydrates-23g |Proteins-34.8g

Ingredients

- A half teaspoon of salt
- Four cups of coarsely crushed honey mustard miniature pretzels
- A half teaspoon of pepper
- A one-third cup of Dijon mustard
- Lemon slices
- Four (Six ounces each) catfish fillets
- A half-cup of all-purpose flour
- Cooking spray
- Two large eggs
- Two tablespoons of 2% milk

Instructions

- Preheat the air fryer to 325 degrees Fahrenheit. Season the catfish with black pepper and salt. In a small bowl, whisk together the mustard, eggs, and milk. Separate the pretzels and flour into two bowls. Coat the fillets in flour, then dunk them in the egg mixture before coating them in pretzels.

- Put fillets in a layer on an oiled tray in the air-fryer basket in batches; spray it with oil, then cook for 10-12 minutes or until the fish flakes with a fork.

- It can be served with some slices of lemon if desired.

Prime Beef Rib Roast

Preparation Time-10 minutes | Cook Time-Two hours | Servings-2 | Difficulty-Hard

Nutritional Facts- Calories-368 | Fats-12g |Carbohydrates-13.8g |Proteins-27.9g

Ingredient

- One (Twelve pounds) bone-in beef rib roast
- Three tablespoons of salt
- One and a half tablespoons of ground black pepper

- One cup of wood chips

Horseradish sauce

- Half cup of sour cream
- A quarter cup of prepared horseradish
- Two tablespoons of Dijon mustard

Instructions

- Season the rib roast with pepper and salt before serving. Refrigerate for at least two hours, if not overnight.
- Remove the rib roast from the refrigerator one hour before cooking. Truss the roast and skewer it onto the rotisserie spit, using the spit forks to secure it. Allow the steak to rest for 5 minutes while the air fryer grill is preheated to 350 degrees F.
- Add the meat ribs to the mix. Set the air fryer to 400 degrees F and cook for about an hour, or until the beef reaches an internal temperature of 120 degrees F.
- Allow the beef to rest once it has been cooked, and while it is resting, combine the ingredients for the horseradish sauce. To carve the beef, first remove the bones from the roast, then slice and serve the roast.

Quick Paella

Preparation Time-8 minutes | Cook Time-18 minutes | Servings-2 | Difficulty-Easy

Nutritional Facts- Calories-345 | Fats-1g | Carbohydrates-65g | Proteins-18g

Ingredients

- One (Ten-ounce) package of thawed frozen cooked rice
- One (Six-ounce) jar of drained and chopped artichoke hearts
- A quarter cup of vegetable broth
- Half teaspoon of turmeric
- Half teaspoon of dried thyme
- One cup of frozen cooked small shrimp
- Half cup of frozen baby peas
- One diced tomato

Instructions

- In a 6-by-6-by-2-inch pan, combine the rice, artichoke hearts, vegetable broth, turmeric, and

thyme, and stir gently.

- Set in the air fryer and bake for 8 to 9 minutes or until the rice is hot.
- Remove from the air fryer and gently stir in the shrimp, peas, and tomato. Cook for 5 to 8 minutes or until the shrimp and peas are hot and the paella is bubbling.
- Substitution tip: If you like intensely flavored food, try using marinated artichoke hearts in this recipe. Be sure you taste the marinade first! For even more flavor, use the liquid in the jar of artichokes in place of the vegetable broth.

Quinoa Arancini

Preparation Time-10 minutes | Cook Time-15 minutes | Servings-2 | Difficulty-Easy

Nutritional Facts- Calories-423 | Fats-12.9g | Carbohydrates-34g | Proteins-21g

Ingredients

- One tablespoon of olive oil
- A half teaspoon of garlic powder
- 1/8 teaspoon of pepper
- Two large eggs, lightly beaten, divided, use
- A quarter cup of shredded Parmesan cheese
- Warmed pasta sauce, optional
- One package of ready-to-serve quinoa (nine ounces) or one and a 3/4 cup of cooked quinoa
- Two teaspoons of dried basil or Two tablespoons of minced fresh basil
- A half teaspoon of salt
- Six cubes (3/4-inch each) part-skim mozzarella cheese
- One cup of seasoned bread crumbs, divided
- Cooking spray

Instructions

- Preheat the air fryer to 375 degrees Fahrenheit. Follow the package directions for quinoa preparation. Then mix one egg, one and a half cups of bread crumbs, basil, oil, Parmesan cheese, and seasonings are mixed in.
- Divide into six equal parts. Form each portion into a ball by wrapping it completely around a cube of cheese.
- In separate shallow bowls, place the remaining half cup of bread crumbs and egg. Then quinoa balls are to be dipped in egg. After that, roll it in

the bread crumbs. Spritz with cooking spray and put on an oiled tray in the air-fryer basket. Cook for 6-8 minutes, or until they are golden brown in color. It should be served with pasta sauce.

Ranch Chicken

Preparation Time-10 minutes | Cook Time-Four hours | Servings-2 | Difficulty-Hard

Nutritional Facts- Calories-465 | Fats-18g |Carbohydrates-1g|Proteins-61.8g

Ingredients

- Three skinless and boneless chicken breasts
- One and a half tablespoons of dry ranch seasoning
- One and a half tablespoons of taco seasoning
- A quarter cup of water
- Two minced cloves of garlic

Instructions

- Place the inner pot in the grill air fryer combo base.
- Add chicken to the inner pot.
- In a small bowl, whisk together the remaining ingredients and pour over the chicken.
- Cover the inner pot with a glass lid.
- Select slow cook mode, then press the temperature button and set the time for 4 hours. Press start.
- When the timer reaches 0, then press the cancel button.
- Shred the chicken using a fork and serve.
- Reuben Beef Rolls with Thousand Island Sauce
- Preparation Time-15 minutes | Cook Time-10 minutes | Servings-2 to 4 | Difficulty-Easy
- Nutritional Facts- Calories-328 | Fats-19g |Carbohydrates-1.5g |Proteins-45g
- Ingredient
- Half pound of chopped cooked corned beef
- Half cup of drained and chopped sauerkraut
- One (eight-ounce) package of softened cream cheese
- Half cup of shredded Swiss cheese
- Twenty slices of prosciutto
- Cooking spray
- Thousand Island Sauce
- A quarter cup of chopped dill pickles

- A quarter cup of tomato sauce
- 1/3 cup of mayonnaise
- Fresh thyme leaves, for garnish
- Two tablespoons of sugar
- 1/8 teaspoon of fine sea salt
- Ground black pepper, to taste
- Instructions
- Spritz the air fry basket with cooking spray.
- Combine the beef, sauerkraut, cream cheese, and Swiss cheese in a large bowl. Stir to mix well.
- Unroll a slice of prosciutto on a clean work surface, and then top with another slice of prosciutto crosswise. Scoop up four tablespoons of the beef mixture in the center.
- Fold the top slice sides over the filling as the ends of the roll, then roll up the long sides of the bottom prosciutto and make it into a roll shape. Overlap the sides by about 1 inch. Repeat with remaining filling and prosciutto.
- Arrange the rolls in the prepared basket, seam side down, and spritz with cooking spray.
- Select Air Fry, Super Convection. Set temperature to 400F (205C) and set time to 10 minutes. Press Start/Stop to begin preheating.
- Once preheated, place the basket in the air fry position. Flip the rolls halfway through.
- When cooking is complete, the rolls should be golden and crispy.
- Meanwhile, merge the ingredients for the sauce in a small bowl. Stir to mix well.
- Serve the rolls with the dipping sauce.

Roast Beef

Preparation Time-10 minutes | Cook Time-30 minutes | Servings-2 | Difficulty-Moderate

Nutritional Facts- Calories-245 | Fats-15g |Carbohydrates-1g |Proteins-24g

Ingredients

- Two lb. of beef roast
- One tablespoon of olive oil
- One teaspoon of steak seasoning

Instructions

- Drizzle roast with oil.
- Sprinkle with steak seasoning.
- Add to the air fryer.

- Select rotisserie.
- Cook at 360 degrees F for 50 minutes.

Roasted Turkey Breast with Bacon and Herb Butter

Preparation Time-10 minutes | Cook Time-One hour and 25 minutes | Servings-2 | Difficulty-Hard

Nutritional Facts- Calories-336 | Fats-9g |Carbohydrates-18g |Proteins-23g

Ingredients

- Three lb. of rinsed and dried turkey breast
- One tablespoon of salt
- One tablespoon of black pepper
- One and a half tablespoons of unsalted butter
- One tablespoon of finely chopped sage leaves
- One tablespoon of finely chopped rosemary leaves
- One tablespoon of finely chopped oregano leaves
- One tablespoon of finely chopped thyme
- Three cooked and crumbled bacon slices

Instructions

- Flavor the turkey breast with salt and pepper on all sides. Transfer them to the crisper tray.
- Place the crisper tray on the pizza rack. Select the roast setting on Emeril Lagasse Air Fryers 360 and Set the temperature at 300F for 60 minutes. Press start.
- Reduce heat to 270F and cook for 15 minutes more or until the internal temperature reaches 165F.
- Meanwhile, combine butter, all herbs, bacon, salt, and pepper in a mixing bowl. Refrigerate until ready to use.
- Serve the turkey with herb butter.

Rosemary Beef Roast

Preparation Time-10 minutes | Cook Time-45 minutes | Servings-2 | Difficulty-Moderate

Nutritional Facts- Calories-302 | Fats-12.9g |Carbohydrates-1.5g |Proteins-45.9g

Ingredients

- Two lbs. of beef roast
- One tablespoon of olive oil
- One teaspoon of rosemary

- One teaspoon of thyme
- A quarter teaspoon of pepper
- One teaspoon of salt

Instructions

- Preheat the air fryer to 360 F.
- Mix together oil, rosemary, thyme, pepper, and salt and rub over the meat.
- Place meat in the air fryer and cook for 45 minutes.
- Serve and enjoy.

Salisbury Steak with Mushroom Gravy

Preparation Time-22 minutes | Cook Time-35 minutes | Servings-2 | Difficulty-Moderate

Nutritional Facts- Calories-167 | Fats-12.9g |Carbohydrates-4g |Proteins-10.5g

Ingredients

For the Steaks

- One tablespoon of dry mustard
- A quarter teaspoon of garlic powder
- Half teaspoon of fine sea salt
- Chopped fresh thyme leaves
- Half pound ground beef (85% lean)
- Two tablespoons of tomato paste
- Half teaspoon of onion powder
- A quarter teaspoon of ground black pepper

For the Mushroom Gravy

- A quarter cup of thinly sliced onions
- 1/3 cup of sliced button mushrooms
- A quarter cup of unsalted butter, melted
- A quarter cup of beef broth
- Half teaspoon of fine sea salt

Instructions

- Combine the onions and mushrooms with the butter in a baking pan and season with salt.
- Turn on the air fryer and place the pan inside. Turn on and off the Power Button. At 390°F, cook for 8 minutes.
- Stir the ingredients halfway during the cooking procedure.
- After they've been cooked, the mushrooms should be tender.

- Leave the stock in the baking pan for another ten minutes to make the gravy.
- Combine all of the ingredients for the steaks, except the thyme leaves, in a large mixing basin. Everything should be well mixed together. Form the mixture into two oval steaks.
- Place the steaks on top of the gravy for 15 minutes. Once the patties have done cooking, they should be golden. Flip the steaks midway through the cooking period.
- Serve the steaks on a dish with gravy on top. Serve with a sprig of fresh thyme on the side.

Salmon and Avocado Salsa

Preparation Time-30 minutes | Cook Time-10 minutes | Servings-2 | Difficulty-Moderate

Nutritional Facts- Calories-301 | Fats-13.8g |Carbohydrates-18g |Proteins-15g

Ingredients

- Two to four salmon fillets
- One tablespoon of olive oil
- Salt and black pepper to the taste
- One teaspoon of ground cumin
- One teaspoon of sweet paprika
- Half teaspoon of chili powder
- One teaspoon of garlic powder

For the salsa

- One chopped small red onion
- One pitted, peeled and chopped avocado
- Two tablespoons of chopped cilantro
- Juice from two limes
- Salt and black pepper to the taste

Instructions

- In a bowl, mix salt, pepper, chili powder, onion powder, paprika and cumin, stir, rub salmon with this mix, drizzle the oil, rub again, transfer to your air fryer and cook at 350 degrees F for 5 minutes on each side.
- Meanwhile, in a bowl, mix avocado with red onion, salt, pepper, cilantro and lime juice and stir.
- Divide fillets among plates, top with avocado salsa and serve.

Salmon and Lemon Relish

Preparation Time-10 minutes | Cook Time-30 minutes | Servings-2 | Difficulty-Easy

Nutritional Facts- Calories-197 | Fats-1g |Carbohydrates-23g |Proteins-19g

Ingredients

- Two boneless salmon fillets
- Pepper and salt as per taste
- One tablespoon of olive oil

For the sauce/relish

- One tablespoon of lemon juice
- One chopped shallot
- One Meyer lemon, cut in wedges and then sliced
- Two tablespoons of chopped parsley
- A quarter cup of olive oil

Instructions

- Season the salmon with pepper and salt, massage with a tablespoon of oil, and place in the air fryer basket. Cook for 20 minutes at 320 degrees F, flipping midway through.
- Meanwhile, combine the lemon juice, shallot, a pinch of salt, and black pepper in a mixing bowl, whisk well, and set aside for 10 minutes.
- In a second dish, whisk together the marinated shallot, parsley, salt, lemon slices, pepper, and a quarter cup of oil.
- Serve the salmon among plates with lemon relish on top.
- Enjoy!

Salmon with Capers and Mash

Preparation Time- minutes | Cook Time- minutes | Servings-2 | Difficulty-Easy

Nutritional Facts- Calories-289 | Fats-16.8g |Carbohydrates-12g |Proteins-18g

Ingredients

- Two skinless and boneless salmon fillets
- One tablespoon of drained capers
- Salt and black pepper to the taste
- Juice from one lemon
- Two teaspoons of olive oil

For the potato mash

- Two tablespoons of olive oil
- One tablespoon of dried dill
- Half pound of chopped potatoes
- Half cup of milk

Instructions

- Put potatoes in a pot, add water to cover, add some salt, bring to a boil over medium-high heat, cook for 15 minutes, drain, transfer to a bowl, mash with a potato masher, add Two tablespoons of oil, dill, salt, pepper and milk, whisk well and leave aside for now.
- Season salmon with salt and pepper, drizzle Two teaspoons of oil over them, rub, transfer to your air fryer's basket, add capers on top, cook at 360 degrees F and cook for 8 minutes.
- Divide salmon and capers among plates, add mashed potatoes on the side, drizzle lemon juice all over and serve.
- Enjoy!

Salmon with Thyme and Mustard

Preparation Time-10 minutes | Cook Time-10 minutes | Servings-2 | Difficulty-Easy

Nutritional Facts- Calories-570 | Fats-27.9g |Carbohydrates-12.9g |Proteins-26g

Ingredients

- Two salmon fillets
- Salt and pepper to taste
- Half teaspoon of dried thyme
- Two tablespoons of mustard
- Two teaspoons of olive oil
- One minced clove of garlic
- One tablespoon of brown sugar

Instructions

- Whisk salt and pepper on both sides of salmon.
- In a bowl, combine the remaining ingredients.
- Spread this mixture on top of the salmon.
- Place the salmon in the air fryer.
- Choose air fry function.
- Cook at 400 F for 10 minutes.

Salsa Beef Meatballs

Preparation Time-10 minutes | Cook Time-10 minutes | Servings-2 | Difficulty-Easy

Nutritional Facts- Calories-348 | Fats-18g |Carbohydrates-1g|Proteins-45g

Ingredient

- One pound of ground beef (85% lean)
- Half cup of salsa
- A quarter cup of red bell peppers
- One large beaten egg
- A quarter cup of chopped onions
- Half teaspoon of chili powder
- One minced clove of garlic
- Half teaspoon of ground cumin
- One teaspoon of fine sea salt
- Lime wedges, for serving
- Cooking spray

Instructions

- Spritz the air fry basket with cooking spray.
- Merge all the ingredients in a large bowl. Stir to mix well.
- Divide and shape the mixture into 1-inch balls. Arrange the balls in the basket and spritz with cooking spray.
- Select Air Fry, Super Convection. Set temperature to 350°F (180°C) and set time to 10 minutes. Press Start/Stop to begin preheating.
- Once preheated, place the basket in the air fry position. Flip the balls with tongs halfway through.
- When cooking is complete, the balls should be well browned.
- Transfer the balls on a plate and squeeze the lime wedges over before serving.

Seafood Tacos

Preparation Time-15 minutes | Cook Time-12 minutes | Servings-2 | Difficulty-Easy

Nutritional Facts- Calories-491 | Fats-28.9g |Carbohydrates-28.9g |Proteins-30g

Ingredients

- One pound of white fish fillets, such as snapper
- One tablespoon of olive oil
- Three tablespoons of lemon juice, divided

- One and a half cups of chopped red cabbage
- Half cup of salsa
- 1/3 cup of sour cream
- Four to six soft flour tortillas
- Two peeled and chopped avocados

Instructions

- Brush the fish with olive oil and sprinkle with One tablespoon of lemon juice. Place in the air fryer basket and air-fry for 9 to 12 minutes or until the fish just flakes when tested with a fork.
- Meanwhile, combine the remaining two tablespoons of lemon juice, cabbage, salsa, and sour cream in a medium bowl.
- When the fish is cooked, remove it from the air fryer basket and break it into large pieces.
- Let everyone assemble their own taco combining the fish, tortillas, cabbage mixture, and avocados.

Seasoned Steak

Preparation Time-10 minutes | Cook Time-10 minutes | Servings-2 | Difficulty-

Nutritional Facts- Calories-260 | Fats-12.9g |Carbohydrates-1.5g |Proteins-34g

Ingredients

- Two sirloin steaks
- Two teaspoons of olive oil
- Two tablespoons of steak seasoning
- Pepper
- Salt

Instructions

- Preheat the air fryer to 350 F.
- Set steak with olive oil and season with steak seasoning, pepper, and salt.
- Spray air fryer basket with cooking spray and place steak in the air fryer basket.
- Cook for 10 minutes. Turn halfway through.
- Slice and serve.

Shrimp Po'boys

Preparation Time-25 minutes | Cook Time-20 minutes | Servings-2 | Difficulty-Moderate

Nutritional Facts- Calories-716 | Fats-20g |Carbohydrates-34g |Proteins-65g

Ingredients

- One pound of peeled and deveined uncooked shrimp (26-30 per pound)
- Four hoagie split buns
- One medium thinly sliced tomato
- One tablespoon of chopped cornichons or dill pickles
- A half teaspoon of garlic powder
- A one-fourth teaspoon of cayenne pepper
- One and a half teaspoons of lemon juice
- One cup of all-purpose flour
- One large egg
- One teaspoon of hot pepper sauce
- A half-cup of mayonnaise
- Cooking spray
- Two cups of shredded lettuce
- One tablespoon of Creole mustard
- A half teaspoon of sea salt
- A half teaspoon of pepper
- One tablespoon of minced shallot
- 1/8 teaspoon of cayenne pepper
- One teaspoon of herb de Provence
- A half-cup of2% milk
- Two cups of sweetened shredded coconut

Instructions

- Mix the ingredients for remoulade in a small bowl. Refrigerate until ready to serve, covered.
- Preheat the air fryer to 375 degrees Fahrenheit. Combine flour, sea salt, herbs de Provence, garlic powder, pepper, and cayenne in a shallow bowl. Whisk together the egg, milk, and hot pepper sauce in a shallow bowl. In a third bowl, place the coconut. Coat both sides of the shrimp in flour and shake off excess. Dip in the egg mixture and then in the coconut, patting it down to help it stick.
- The shrimp is to be arranged in a single layer on a greased tray in the air-fryer basket in batches; spritz with cooking spray. Cook for 3-4 minutes on each side, or until the coconut turns light brown and the shrimp are pink.
- Then Spread the cut side of the buns. Put shrimp, lettuce, and tomato to the top.

Simple and Easy Slow Cook Chicken

Preparation Time-10 minutes | Cook Time-Four hours | Servings-2 | Difficulty-Hard

Nutritional Facts- Calories-550 | Fats-12.9g |Carbohydrates-18g |Proteins-78g

Ingredients

- One and a quarter lbs. of boneless chicken
- Eight ounces of salsa
- Seven ounces of condensed cheddar soup

Instructions

- Place the inner pot in the grill air fryer combo base.
- Add all ingredients into the inner pot and mix well.
- Cover the inner pot with a glass lid.
- Select slow cook mode, then press the temperature button and set the time for 4 hours. Press start.
- When the timer reaches 0, then press the cancel button.
- Shred the chicken using a fork and serve.

Simple Creole Cornish Hens

Preparation Time-10 minutes | Cook Time-40 minutes | Servings-2 | Difficulty-Moderate

Nutritional Facts- Calories-231 | Fats-12.9g |Carbohydrates-9.9g |Proteins-23g

Ingredients

- Half tablespoon of Creole seasoning
- Half tablespoon of garlic powder
- Half tablespoon of onion powder
- Half tablespoon of freshly ground black pepper
- Half tablespoon of paprika
- Two tablespoons of olive oil
- Two Cornish hens
- Cooking spray

Instructions

- Spritz the air fry basket with cooking spray.
- In a small bowl, merge the garlic powder, onion powder, Creole seasoning, paprika, and pepper.
- Pat, the Cornish hens, dry and brush each hen all over with the olive oil. Rub each hen with the seasoning mixture. Place the Cornish hens in the air fry basket.
- Place the basket on the air fry position.
- Select Air Fry. Set the temperature to 375F (190C) and set the time to 30 minutes.
- After 15 minutes, detach the basket from the air fryer grill. Flip the hens over and baste them with any drippings collected in the bottom drawer of the air fryer grill. Return the basket to the air fryer grill and continue cooking.
- When cooking is complete, a thermometer inserted into the thickest part of the hens should reach at least 165F (74C).
- Let the hens rest before carving.

Simple Salmon Patties

Preparation Time-10 minutes | Cook Time-10 minutes | Servings-2 | Difficulty-Easy

Nutritional Facts- Calories-351 | Fats-15.9g |Carbohydrates-4g |Proteins-45g

Ingredients

- Fourteen ounces of salmon
- Half diced onion
- One lightly beaten egg
- One teaspoon of dill
- Half cup of almond flour

Instructions

- Spray air fryer basket with cooking spray.
- Set all ingredients into the bowl and mix until well combined.
- Spray air fryer basket with cooking spray.
- Make patties from the salmon mixture and place them into the air fryer basket.
- Cook at 370 F for 5 minutes.
- Turn patties to another side and cook for 5 minutes more.
- Serve and enjoy.

Slow-cooked Chicken Cacciatore

Preparation Time-10 minutes | Cook Time-Five hours | Servings-2 | Difficulty-Hard

Nutritional Facts- Calories-673 | Fats-27g |Carbohydrates-39g |Proteins-72g

Ingredients

- One and 3/4 lb. of chicken thighs
- One cherry pepper
- One small chopped onion
- Six ounces of cremini mushrooms
- One medium red pepper
- Fourteen ounces of tomato paste
- One tablespoon of capers
- One fresh rosemary sprig
- One garlic clove
- One cup of chicken broth
- Pepper
- Salt

Instructions

- Place the inner pot in the grill air fryer combo base.
- Whisk together tomato paste and broth in a bowl.
- Season chicken with pepper and salt.
- Place season chicken into the inner pot.
- Add remaining ingredients to the inner pot, then pour tomato paste mixture over chicken.
- Cover the inner pot with a glass lid.
- Select slow cook mode, then press the temperature button and set the time for 5 hours. Press start.
- When the timer reaches 0, then press the cancel button.
- Serve and enjoy.

Spicy Chicken Thighs

Preparation Time-55 minutes | Cook Time-25 minutes | Servings-2 | Difficulty-Hard

Nutritional Facts- Calories-180 | Fats-12g | Carbohydrates-1g | Proteins-27g

Ingredients

- A quarter cup of extra-virgin olive oil
- Two tablespoons of chili garlic sauce
- Thinly sliced green onions for garnish
- Juice of one lime
- Two teaspoons of. freshly grated ginger
- One-third cup of low-sodium soy sauce
- Two tablespoons of honey
- Four (about 2 lb.) bone-in skin-on chicken thighs
- Toasted sesame seeds for garnish

- Two cloves minced garlic

Instructions

- Combine the soy sauce, oil, butter, ginger, chili garlic sauce, lime juice and garlic in a large bowl. Reserve half a cup of marinade. To bowl, add chicken thighs and toss to cover. Cover for at least 30 minutes and refrigerate.
- Take two thighs from the marinade and put them in the air fryer basket. Cook for 15 to 20 minutes at 400 ° F before the thighs are cooked to an internal temperature of 165 ° F. Move the thighs to a plate. Repeat for the thighs that remain.
- Meanwhile, bring the reserved marinade to a boil in a shallow saucepan over medium heat. Reduce the heat and cook for 4 to 5 minutes until the sauce thickens slightly.
- Brush the sauce on the thighs and garnish before serving with sesame seeds and green onions.

Spicy Turkey Breast

Preparation Time-5 minutes | Cook Time-40 minutes | Servings-2 | Difficulty-Moderate

Nutritional Facts- Calories-263 | Fats-7.2g | Carbohydrates-12g | Proteins-39g

Ingredients

- Two pounds turkey breast
- Two teaspoons of taco seasonings
- One teaspoon of ground cumin
- One teaspoon of red pepper flakes
- Salt and ground black pepper, to taste

Instructions

- Preheat the air fryer to 356 degrees Fahrenheit. Set the air fryer basket with cooking spray.
- On a clean work surface, rub the turkey breast with taco seasoning, ground cumin, red pepper flakes, salt, and black pepper.
- Arrange the turkey in the preheated air fryer and cook for 40 minutes or until the internal temperature of the turkey reads at least 165F (74C). Flip the turkey breast halfway through the cooking time.
- Remove the turkey from the basket. Set to cool for 15 minutes before slicing to serve.

Steak with Mashed Cauliflower

Preparation Time-15 minutes | Cook Time-13 minutes | Servings-2 | Difficulty-Easy

Nutritional Facts- Calories-292 | Fats-13.8g |Carbohydrates-1.5g |Proteins-39g

Ingredients

- Two rib-eye steaks
- Salt and pepper to taste
- Two tablespoons of butter
- Two cups of cauliflower florets, roasted
- A quarter cup of almond milk

Instructions

- Choose grill setting in your air fryer.
- Set it to 400 degrees F.
- Set both sides of steak with salt and pepper.
- Add the steaks to the air fryer.
- Cook for 12 minutes, flipping halfway through.
- Add cauliflower florets to a food processor.
- Stir in almond milk, salt and pepper.
- Pulse until smooth.
- Serve steaks with mashed cauliflower.

Stuffed Beef Tenderloin with Feta Cheese

Preparation Time-10 minutes | Cook Time-10 minutes | Servings-2 | Difficulty-Easy

Nutritional Facts- Calories-321 | Fats-10.8g |Carbohydrates-1g|Proteins-30g

Ingredient

- One and a half pounds of pounded beef tenderloin
- Three teaspoons of sea salt
- One teaspoon of ground black pepper
- Two ounces of creamy goat cheese
- Half cup of crumbled feta cheese
- A quarter cup of finely chopped onions
- Two cloves of minced garlic
- Cooking spray

Instructions

- Spritz the air fry basket with cooking spray.
- Unfold the beef tenderloin on a clean work surface. Rub the salt and pepper all over the beef tenderloin to season.

- Make the filling for the stuffed beef tenderloins: Combine the goat cheese, feta, onions, and garlic in a medium bowl. Stir until well blended.
- Spoon the mixture in the center of the tenderloin. Roll the tenderloin up tightly like rolling a burrito and use some kitchen twine to tie the tenderloin.
- Arrange the tenderloin in the air fry basket.
- Select Air Fry, Super Convection. Set temperature to 400F (205C) and set time to 10 minutes. Press Start/Stop to begin preheating.
- Once preheated, place the basket in the air fry position. Flip the tenderloin halfway through.
- When cooking is complete, the instant-read thermometer inserted in the center of the tenderloin should register 135F (57C) for medium-rare.
- Transfer to a platter and serve immediately.

Sumptuous Beef and Pork Sausage Meatloaf

Preparation Time-10 minutes | Cook Time-25 minutes | Servings-2 | Difficulty-Easy

Nutritional Facts- Calories-317 | Fats-23g |Carbohydrates-1.5g |Proteins-45g

Ingredient

- 1/3 pound of ground chuck
- Four ounces of ground pork sausage
- Two beaten eggs
- One cup of grated Parmesan cheese
- One cup of chopped shallot
- Three tablespoons of plain milk
- One tablespoon of oyster sauce
- One tablespoon of fresh parsley
- One teaspoon of garlic paste
- One teaspoon of chopped porcini mushrooms
- Half teaspoon of cumin powder
- Seasoned salt and crushed red pepper flakes to taste

Instructions

- In a large bowl, merge all the ingredients until well blended.
- Place the meat mixture in the baking pan. Use a spatula to press the mixture to fill the pan.
- Select Bake, Super Convection, set the temperature to 360 degrees F (182C) and set time

- to 25 minutes. Press Start/Stop to begin preheating.
- Once preheated, place the pan in the bake position.
- When cooking is complete, the meatloaf should be well browned.
- Let the meatloaf rest for 5 minutes. Transfer to a serving dish and slice. Serve warm.

Super Lemony Chicken Breasts

Preparation Time-5 minutes | Cook Time-35 minutes | Servings-2 | Difficulty-Moderate

Nutritional Facts- Calories-233 | Fats-7.8g |Carbohydrates-4g |Proteins-35.4g

Ingredients

- Three (Eight-ounce) boneless, skinless, halved, rinsed chicken breasts
- One cup of dried bread crumbs
- A quarter cup of olive oil
- A quarter cup of chicken broth
- Zest of one lemon
- Three medium minced garlic cloves
- Half cup of fresh lemon juice
- Half cup of water
- A quarter cup of minced fresh oregano
- One medium lemon
- A quarter cup of minced fresh parsley, divided
- Cooking spray

Instructions

- Place the bread crumbs in a shadow dish and roll the chicken breasts in them to coat them.
- Spray a skillet with cooking spray and brown the coated chicken breasts for 3 minutes on each side over medium heat. In a baking pan, place the browned chicken.
- Combine the remaining ingredients in a small bowl, excluding the lemon and parsley. Over the chicken, pour the sauce.
- Preheat the oven to 350°F. Place the pan on the bake setting.
- Bake is the option to choose. Preheat the oven to 325°F (163C).
- Remove the pan from the air fryer grill and set it aside. Turn the breasts over. Continue to cook on the air fryer grill with the pan.

- When the chicken is done, it should no longer be pink.
- Place the chicken on a serving plate and pour the sauce over it. Serve with parsley and lemon on the side.

Tabasco Shrimp

Preparation Time-10 minutes | Cook Time-10 minutes | Servings-2 | Difficulty-Easy

Nutritional Facts- Calories-201 | Fats-6g |Carbohydrates-12.9g |Proteins-7.8g

Ingredients

- One pound of peeled and deveined shrimp
- One teaspoon of red pepper flakes
- Two tablespoons of olive oil
- One teaspoon of Tabasco sauce
- Two tablespoons of water
- One teaspoon of dried oregano
- Salt and black pepper to the taste
- Half teaspoon of dried parsley
- Half teaspoon of smoked paprika

Instructions

- In a bowl, mix oil with water, Tabasco sauce, pepper flakes, oregano, parsley, salt, pepper, paprika and shrimp and toss well to coat.
- Transfer shrimp to your preheated air fryer at 370 degrees F and cook for 10 minutes, shaking the fryer once.
- Divide shrimp among plates and serve with a side salad.

Teriyaki Beef Short Ribs with Pomegranate

Preparation Time-15 minutes | Cook Time-One hour | Servings-2 | Difficulty-Hard

Nutritional Facts- Calories-333 | Fats-23g |Carbohydrates-4g |Proteins-31.8g

Ingredient

- One cup of tamari soy sauce or dark soy sauce
- Half cup of packed brown sugar
- A quarter cup of pomegranate molasses
- Three finely chopped scallions
- Four cloves of minced garlic
- One tablespoon of oyster sauce

- Two teaspoons of Worcestershire sauce
- Two teaspoons of mirin
- One teaspoon of vegetable oil
- One teaspoon of grated fresh ginger
- One teaspoon of Asian chili sauce
- Six beef short ribs
- Chopped scallion for garnish
- 1/3 cup of pomegranate seeds for garnish

Instructions

- Merge the marinade ingredients in a saucepan and simmer over medium heat for 3 to 5 minutes, until the sugar has dissolved, stirring occasionally. Remove from the heat and let the mixture cool for 30 minutes. Divide the marinade into two equal portions. Store one half in the refrigerator for basting. Use the remaining half as the marinade.
- Trim off any excess fat or straggling meat from the surface of the ribs. Do not attempt to remove any internal fat. Place the ribs in a resealable plastic bag and add the marinade. Using tongs, gently turn the ribs to coat. Secure the bag and place it in the refrigerator for 6 to 12 hours.
- Prepare the grill for medium heat with indirect cooking.
- Set a tumbling basket on a large cutting board. This will keep your floors and countertop clean. Remove the ribs from the bag and place them in the basket. Discard any marinade left in the bag. Secure the basket.
- Place the basket on the preheated grill with a drip pan underneath, making sure that it doesn't get in the way of the basket as it turns. Cook for 1 to 11/2 hours, or until the ribs have rendered the majority of their fat and have reached an internal temperature of 170F (77C) to 180F (82C).
- Heat the reserved marinade in a bowl in the microwave for 1 minute. Stir. Begin basting with this mixture during the last 20 to 30 minutes of cooking time.
- Remove the basket from the grill and place it on a heat-resistant cutting board. Let the ribs rest for 5 minutes or so. Carefully open the basket and plate the ribs. Serve garnished with chopped scallion and pomegranate seeds.

Thai Chicken Drumsticks with Beans

Preparation Time-5 minutes | Cook Time-25 minutes | Servings-2 | Difficulty-Easy

Nutritional Facts- Calories-180 | Fats-6g | Carbohydrates-1g | Proteins-26g

Ingredients

- Four skin-on chicken drumsticks
- One teaspoon of kosher salt, divided
- Half pound of trimmed green beans
- Two minced cloves of garlic
- Two tablespoons of vegetable oil
- 1/3 cup of Thai sweet chili sauce

Instructions

- Salt the drumsticks on all sides with a half teaspoon of kosher salt. Let sit for a few minutes, then blot dry with a paper towel. Place on a baking pan.
- Place the pan on the toast position.
- Select Toast, set temperature to 375F (190C), and set time to 25 minutes.
- While the chicken cooks, place the green beans in a large bowl. Add the remaining kosher salt, oil, and garlic. Toss to coat.
- After 15 minutes, detach the pan from the air fryer grill. Brush the drumsticks with the sweet chili sauce. Place the green beans in the pan. Return the pan to the air fryer grill and continue cooking.
- When cooking is complete, the green beans should be sizzling and browned in spots, and the chicken cooked through, reading 165F (74C) on a meat thermometer. Serve the chicken with the green beans on the side.

Thai Curry Beef Meatballs

Preparation Time-5 minutes | Cook Time-15 minutes | Servings-2 | Difficulty-Easy

Nutritional Facts- Calories-338 | Fats-28.9g | Carbohydrates-4g | Proteins-52.8g

Ingredient

- One pound of ground beef
- One tablespoon of sesame oil
- Two teaspoons of chopped lemongrass
- One teaspoon of red Thai curry paste

- One teaspoon of Thai seasoning blend
- Juice and zest of half lime
- Cooking spray

Instructions

- Spritz the air fry basket with cooking spray.
- In a medium bowl, merge all the ingredients until well blended.
- Shape the meat mixture into 24 meatballs and arrange them in the basket.
- Select Air Fry, Super Convection. Set temperature to 380F (193C) and set time to 15 minutes. Press Start/Stop to begin preheating.
- Once preheated, place the basket in the air fry position. Flip the meatballs.
- When cooking is processed, the meatballs should be browned.
- Transfer the meatballs to plates. Let cool for 5 minutes before serving.

Thai Game Hens with Vegetable Salad

Preparation Time-25 minutes | Cook Time-25 minutes | Servings-2 | Difficulty-Moderate

Nutritional Facts- Calories-189 | Fats-6g |Carbohydrates-7.8g |Proteins-25g

Ingredients

- Two Cornish game hens (one and a quarter pound), giblets discarded
- One tablespoon of fish sauce
- Six tablespoons of chopped fresh cilantro
- Two teaspoons of lime zest
- One teaspoon of ground coriander
- Two minced cloves of garlic
- Two tablespoons of packed light brown sugar
- Two teaspoons of vegetable oil
- Salt and ground black pepper, to taste
- One English cucumber
- One stemmed, deseeded, and minced Thai chili
- Two tablespoons of chopped dry-toasted peanuts
- One small thinly sliced shallot
- One tablespoon of lime juice
- Lime wedges, for serving
- Cooking spray

Instructions

- Place a game hen on a clean work area, remove the backbone with kitchen shears, and flatten the hen breast with a pounding mallet. The breast should be cut in half. Carry on with the remaining game hens in the same manner.
- Remove the skin from the game chickens' breast and thighs with your fingertips, then pat them dry and pierce roughly ten holes in their fat deposits. Under the hens, tuck the wings.
- In a small mixing bowl, combine two teaspoons fish sauce, coriander, lime zest, a quarter cup cilantro, four teaspoons sugar, garlic, one teaspoon vegetable oil, half teaspoon salt, and 1/8 teaspoon crushed black pepper. Stir everything together thoroughly.
- Allow the game hens to marinade for 10 minutes after rubbing the fish sauce mixture under their skin on the breast and thighs.
- Using cooking spray, spritz the air fry basket.
- Place the marinated game hens skin side down in the basket.
- Set the basket to the air fry setting.
- Choose Air Fry. Preheat oven to 400 degrees F (205 degrees C) and bake for 25 minutes. Halfway through the cooking period, flip the game hens.
- When the hens are done cooking, their skin should be golden brown and their internal temperature should be at least 165 degrees F. (74C).
- In a large mixing bowl, combine all of the remaining ingredients, except the lime wedges, and season with salt and black pepper. Toss well to combine.
- Place the birds on a big plate, then set aside the salad and squeeze the lime over the top before serving.

Thai Shrimp

Preparation Time-10 minutes | Cook Time-10 minutes | Servings-2 | Difficulty-Easy

Nutritional Facts- Calories-156 | Fats-1.5g |Carbohydrates-6g |Proteins-25g

Ingredients

- One lb. of peeled and deveined shrimp
- One teaspoon of toasted sesame seeds

- Two minced cloves of garlic
- Two tablespoons of soy sauce
- Two tablespoons of Thai chili sauce
- One tablespoon of arrowroot powder
- One tablespoon of sliced green onion
- 1/8 teaspoon of minced ginger

Instructions

- Spray air fryer basket with cooking spray.
- Toss shrimp with arrowroot powder and place them into the air fryer basket.
- Cook shrimp at 350 degrees F for 5 minutes. Shake basket well and cook for 5 minutes more.
- Meanwhile, in a bowl, mix together soy sauce, ginger, garlic, and chili sauce.
- Add shrimp to the bowl and toss well.
- Garnish with green onions and sesame seeds.
- Serve and enjoy.

Thyme and Parsley Salmon

Preparation Time-10 minutes | Cook Time-15 minutes | Servings-2 | Difficulty-Easy

Nutritional Facts- Calories-241 | Fats-9g |Carbohydrates-20g |Proteins-31g

Ingredients

- Two boneless salmon fillets
- Juice from one lemon
- One chopped yellow onion
- Two sliced tomatoes
- Two thyme springs
- Two parsley springs
- Two tablespoons of extra virgin olive oil
- Salt and black pepper to the taste

Instructions

- Drizzle one tablespoon of oil in a pan that fits your air fryer, add a layer of tomatoes, salt and pepper, drizzle one more tablespoon of oil, add fish, season them with salt and pepper, drizzle the rest of the oil, add thyme and parsley springs, onions, lemon juice, salt and pepper, place in your air fryer's basket and cook at 360 degrees F for 12 minutes shaking once.
- Divide everything among plates and serve right away.
- Enjoy!

Tilapia and Chives Sauce

Preparation Time-10 minutes | Cook Time-10 minutes | Servings-2 | Difficulty-Easy

Nutritional Facts- Calories-261 | Fats-7.8g |Carbohydrates-24g |Proteins-21.9g

Ingredients

- Four medium tilapia fillets
- Cooking spray
- Salt and black pepper to the taste
- Two teaspoons of honey
- A quarter cup of Greek yogurt
- Juice from one lemon
- Two tablespoons of chopped chives

Instructions

- Season fish with salt and pepper, spray with cooking spray, place in preheated air fryer 350 degrees F and cook for 8 minutes, flipping halfway.
- Meanwhile, in a bowl, mix yogurt with honey, salt, pepper, chives and lemon juice and whisk really well.
- Divide air fryer fish among plates, drizzle yogurt sauce all over and serve right away.

Trout and Butter Sauce

Preparation Time- 10 minutes | Cook Time- 10 minutes | Servings-2 | Difficulty-Easy

Nutritional Facts- Calories-272 | Fats-12g |Carbohydrates-27g |Proteins-21g

Ingredients

- Two boneless trout fillets
- Salt and black pepper to the taste
- Two teaspoons of grated lemon zest
- Three tablespoons chopped of chives
- Three tablespoons of butter
- Two tablespoons of olive oil
- Two teaspoons of lemon juice

Instructions

- Season trout with salt and pepper, drizzle the olive oil, rub, transfer to your air fryer and cook at 360 degrees F for 10 minutes, flipping once.
- Meanwhile, heat up a pan with the butter over medium heat, add salt, pepper, chives, lemon

juice and zest, whisk well, cook for 1-2 minutes and take off heat

- Divide fish fillets among plates, drizzle butter sauce all over and serve.
- Enjoy!

Trout Fillet and Orange Sauce

Preparation Time- 10 minutes | Cook Time-10 minutes | Servings-2 | Difficulty-Easy

Nutritional Facts- Calories-239 | Fats-9.9g |Carbohydrates- 18g |Proteins- 23g

Ingredients

- Two skinless and boneless trout fillets
- Two chopped spring onions
- One tablespoon of olive oil
- One tablespoon of minced ginger
- Salt and black pepper to the taste
- Juice and zest from one orange

Instructions

- Season trout fillets with salt, pepper, rub them with the olive oil, place in a pan that fits your air fryer, add ginger, green onions, orange zest and juice, toss well, place in your air fryer and cook at 360 degrees F for 10 minutes.
- Divide fish and sauce among plates and serve right away.
- Enjoy!

Tuna Veggie Stir-Fry

Preparation Time-15 minutes | Cook Time-14 minutes | Servings-2 | Difficulty-Easy

Nutritional Facts- Calories-201 | Fats-10.8g |Carbohydrates-12.9g |Proteins-16.8g

Ingredients

- One tablespoon of olive oil
- One chopped red bell pepper
- One cup of green beans
- One sliced onion
- Two sliced cloves of garlic
- Two tablespoons of low-sodium soy sauce
- One tablespoon of honey
- Half pound of cubed fresh tuna

Instructions

- In a 6-inch metal bowl, combine the olive oil, pepper, green beans, onion, and garlic.
- Cook in the air fryer for 4 to 6 minutes, stirring once, until crisp and tender. Add soy sauce, honey, and tuna, and stir.
- Cook for another 3 to 6 minutes, stirring once until the tuna is cooked as desired. Tuna can be served rare or medium-rare, or you can cook it until well done.

Turkey Quarters and Veggies

Preparation Time-10 minutes | Cook Time-35 minutes | Servings-2 | Difficulty-Moderate

Nutritional Facts- Calories-362 | Fats-12.9g |Carbohydrates-21.9g |Proteins-18g

Ingredients

- One chopped yellow onion
- One chopped carrot
- Three minced garlic cloves
- Two pounds turkey quarters
- One chopped celery stalk
- One cup of chicken stock
- Two tablespoons of olive oil
- Two bay leaves
- Half teaspoon of dried rosemary
- Half teaspoon of dried sage
- Half teaspoon of dried thyme
- Salt and black pepper to the taste

Instructions

- Rub turkey quarters with salt, pepper, half of the oil, thyme, sage, rosemary and thyme, put in your air fryer and cook at 360 degrees F for 20 minutes.
- In a pan that fits your air fryer, mix the onion with carrot, garlic, celery, the rest of the oil, stock, bay leaves, salt and pepper and toss.
- Add turkey, introduce everything in your air fryer and cook at 360 degrees F for 14 minutes more.
- Divide everything among plates and serve.

Chapter 4-Air Fried Snacks and Appetizers Recipes

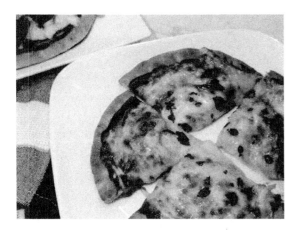

6 Minute Pita Bread Cheese Pizza

Preparation Time-10 minutes | Cook Time-35 minutes | Servings-2 | Difficulty-Moderate

Nutritional Facts- Calories-283 | Fats-15g|Carbohydrates-13.8g|Proteins-23g

Ingredients

- One Pita Bread
- One Tablespoon of Pizza Sauce
- One Tablespoon of thinly sliced Yellow/Brown Onion
- Half teaspoon of Minced Fresh Garlic
- A quarter cup of Mozzarella Cheese
- One Stainless Steel Short Legged Trivet
- One drizzle Extra Virgin Olive Oil
- Seven or more slices of Pepperoni
- A quarter cup of Sausage

Instructions

- Use the spoon and swirl pizza sauce on the pita bread. Insert your favorite cheese and toppings. On top of the pizza, apply a little more drizzle of extra virgin olive oil.
- Place a trivet over Pita Bread in the Air Fryer. Cook for 6 minutes at 350 degrees F. Finally, remove from the Air Fryer cautiously and cut.

Apple Chips

Preparation Time-10 minutes | Cook Time-20 minutes | Servings-2 | Difficulty-Easy

Nutritional Facts- Calories-178 | Fats-6.9g |Carbohydrates-13.8g |Proteins-4g

Ingredients

- Four medium-sized apples
- One tablespoon of Extra Virgin Avocado Oil
- One tablespoon of Cinnamon

Instructions

- Apples are to be thinly cut using a mandolin (or something similar).
- Toss your sliced apples in oil using the chosen balanced oil. Sprinkle the apples in cinnamon after you've applied the oil.
- Load it into the air fryer and cook at 200c/400F for 15 minutes.
- Adjust the cooking time to four hours and a temperature to 30C/85F if using the air fryer oven.

Artichoke Turkey Pizza

Preparation Time-10 minutes | Cook Time-20 minutes | Servings-2 | Difficulty-Easy

Nutritional Facts- Calories-196 | Fats-6.9g |Carbohydrates-27.9g |Proteins-7.8g

Ingredients

- Two cups of chopped cooked turkey
- One to a half cup of mozzarella cheese
- Two baked pizza crust
- One can of black olives
- One can of diced tomatoes with garlic, oregano, and basil
- Half cup of shredded parmesan cheese
- One can of artichoke hearts

Instructions

- Place the pizza crusts on a working surface.
- Place turkey, olive, tomatoes mix, parmesan cheese, olives, and artichokes on them.
- Transfer the pizza crusts to the Air Fryer Grill pan.
- Set the Air Fryer Grill to the pizza function.
- Cook for 10 minutes at 450 degrees F.
- Serve immediately.

Artichoke with Red Pepper Pizza

Preparation Time-10 minutes | Cook Time-20 minutes | Servings-2 | Difficulty-Easy

Nutritional Facts- Calories-359 | Fats-18g |Carbohydrates-43g |Proteins-12g

Ingredients

- One teaspoon of dried basil
- One can of artichoke hearts
- One cup of mozzarella cheese
- One cup of red bell pepper
- Five cloves of garlic
- Cracked pepper
- One tablespoon of olive oil
- One pizza shell
- One teaspoon of oregano
- One jar of sliced mushroom

Instructions

- Mix artichoke hearts, basil, bell pepper, garlic, and cracked pepper in a bowl.
- Add oregano, mushroom, and olive oil.
- Place the mixture on the pizza shell
- Transfer the pizza shell to Air Fryer Grill pan.
- Set the Air Fryer Grill to the pizza function.
- Cook for about 20 minutes at 350 degrees F.
- Serve immediately

Asparagus galette

Preparation Time-10 minutes | Cook Time-30 minutes | Servings-2 | Difficulty-Easy

Nutritional Facts- Calories-117 | Fats-1g|Carbohydrates-16.8g |Proteins-1g

Ingredients

- Two cups of minced asparagus
- Three teaspoons of finely chopped ginger
- Two tablespoons of fresh coriander leaves
- Three finely chopped green chilies
- Two tablespoons of lemon juice
- Salt and pepper to taste

Instructions

- Mix the ingredients in a clean bowl.
- Mold this mixture into round and flat galettes.
- Wet the galettes slightly with water.

- Preheat the Air Fryer at 160 degrees Fahrenheit for 5 minutes. Place the galettes in the fry basket and let them cook for another 25 minutes at the same temperature. Keep rolling them over to get a uniform cook.
- Serve either with mint chutney or ketchup.

Asparagus Wrapped Filo

Preparation Time-10 minutes | Cook Time-30 minutes | Servings-2 | Difficulty-Moderate

Nutritional Facts- Calories-112 | Fats-7.8g |Carbohydrates-4.8g |Proteins-9.9g

Ingredients

- Twelve slices of prosciutto
- Twenty-four asparagus stalks
- Twelve filo sheets
- One stick of butter

Instructions

- Unroll the filo sheets on a cutting board and cut each sheet into four equal rectangles.
- Place half of the cut filo pieces on the counter, brush these leaves with the melted butter, and top each buttered sheet with a second cut filo piece.
- Set a slice of prosciutto on one end of each leaf and then the stem end of an asparagus stalk on top of each leaf. Roll up the filo, the prosciutto and the asparagus.
- Position the rolled sheets on 2 Air Flow racks. Place the racks on the bottom and middle shelves of the Power Air fryer.
- Press the power button then the bake button (350F) and decrease the cooking time to 15 minutes. Rotate the racks after 7 minutes.

Avocado Fries

Preparation Time-10 minutes | Cook Time-10 minutes | Servings-2 | Difficulty-Easy

Nutritional Facts- Calories-60 | Fats-1g |Carbohydrates-9.9g |Proteins-1.5g

Ingredients

- Half teaspoon of salt
- Aquafaba from one fifteen ounces can of white beans or garbanzo beans
- Half cup of panko breadcrumbs
- One peeled pitted and sliced Haas avocado

Instructions

- Toss the panko and salt together in a shallow bowl. Into another shallow bowl, put the aquafaba.
- In the aquafaba and then in the panko, dredge the avocado slices and obtain a clean, even coating.
- Arrange the slices in your air fryer basket in a single layer. The single layer is important. Air fry at 390F for 10 minutes (do not preheat), shaking well 5 minutes later.
- Serve with your favorite dipping sauce instantly.

Avocado Toast

Preparation Time-10 minutes | Cook Time-30 minutes | Servings-2 | Difficulty-Moderate

Nutritional Facts- Calories-233 | Fats-7.8g |Carbohydrates-3.18g |Proteins-35.4g

Ingredients

- Juice of one lime
- One teaspoon of salt
- A quarter cup of feta
- One tablespoon of cilantro
- Salt
- One ripe avocado
- Two slice grain bread
- Four slices of Tomato
- Balsamic glaze

Instructions

- Mash the two avocados with lime juice and salt.
- Position the grain bread slices on an Air Flow rack. Position the rack on the center shelf of the appliance.
- Press the power button, raise the cooking temperature to 375 degrees F and reduce the cooking time to 7 minutes. Flip the bread after 4 minutes.
- Spread the mashed avocado on each toast.
- Place two tomato slices on each toast.
- Sprinkle the feta cheese on the toast.
- Season the toasts with salt. Drizzle with balsamic glaze and sprinkle cilantro on top of toast.
- Garnish with the last avocado.

Bacon Cheeseburger Pizza

Preparation Time-10 minutes | Cook Time-20 minutes | Servings-2 | Difficulty-Easy

Nutritional Facts- Calories-322 | Fats-12g |Carbohydrates-42g |Proteins-16.8g

Ingredients

- Six bacon strips
- Half pound of ground beef
- One teaspoon of pizza seasoning
- Two cups of mozzarella cheese
- Two baked-bread crusts
- Twenty slices of dill pickles
- One chopped small onion
- Two cups of shredded cheddar cheese
- Eight ounces of pizza sauce

Instructions

- Set onion and beef over medium heat for about 5 minutes.
- Drain the meat.
- Add bacon, seasonings, sauce, cheeses, and pickles.
- Place the bread crusts on a working surface.
- Place the ingredients on them.
- Transfer it to the Air Fryer Grill pan
- Set the Air Fryer Grill to the pizza function.
- Cook for 10 minutes at 450 degrees F.

Bacon Lettuce Tomato Pizza

Preparation Time-10 minutes | Cook Time-20 minutes | Servings-2 | Difficulty-Easy

Nutritional Facts- Calories-132 | Fats-7.8g |Carbohydrates-9g |Proteins-7.8g

Ingredients

- Six slices of plum tomatoes
- One cup of torn romaine lettuce
- 1/3 cup of mayonnaise
- Eight slices of bacon
- Two bread shell
- One cup of mozzarella cheese

Instructions

- Spread the bread shell on a working surface.

- Put mayonnaise, cheese, bacon, and tomatoes on the bread shells.
- Transfer to the Air Fryer Grill pan.
- Set the Air Fryer Grill to the pizza function.
- Cook for 17 minutes at 450 degrees F.
- Serve immediately.

Bacon-Wrapped Avocado

Preparation Time-15 minutes | Cook Time-10 minutes | Servings-2 | Difficulty-Easy

Nutritional Facts- Calories-103 | Fats-4.8g |Carbohydrates-1.5g |Proteins-6g

Ingredients

- Two avocados
- Sixteen thin strips of bacon
- A quarter cup of ranch dressing for serving

Instructions

- Slice every avocado into eight wedges of equal size. Wrap each wedge with a bacon strip and, if necessary, cut the bacon.
- Working in batches, place in a single layer in an air fryer basket. Cook for 8 minutes at 400 °F until the bacon is fried and crispy.
- Serve warm along with the ranch.

Baked Smoked Trout and Frittata

Preparation Time-10 minutes | Cook Time-10 minutes | Servings-2 | Difficulty-Easy

Nutritional Facts- Calories-184 | Fats-10.8g |Carbohydrates-4.8g |Proteins-12g

Ingredients

- Two tablespoons of olive oil
- One sliced
- One beaten egg
- Half tablespoon of horseradish sauce
- Four tablespoons of crème fraiche
- One cup of diced smoked trout
- Two tablespoons of chopped fresh dill
- Cooking spray

Instructions

- Spritz a baking pan with cooking spray.
- Warm the olive oil in a nonstick skillet over medium heat until shimmering.

- Add the onion and sauté for 3 minutes or until translucent.
- Combine the egg, crème Fraiche, and horseradish sauce in a large bowl. Stir to mix well, and then mix in the smoked trout, sautéed onion, and dill.
- Set the mixture in the prepared baking pan.
- Bring the pan to the bake position.
- Select Bake, set temperature to 350°F (180°C) and set time to 14 minutes. Stir the mixture halfway through.
- When cooking is complete, the egg should be set, and the edges should be lightly browned.
- Serve immediately.

Banana Snack

Preparation Time-10 minutes | Cook Time-5 minutes | Servings-2 | Difficulty-Easy

Nutritional Facts- Calories-71 | Fats-4g |Carbohydrates-10.8g |Proteins-1.5g

Ingredients

- Eight baking cups of crust
- A quarter cup of peanut butter
- 3⁄4 cup of chocolate chips
- One banana, peeled and sliced
- One tablespoon of vegetable oil

Instructions

- Put chocolate chips in a small pot, heat up over low heat, stir until it melts and take off the heat.
- In a bowl, mix peanut butter with coconut oil and whisk well.
- Spoon one teaspoon of chocolate mix in a cup of, add one banana slice and top with one teaspoon of butter mix
- Repeat with the rest of the cups, place them all into a dish that fits your air fryer, cook at 320 degrees F for 5 minutes, transfer to a freezer and keep there until you serve them as a snack.
- Enjoy!

Basic Zucchini Chips

Preparation Time-10 minutes | Cook Time-One hour | Servings-2 | Difficulty-

Nutritional Facts- Calories-45 | Fats-1g|Carbohydrates-1g|Proteins-6.9g

Ingredients

One thinly sliced zucchini

- Salt and black pepper to the taste
- Two tablespoons of olive oil
- Two tablespoons of balsamic vinegar

Instructions

- In a bowl, mix oil with vinegar, salt and pepper and whisk well.
- Add zucchini slices, toss to coat well, introduce in your air fryer and cook at 200 degrees F for 1 hour.
- Serve zucchini chips cold as a snack.
- Enjoy!

Beef Steak fingers

Preparation Time-10 minutes | Cook Time-25 minutes | Servings-2 | Difficulty-Easy

Nutritional Facts- Calories-167 | Fats-6g |Carbohydrates-9g |Proteins-15g

Ingredients

- One lb. of boneless beef steak cut into fingers
- Two cups of dry breadcrumbs
- Two teaspoons of oregano
- Two teaspoons of red chili flakes

Marinade

- Two tablespoons of ginger-garlic paste
- Four tablespoons of lemon juice
- Two teaspoons of salt
- One teaspoon of pepper powder
- One teaspoon of red chili powder
- Six tablespoons of cornflour
- Four eggs

Instructions

- Mix all the ingredients for the marinade and put the beef fingers inside, and let it rest overnight.
- Mix the breadcrumbs, oregano and red chili flakes well and place the marinated fingers on this mixture. Cover it with plastic wrap and leave it till right before you serve to cook.
- Preheat the Air fryer at 160 degrees Fahrenheit for 5 minutes. Place the fingers in the fry basket and close it. Let them cook at the same temperature for another 15 minutes or so. Toss

the fingers well so that they are cooked uniformly.

Beef Stew

Preparation Time-10 minutes | Cook Time-20 minutes | Servings-2 | Difficulty-Easy

Nutritional Facts- Calories-260 | Fats-4.8g |Carbohydrates-24g |Proteins-21.9g

Ingredients

- Two pounds beef meat, cut into medium chunks
- Two chopped carrots
- Four chopped potatoes
- Salt and black pepper to the taste
- One quart veggie stock
- Half teaspoon of smoked paprika
- A handful chopped thyme

Instructions

- In a dish that fits your air fryer, mix beef with carrots, potatoes, stock, salt, pepper, paprika and thyme, stir, place in the air fryer's basket and cook at 375 degrees F for 20 minutes.
- Divide into bowls and serve right away for lunch.
- Enjoy!

Beef Wontons

Preparation Time-10 minutes | Cook Time-25 minutes | Servings-2 | Difficulty-Easy

Nutritional Facts- Calories-164 | Fats-7.8g |Carbohydrates-12g |Proteins-15.9g

Ingredients

For dough

- One and a half cups of all-purpose flour
- Two teaspoons of salt
- Five tablespoons of water

For filling

- Two cups of minced beef steak
- Two tablespoons of oil
- Two teaspoons of ginger-garlic paste
- Two teaspoons of soya sauce
- Two teaspoons of vinegar

Instructions

- Knead the dough and cover it with plastic wrap, and set it aside. Next, cook the ingredients for the filling and try to ensure that the beef is covered well with the sauce.
- Roll the dough and place the filling in the center. Now, wrap the dough to cover the filling and pinch the edges together.
- Preheat the Air fryer at 200° F for 5 minutes. Place the wontons in the fry basket and close it. Let them cook at the same temperature for another 20 minutes.
- Recommended sides are chili sauce or ketchup.

Best-Ever Mozzarella Sticks

Preparation Time-15 minutes | Cook Time-2 hours and 25 minutes | Servings-2 | Difficulty-Hard

Nutritional Facts- Calories-230 | Fats-6.9g |Carbohydrates-9.9g |Proteins-4g

Ingredients

Two mozzarella sticks
One beaten egg
One tablespoon of all-purpose flour
Half cup of Panko bread crumbs
Kosher salt
Freshly cracked black pepper
Warm marinara, for serving

Instructions

- Freeze sticks of mozzarella until completely frozen for at least 2 hours.
- Establish a breading station after 3 hours: Put panko, eggs, and flour in three different shallow bowls. With pepper and salt, season the panko generously.
- Frozen mozzarella sticks are covered in flour, then soaked in eggs, then panko, back in the egg, finally back in the panko.
- Arrange in the air fryer's basket frozen sticks of breaded mozzarella in an even layer. Cook for 6 minutes at 400 ° F, or until the exterior is golden and crisp and melted in the middle.
- It can be served with warm marinara sauce.

Blooming Onion

Preparation Time-10 minutes | Cook Time-45 minutes | Servings-2 | Difficulty-Moderate

Nutritional Facts- Calories-161 | Fats-7.8g |Carbohydrates-15g |Proteins-7.8g

Ingredients

- One large yellow onion
- A half teaspoon of garlic powder
- A quarter teaspoon of dried oregano
- Kosher salt
- Two eggs
- Half cup of breadcrumbs
- Two teaspoons of paprika
- One teaspoon of garlic powder
- One teaspoon of onion powder
- One teaspoon of kosher salt
- One and a half tablespoons of extra-virgin olive oil
- 2/3 cup of mayonnaise
- Two tablespoons of ketchup
- One teaspoon of horseradish
- A half teaspoon of paprika

Instructions

- Cut the onion stem off and arrange the onion on the flat side. Cut an inch from the root into 12 to 16 sections, being careful not to cut all the way. To remove petals, turn over and softly pull sections of onion out.
- Whisk the eggs and one tablespoon of water together in a shallow bowl. Whisk the breadcrumbs and spices together in another small bowl. Dip the onion into the egg wash, then dredge it in the breadcrumb paste, then cover it completely with a spoon. Sprinkle the onion with some oil.
- Place in the air fryer basket and cook at 375 ° F until the onion is tender, 20 to 25 minutes all the way through. Drizzle as needed with more oil.
- Meanwhile, make a sauce: stir together horseradish, mayonnaise, ketchup, paprika, garlic powder and dried oregano in a medium bowl, with salt, season.
- For dipping, serve the onion with sauce.

Bourbon French toast

Preparation Time-15 minutes | Cook Time-6 minutes | Servings-2 | Difficulty-Easy

Nutritional Facts- Calories-67 | Fats-7.8g |Carbohydrates-1g |Proteins-17g

Ingredients

- One large egg
- One tablespoon of water
- 1/3 cup of whole milk
- One tablespoon of melted butter
- One tablespoon of bourbon
- One teaspoon of vanilla extract
- Four (1-inch-thick) French bread slices
- Cooking spray

Instructions

- Set the air fryer basket with parchment paper and spray it with cooking spray.
- Beat the eggs with the water in a shallow bowl until combined. Add the milk, melted butter, bourbon, and vanilla and stir to mix well.
- Dredge four slices of bread in the batter, turning to coat both sides evenly. Transfer the bread slices onto the parchment paper.
- Slide the basket into the air fryer. Cook at the corresponding preset mode or Air Fry at 320F (160C) for 6 minutes.
- Flip the slices halfway through the cooking time.
- When cooking is complete, the bread slices should be nicely browned.
- Detach from the air fryer to a plate and serve warm.

Broccoli and Tomatoes Air Fried Stew

Preparation Time-10 minutes | Cook Time-20 minutes | Servings-2 | Difficulty-Easy

Nutritional Facts- Calories-155 | Fats-4g |Carbohydrates-9g |Proteins-7.8g

Ingredients

- One broccoli head, florets separated
- Two teaspoons of coriander seeds
- One tablespoon of olive oil
- One chopped yellow onion
- Salt and black pepper to the taste
- A pinch of crushed red pepper
- One small chopped ginger piece
- One minced garlic clove
- Sixteen ounces of pureed canned tomatoes

Instructions

- Heat up a pan that fits your air fryer with the oil over medium heat, add onions, salt, pepper and red pepper, stir and cook for 7 minutes.
- Add ginger, garlic, coriander seeds, tomatoes and broccoli, stir, introduce in your air fryer and cook at 360 degrees F for 12 minutes.
- Divide into bowls and serve.
- Enjoy!

Broccoli Fritters

Preparation Time-10 minutes | Cook Time-15 minutes | Servings-2 | Difficulty-Easy

Nutritional Facts- Calories-285 | Fats-21.9g |Carbohydrates-6.9g |Proteins-20g

Ingredients

- Three cups of steamed & chopped broccoli florets
- Two cups of shredded cheddar cheese
- A quarter cup of almond flour
- Two lightly beaten eggs
- Two minced cloves of garlic

Instructions

- Line air fryer basket with parchment paper.
- Add all ingredients into the mixing bowl and mix until well combined.
- Make patties from the broccoli mixture and place them in the air fryer basket.
- Cook at 375 degrees F for 15 minutes. Turn patties halfway through.

Broccoli Hash

Preparation Time-30 minutes | Cook Time-10 minutes | Servings-2 | Difficulty-Moderate

Nutritional Facts- Calories-183 | Fats-1g |Carbohydrates-4.8g |Proteins-7.8g

Ingredients

- Ten ounces of halved mushrooms
- One broccoli head, florets separated
- One minced garlic clove
- One tablespoon of balsamic vinegar

- One chopped yellow onion
- One tablespoon of olive oil
- Salt and black pepper
- One teaspoon of dried basil
- One peeled and pitted avocado
- A pinch of red pepper flakes

Instructions

- In a bowl, mix mushrooms with broccoli, onion, garlic and avocado.
- In another bowl, mix vinegar, oil, salt, pepper and basil and whisk well.
- Pour this over the veggies, toss to coat, leave aside for 30 minutes, transfer to your air fryer's basket and cook at 350 degrees F for 8 minutes.
- Divide among plates and serve with pepper flakes on top.
- Enjoy!

Broccoli Stuffed Peppers

Preparation Time-11 minutes | Cook Time-42 minutes | Servings-2 | Difficulty-Moderate

Nutritional Facts- Calories-290 | Fats-20g | Carbohydrates-13.8g | Proteins-12g

Ingredients

- Half cup of grated cheddar cheese
- Half teaspoon of garlic powder
- A quarter cup of crumbled feta cheese
- Four eggs
- Two bell peppers cut in half and remove seeds
- One teaspoon of dried thyme
- Half cup of cooked broccoli
- Half teaspoon of salt
- A quarter teaspoon of pepper

Instructions

- Preheat the oven to 325 degrees Fahrenheit.
- Fill halved bell peppers with feta and broccoli.
- In a mixing bowl, whisk up the egg and seasonings, then pour into the pepper halves halved over the feta and broccoli.
- Cook for 35-40 minutes in the air fryer basket with halved bell peppers.
- Cook until the shredded cheddar cheese has melted on top.
- Serve and have fun.

Brussels Sprout Chips

Preparation Time-10 minutes | Cook Time-15 minutes | Servings-2 | Difficulty-Easy

Nutritional Facts- Calories-175 | Fats-4.8g | Carbohydrates-1g | Proteins-26g

Ingredients

- Two cups of thinly sliced Brussels sprouts
- One tablespoon of olive oil
- One teaspoon of garlic powder
- Salt and pepper to taste
- Two tablespoons of grated Parmesan cheese

Instructions

- Toss the Brussels sprouts in oil.
- Sprinkle with garlic powder, salt, pepper and Parmesan cheese.
- Choose bake function.
- Add the Brussels sprouts to the air fryer.
- Cook at 350 degrees F for 8 minutes.
- Flip and cook for seven more minutes.

Buffalo Cauliflower

Preparation Time-5 minutes | Cook Time-25 minutes | Servings-2 | Difficulty-Easy

Nutritional Facts- Calories-227 | Fats-10.8g | Carbohydrates-12g | Proteins-20g

Ingredients

- One large head cauliflower
- A quarter teaspoon of cayenne pepper
- A half-cup of Cayenne Pepper Sauce
- Two cloves minced garlic
- A quarter teaspoon of chili powder
- A quarter teaspoon of paprika
- One cup of unbleached all-purpose flour
- One teaspoon of vegan chicken bouillon granules
- A quarter teaspoon of dried chipotle chili flake
- One cup of soy milk
- canola oil spray
- Two tablespoons of non-dairy butter

Instructions

- Slice the cauliflower into parts that are bite-size. Rinse the cauliflower pieces and drain them.

- Combine in a large bowl the chili powder, flour, bouillon granules, cayenne, paprika, and chipotle flakes. Whisk in the milk slowly until a thick batter develops.
- Spray with canola oil the air fryer basket and preheat the air fryer for 10 minutes to 390 °F.
- Throw the cauliflower in the batter while the air fryer is preheating. Move the battered cauliflower to the bowl of an air fryer. Cook it at 390 ° F for 20 minutes. Turn the pieces of cauliflower after 10 minutes using tongs (do not be worried if they stick).
- Heat the garlic, butter and hot sauce over medium-high heat in a shallow saucepan after turning the cauliflower. Bring the mixture to a boil, cook, reduce the heat, and cover it.
- Move it to a wide bowl once the cauliflower is baked. Over the cauliflower, pour the sauce and toss gently with tongs. Immediately serve.

Calamari and Shrimp Snack

Preparation Time-10 minutes | Cook Time-20 minutes | Servings-2 | Difficulty-Easy

Nutritional Facts- Calories-278 | Fats-21g |Carbohydrates-9.9g |Proteins-16.8g

Ingredients

- Eight ounces of calamari, cut into medium rings
- Eight ounces of peeled and deveined shrimp
- One egg
- Three tablespoons of white flour
- One tablespoon of olive oil
- Two tablespoons of chopped avocado
- One teaspoon of tomato paste
- One tablespoon of mayonnaise
- A splash of Worcestershire sauce
- One teaspoon of lemon juice
- Salt and black pepper to the taste
- Half teaspoon of turmeric powder

Instructions

- In a bowl, whisk the egg with oil, add calamari rings and shrimp and toss to coat.
- In another bowl, mix flour with salt, pepper and turmeric and stir.
- Dredge calamari and shrimp in this mix, place them in your air fryer's basket and cook at 350 degrees F for 9 minutes, flipping them once.

- Meanwhile, in a bowl, mix avocado with mayo and tomato paste and mash using a fork.
- Add Worcestershire sauce, lemon juice, salt and pepper and stir well.
- Arrange calamari and shrimp on a platter and serve with the sauce on the side.
- Enjoy!

Canadian bacon with Cheesy English Muffins

Preparation Time-5 minutes | Cook Time-10 minutes | Servings-2 | Difficulty-Easy

Nutritional Facts- Calories-261 | Fats-12.9g |Carbohydrates-20g |Proteins-12g

Ingredients

- Two English muffins
- Four slices of Canadian bacon
- Two slices of cheese
- Cooking oil

Instructions

- Split each English muffin. Assemble the breakfast sandwiches by layering two slices of Canadian bacon and one slice of cheese onto each English muffin bottom. Put the other half on top of the English muffin. Place the sandwiches in the air fryer. Spray the top of each with cooking oil. Cook for 4 minutes
- Open the air fryer and flip the sandwiches. Cook for an additional 4 minutes
- Cool before serving.

Cauliflower Bars

Preparation Time-10 minutes | Cook Time- 25 minutes | Servings-2 | Difficulty-Easy

Nutritional Facts- Calories-60 | Fats-1.5g |Carbohydrates-4.8g |Proteins-17g

Ingredients

- Half cauliflower head, florets separated
- Half cup of shredded mozzarella
- A quarter cup of egg whites
- One teaspoon of Italian seasoning
- Salt and black pepper to the taste

Instructions

- Put cauliflower florets in your food processor, pulse well, spread a baking sheet that fits the air fryer, introduce in the fryer and cook at 360 degrees F for 10 minutes.
- Transfer cauliflower to a bowl, add salt, pepper, cheese, egg whites and Italian seasoning, stir really well, spread this into a rectangle pan that fits your air fryer, press well, introduce in the fryer and cook at 360 degrees F for 15 minutes more.
- Cut into 12 bars, arrange them on a platter and serve as a snack
- Enjoy!

Cauliflower Snack

Preparation Time-10 minutes | Cook Time-15 minutes | Servings-2 | Difficulty-Easy

Nutritional Facts- Calories-241 | Fats-4g |Carbohydrates-15g |Proteins-4g

Ingredients

- Two cups of cauliflower florets
- One cup of panko bread crumbs
- A quarter cup of melted butter
- A quarter cup of buffalo sauce
- Mayonnaise for serving

Instructions

- In a bowl, mix buffalo sauce with butter and whisk well.
- Dip cauliflower florets in this mix and coat them in panko bread crumbs.
- Place them in your air fryer's basket and cook at 350 degrees F for 15 minutes.
- Arrange them on a platter and serve with mayo on the side.
- Enjoy!

Cauliflower Tots

Preparation Time-5 minutes | Cook Time-30minutes | Servings-2 | Difficulty-Easy

Nutritional Facts- Calories-227| Fats-10.8g|Carbohydrates-12g|Proteins-20g

Ingredients

- A quarter cup of shredded cheddar

- A quarter cup of ketchup
- One tablespoon of Sriracha
- Half of freshly grated Parmesan
- 2/3 cup of panko breadcrumbs
- Two tablespoons of freshly chopped chives
- Cooking spray
- Two cups of cauliflower florets, steamed
- One lightly beaten egg
- Kosher salt
- Freshly ground black pepper

Instructions

- Process steamed cauliflower In a food processor till riced. Put riced cauliflower on a clean kitchen towel. Then squeeze to drain water.
- Move cauliflower to a big bowl with panko, egg, cheddar, Parmesan and chives. Now mix till combined. Season with pepper and salt as per the requirement.
- One tablespoon of the mixture is to be spooned and rolled into a tater-tot shape using your hands. Working in batches. Now, these have to be arranged in a single layer in the air fryer basket.
- Then cook for ten minutes at 375° F or until tots turn golden.
- Prepare spicy ketchup by combining ketchup and Sriracha in a small serving bowl. Stir well to mix.
- Enjoy warm cauliflower tots along with spicy ketchup.

Cheesy Bread

Preparation Time-10 minutes | Cook Time-20 minutes | Servings-2 to 4 | Difficulty-Easy

Nutritional Facts- Calories-226 | Fats-7.8g |Carbohydrates-31.8g |Proteins-7.8g

Ingredients

- Four cloves of garlic
- One cup of mozzarella cheese
- Eight slices of bread
- Six teaspoons of sun-dried tomatoes
- Five tablespoons of melted butter

Instructions

- Set the bread slices on a flat surface.
- Put butter on it, garlic, and tomato paste.
- Add cheese

- Place the bread on the Air Fryer Grill pan.
- Set the Air Fryer Grill to toast/bagel function.
- Cook for 8 minutes a 350F.

Cheesy Brussels Sprout

Preparation Time-10 minutes | Cook Time-10 minutes | Servings-2 | Difficulty-Easy

Nutritional Facts- Calories-75 | Fats-4.8g | Carbohydrates-7.8g | Proteins-6g

Ingredients

- Juice of one lemon
- Two tablespoons of butter
- One pound of Brussel sprout
- Three tablespoons of grated parmesan
- Black pepper and salt

Instructions

- Place the Brussel sprout on the Air Fryer Grill pan.
- Set the Air Fryer Grill to the air fry function.
- Cook for 8 minutes at 350 degrees F.
- Heat butter in a pan over medium heat, add pepper, lemon juice, and salt.
- Add Brussel sprout and parmesan.
- Serve immediately.
- If desired, serve with mint chutney

Cheesy Chicken Divan

Preparation Time-10 minutes | Cook Time-25 minutes | Servings-2 | Difficulty-Easy

Nutritional Facts- Calories-264 | Fats-4g | Carbohydrates-24g | Proteins-31.8g

Ingredients

- Four chicken breasts
- Salt and ground black pepper, to taste
- One head of broccoli, cut into florets
- Half cup of cream of mushroom soup
- One cup of shredded Cheddar cheese
- Half cup of croutons
- Cooking spray

Instructions

- Spritz the air fry basket with cooking spray.
- Put the chicken breasts in the air fry basket and sprinkle with salt and ground black pepper.

- Place the basket on the air fry position.
- Select Air Fry. Set temperature to 390F (199C) and set time to 14 minutes. Flip the breasts halfway through the cooking time.
- When cooking is complete, the breasts should be well browned and tender.
- Remove the breasts from the air fryer grill and allow them to cool for a few minutes on a plate, and then cut the breasts into bite-size pieces.
- Combine the chicken, broccoli, mushroom soup, and Cheddar cheese in a large bowl. Stir to mix well.
- Spritz a baking pan with cooking spray. Pour the chicken mixture into the pan. Spread the croutons over the mixture.
- Place the pan on the bake position.
- Select Bake. Set time to 10 minutes.
- When cooking is complete, the croutons should be lightly browned, and the mixture should be set.
- Remove the baking pan from the air fryer grill and serve immediately.

Cheesy Chile Toast

Preparation Time-5 minutes | Cook Time-5 minutes | Servings-2 | Difficulty-Easy

Nutritional Facts- Calories-147 | Fats-4.8g | Carbohydrates-9.9g | Proteins-15.9g

Ingredients

- Four tablespoons of grated Parmesan cheese
- Four tablespoons of grated Mozzarella cheese
- Four teaspoons of salted butter
- Fifteen to twenty thin slices of Serrano chili or jalapeño
- Four slices of sourdough bread
- One teaspoon of black pepper

Instructions

- Place the crisper tray on the bake position. Select Bake, set the temperature to 325F (163C), and set the time to 5 minutes.
- In a small bowl, merge together the Parmesan, Mozzarella, butter, and chilies.
- Scatter half the mixture onto one side of each slice of bread. Sprinkle with pepper. Place the slices, cheese side up, in the crisper tray.

- Bake for 5 minutes, or until the cheese has melted and started to brown slightly.
- Serve immediately.

Cheesy Crab Toasts

Preparation Time-10 minutes | Cook Time-5 minute | Servings-2 | Difficulty-Easy

Nutritional Facts- Calories-374 | Fats-15.9g |Carbohydrates-37.8g |Proteins-21g

Ingredients

- One (Six ounces) can flake well-drained crab meat
- Three tablespoons of light mayonnaise
- A quarter cup of shredded Parmesan cheese
- A quarter cup of shredded Cheddar cheese
- One teaspoon of Worcestershire sauce
- Half teaspoon of lemon juice
- One loaf artisan bread, French bread, or baguette, cut into 3/8inch-thick slices

Instructions

- Place the crisper tray on the bake position. Select Bake, set the temperature to 360 degrees F (182C), and set the time to 5 minutes.
- In a large bowl, merge together all the ingredients except the bread slices.
- On a clean work surface lay the bread slices. Spread one to two tablespoons of crab mixture onto each slice of bread.
- Arrange the bread slices in the crisper tray in a single layer. You'll need to work in batches to avoid overcrowding.
- Bake for 5 minutes until the tops are lightly browned.
- Bring to a plate and repeat with the remaining bread slices.
- Serve warm.

Cheesy Ham Toast

Preparation Time-5 minutes | Cook Time-8 minutes | Servings-2 | Difficulty-Easy

Nutritional Facts- Calories-184 | Fats-10.8g |Carbohydrates-4.8g |Proteins-12g

Ingredients

- Two slices of bread

- One teaspoon of butter
- Two eggs
- Salt and ground black pepper, to taste
- Four teaspoons of diced ham
- Two tablespoons of Cheddar cheese

Instructions

- Set a clean work surface; use a 2 1/2-inch biscuit cutter to make a hole in the center of the bread slice with about 1/2-inch of bread remaining.
- Scatter the butter on both sides of the bread slice. Set the egg into the hole and season with salt and pepper to taste. Transfer the bread to the air fryer basket.
- Slide the basket into the air fryer. Cook at the corresponding preset mode or Air Fry at 325F (163C) for 6 minutes.
- After 5 minutes, detach from the air fryer. Set the cheese and diced ham on top and continue cooking for an additional 1 minute.
- When cooking is processed, the egg should be set, and the cheese should be melted. Remove the toast from the air fryer to a plate and let cool for 5 minutes.

Cheesy Mushrooms and Spinach Frittata

Preparation Time-12 minutes | Cook Time-15 minutes | Servings-2 | Difficulty-

Nutritional Facts- Calories-233 | Fats-7.8g |Carbohydrates-4g |Proteins-39g

Ingredients

- One cup of chopped mushrooms
- Two cups of chopped spinach
- Four lightly beaten eggs
- Three ounces of crumbled feta cheese
- Two tablespoons of heavy cream
- A handful of chopped fresh parsley
- Salt and ground black pepper, to taste
- Cooking spray

Instructions

- Spritz a baking pan with cooking spray.
- Set together all the ingredients in a large bowl. Stir to mix well.
- Whisk the mixture in the prepared baking pan.
- Place the pan on the bake position.

- Select Bake, set temperature to 356 degrees Fahrenheit and set time to 8 minutes. Stir the mixture halfway through.
- When cooking is complete, the eggs should be set.
- Serve immediately.

Cheesy Mustard and Ham Rounds

Preparation Time-35 minutes | Cook Time-10 minutes | Servings-2 | Difficulty-Moderate

Nutritional Facts- Calories-199 | Fats-6.9g |Carbohydrates-12.9g |Proteins-20g

Ingredients

- One cup of grated gruyere cheese
- Two slices of ham
- One tablespoon of mustard
- One sheet of pre-rolled puff pastry

Instructions

- Cover your workbench with flour and put the pastry on it.
- Add the ham, mustard and cheese evenly on the pastry and roll up beginning from the shorter edge.
- Cover with cling film and place in the freezer until firm for 30 minutes. Remove, and slice into 1-cm small thick circles.
- Heat your air fryer to 370°F and cook the rounds in it until golden brown for 10 minutes.

Chicken galette

Preparation Time-10 minutes | Cook Time-30 minutes | Servings-2 | Difficulty-Easy

Nutritional Facts- Calories-165 | Fats-9g |Carbohydrates-7.8g |Proteins-13.8g

Ingredients

- Two tablespoons of garam masala
- One lb. of minced chicken
- Three teaspoons of finely chopped ginger
- Two tablespoons of fresh coriander leaves
- Three finely chopped green chilies
- Two tablespoons of lemon juice
- Salt and pepper to taste

Instructions

- Mix the ingredients in a clean bowl.

- Mold this mixture into round and flat galettes.
- Wet the galettes slightly with water.
- Preheat the Air Fryer at 160 degrees Fahrenheit for 5 minutes. Place the galettes in the fry basket and let them cook for another 25 minutes at the same temperature. Keep rolling them over to get a uniform cook.
- Serve either with mint chutney or ketchup.

Chicken Wings and Mint Sauce

Preparation Time-20 minutes | Cook Time-18 minutes | Servings-2 | Difficulty-Moderate

Nutritional Facts- Calories-300 | Fats-15g |Carbohydrates-27g |Proteins-15.9g

Ingredients

- Eight chicken wings halved
- One tablespoon of turmeric powder
- One tablespoon of ground cumin
- One tablespoon of grated ginger
- One tablespoon of ground coriander
- One tablespoon of sweet paprika
- Salt and black pepper to the taste
- Two tablespoons of olive oil

For the mint sauce

- Juice from 1/2 lime
- One cup of mint leaves
- One small ginger piece, chopped
- 3/4 cup of cilantro
- One tablespoon of olive oil
- One tablespoon of water
- Salt and black pepper to the taste
- One chopped Serrano pepper

Instructions

- In a bowl, mix one tablespoon of ginger with cumin, coriander, paprika, turmeric, salt, pepper, cayenne and Two tablespoons of oil and stir well. Add chicken wings pieces to this mix, toss to coat well and keep in the fridge for 10 minutes.
- Transfer chicken to your air fryer's basket and cook at 370 degrees F for 16 minutes, flipping them halfway.
- In your blender, mix mint with cilantro, one small ginger piece, juice from 1/2 lime, One

tablespoon of olive oil, salt, pepper, water and Serrano pepper and blend very well.

- Divide chicken wings among plates, drizzle the mint sauce all over and serve.
- Enjoy!

Chickpea Fritters with Sweet-Spicy Sauce

Preparation Time-10 minutes | Cook Time-25 minutes | Servings-2 | Difficulty-

Nutritional Facts- Calories-121 | Fats-1g | Carbohydrates-6.9g | Proteins-17g

Ingredients

- Two tablespoons of sugar
- A half teaspoon of salt
- A half teaspoon of crushed red pepper flakes
- One teaspoon of ground cumin
- A half teaspoon of garlic powder
- One large egg
- A half-cup of chopped fresh cilantro
- One cup of plain yogurt
- One tablespoon of honey
- A half teaspoon of pepper
- One can (15 ounces) chickpeas or garbanzo beans, rinsed and drained
- A half teaspoon of salt
- A half teaspoon of ground ginger
- A half teaspoon of baking soda
- Two thinly sliced green onions

Instructions

- Preheat the air fryer to 400 degrees Fahrenheit. Mix the ingredients in a small bowl and set aside until ready to serve.
- In a food processor, combine chickpeas and seasonings and process till finely ground. Then pulse in the egg as well as baking soda until well combined. Toss in the cilantro as well as green onions in a mixing bowl.
- Put a rounded tablespoon of bean mixture onto a greased tray in the air-fryer basket in batches. Now cook for 5-6 minutes, or until lightly browned.
- It can be served with sauce.

Clams galette

Preparation Time-10 minutes | Cook Time-30 minutes | Servings-2 | Difficulty-Easy

Nutritional Facts- Calories-148 | Fats-6.9g | Carbohydrates-6.9g | Proteins-13.8g

Ingredients

- Two tablespoons of garam masala
- One lb. minced clam
- Three teaspoons of finely chopped ginger
- Two tablespoons of fresh coriander leaves
- Three finely chopped green chilies
- One and a half tablespoons of lemon juice
- Salt and pepper to taste

Instructions

- Mix the ingredients in a clean bowl.
- Mold this mixture into round and flat galettes.
- Wet the galettes slightly with water.
- Preheat the Air Fryer at 160 degrees Fahrenheit for 5 minutes. Place the galettes in the fry basket and let them cook for another 25 minutes at the same temperature. Keep rolling them over to get a uniform cook.
- Serve either with mint chutney or ketchup.

Classic French Fries

Preparation Time-5 minutes | Cook Time-25 minutes | Servings-2 | Difficulty-Easy

Nutritional Facts- Calories-283 | Fats-4g | Carbohydrates-16.8g | Proteins-23g

Ingredients

- Two russet potatoes, peeled and cut into 1/2-inch sticks
- Two teaspoons of olive oil
- Salt, to taste
- A quarter cup of ketchup for serving

Instructions

- Set a pot of salted water to a boil. Put the potato sticks into the pot and blanch for 4 minutes.
- Rinse the potatoes under running cold water and pat dry with paper towels.
- Put the potato sticks in a large bowl and drizzle with olive oil. Toss to coat well.
- Transfer the potato sticks to the air fry basket.

- Place the basket on the air fry position.
- Select Air Fry, set the temperature to 400 degrees F (205C) and set time to 25 minutes. Stir the potato sticks and sprinkle with salt halfway through.
- When processed, the potato sticks will be crispy and golden brown. Detach the French fries from the air fryer grill and serve with ketchup.

Classic Hash Browns

Preparation Time-15 minutes | Cook Time-20 minutes | Servings-2 | Difficulty-Moderate

Nutritional Facts- Calories-150 | Fats-4g |Carbohydrates-34g |Proteins-1g

Ingredients

- Two russet potatoes
- One teaspoon of paprika
- Salt
- Pepper
- Cooking oil

Instructions

- Using a vegetable peeler, peel the potatoes. Shred the potatoes with a cheese grater. If your grater has holes of varying sizes, use the section with the largest holes.
- In a large dish of cold water, toss the shredded potatoes. Allow for 5 minutes of resting time. Stir to help the starch dissolve.
- Using paper towels or napkins, pat dry the potatoes. Make sure the potatoes are totally dry before cooking them.
- Season the potatoes to taste with salt, paprika, and pepper.
- Transfer the potatoes to the air fryer after spraying them with cooking oil. Cook for 20 minutes, shaking the basket every 5 minutes throughout that time (a total of 4 times).
- Allow cooling before serving.

Clean Eating Air Fryer Cheese Sticks

Preparation Time-10 minutes | Cook Time-22 minutes | Servings-2 | Difficulty-Easy

Nutritional Facts- Calories-90 | Fats-1g|Carbohydrates-13.8g |Proteins-1.5g

Ingredients

- A quarter cup of grated parmesan cheese
- One teaspoon of garlic powder
- A quarter cup of whole wheat flour
- Six snack-size cheese sticks
- One teaspoon of Italian Seasoning
- Two large eggs
- A quarter teaspoon of ground rosemary

Instructions

- Unwrap the sticks of cheese and set them aside.
- With a fork, crack and beat the eggs in a small bowl that is broad enough to match the length of the cheese sticks.
- Blend the flour, cheese and seasonings in another bowl (or plate).
- Roll the sticks of cheese into the egg and then into the batter. Repeat until it is well covered all around the cheese sticks.
- Place them in your air fryer's basket, ensuring they do not touch.
- Cook as directed by your air fryer. The temperature should be 370 degrees F and fry for 6-7 minutes.
- Serve with clean marinara.

Coconut Chicken Bites

Preparation Time-10 minutes | Cook Time-15 minutes | Servings-2 to 4 | Difficulty-Easy

Nutritional Facts- Calories-252 | Fats-4.8g |Carbohydrates-13.8g |Proteins-24g

Ingredients

- Two teaspoons of garlic powder
- Two eggs
- Salt and black pepper to the taste
- 3⁄4 cup of panko bread crumbs
- 3⁄4 cup of shredded coconut
- Cooking spray
- Eight chicken tenders

Instructions

- In a bowl, mix eggs with salt, pepper and garlic powder and whisk well.
- In another bowl, mix coconut with panko and stir well.

- Dip chicken tenders in eggs mix and then coat in coconut one well.
- Spray chicken bites with cooking spray, place them in your air fryer's basket and cook them at 350 degrees F for 10 minutes.
- Arrange them on a platter and serve as an appetizer.
- Enjoy!

Cod Fish Nuggets

Preparation Time-5 minutes | Cook Time-20 minutes | Servings-2 | Difficulty-Easy

Nutritional Facts- Calories-334 | Fats-9.9g |Carbohydrates-7.8g |Proteins-31.8g

Ingredients

- One lb. of Cod fillet
- Three eggs
- Four tablespoons of Olive oil
- One cup of Almond flour
- One cup of Gluten-free breadcrumbs

Instructions

- Warm the Air Fryer at 390Fahrenheit.
- Slice the cod into nuggets.
- Prepare three bowls. Whisk the eggs in one. Combine the salt, oil, and breadcrumbs in another. Sift the almond flour into the third one.
- Cover each of the nuggets with flour, dip in the eggs and the breadcrumbs.
- Arrange the nuggets in the basket and set the timer for 20 minutes.
- Serve the fish with your favorite dips or sides.

Cornflakes Toast Sticks

Preparation Time-10 minutes | Cook Time-7 minutes | Servings-2 | Difficulty-Easy

Nutritional Facts- Calories-421 | Fats-9.9g |Carbohydrates-34g |Proteins-41g

Ingredients

- One egg
- Half cup of milk
- 1/8 teaspoon of salt
- Half teaspoon of pure vanilla extract
- 1/3 cup of crushed cornflakes

- Four slices sandwich bread, each slice cut into four strips
- Maple syrup, for dipping
- Cooking spray

Instructions

- Place the crisper tray in the air fry position. Select Air Fry, set the temperature to 390 degrees F (199C) and set the time to 6 minutes.
- In a small bowl, set together with the eggs, milk, salt, and vanilla.
- Put the cornflakes on a plate or in a shallow dish.
- Dunk the bread strips in egg mixture, shake off excess, and roll in cornflake crumbs.
- Spray all sides of bread strips with oil.
- Put bread strips in a crisper tray in a single layer.
- Air fry for 6 minutes or until golden brown.
- Repeat the steps to air fry the remaining French toast sticks.
- Serve with maple syrup.

Crab Wontons

Preparation Time-10 minutes | Cook Time-10 minutes | Servings-2 | Difficulty-Easy

Nutritional Facts- Calories-345 | Fats-1g|Carbohydrates-65g |Proteins-18g

Ingredients

- Twenty-four wonton wrappers, thawed if frozen
- Cooking spray

Filling

- Five ounces of drained and dry lump crabmeat
- Four ounces of softened cream cheese
- Two sliced scallions
- One and a half teaspoons of toasted sesame oil
- One teaspoon of Worcestershire sauce
- Kosher salt and black pepper, to taste

Instructions

- Set the air fryer basket with cooking spray.
- In a medium-size bowl, place all the ingredients for the filling and stir until well mixed. Prepare a small bowl of water alongside.
- On a clean work surface, lay the wonton wrappers. Scoop One teaspoon of the filling in the center of each wrapper. Wet the edges with a touch of water. Fold each wonton wrapper

diagonally in half over the filling to form a triangle.

- Arrange the wontons in the basket. Spritz the wontons with cooking spray.
- Slide the basket into the air fryer. Cook at the corresponding preset mode or Air Fry at 356 degrees F for 10 minutes.
- Flip the wontons halfway through the cooking time.
- When cooking is complete, the wontons will be crispy and golden brown.
- Serve immediately.

Creamy Chicken Stew

Preparation Time-10 minutes | Cook Time-25 minutes | Servings-2 | Difficulty-Easy

Nutritional Facts- Calories-279 | Fats-10.8g |Carbohydrates-23g |Proteins-15g

Ingredients

- One and a half cups of canned cream of celery soup
- Six chicken tenders
- Salt and black pepper to the taste
- Two chopped potatoes
- One bay leaf
- One chopped thyme spring
- One tablespoon of milk
- One egg yolk
- Half cup of heavy cream

Instructions

- In a bowl, mix chicken with cream of celery, potatoes, heavy cream, bay leaf, thyme, salt and pepper, toss, pour into your air fryer's pan and cook at 320 degrees F for 25 minutes.
- Leave your stew to cool down a bit, discard bay leaf, divide among plates and serve right away.
- Enjoy!

Crispy Bacon in the Air Fryer

Preparation Time-10 minutes | Cook Time-5 minutes | Servings-2-4 | Difficulty-Easy

Nutritional Facts- Calories-177 | Fats-7.8g |Carbohydrates-1g|Proteins-20g

Ingredients

- A quarter-pound of Bacon

Instructions

- Add bacon uniformly into the air fryer basket. This can require two batches to cook all the bacon, depending on the size.
- Cook for 5 minutes at 350 degrees F.
- Flip the bacon and cook for an additional five minutes or until the crispiness you prefer.
- Remove the bacon with tongs and put it on a plate lined with paper towels.
- Allow it to cool and serve.

Crispy Baked Tofu

Preparation Time-15 minutes | Cook Time-20 minutes | Servings-2-4 | Difficulty-Easy

Nutritional Facts- Calories-332 | Fats-8.7g |Carbohydrates-23.1g |Proteins-12.9g

Ingredients

- One cup of whole wheat flour
- One package (Sixteen ounces) extra-firm tofu, chopped into eight slices
- 3/4 cup of raw cashews
- Two cups of pretzel sticks
- One tablespoon of extra virgin olive oil
- Two teaspoons of chili powder
- One cup of unsweetened almond milk
- Two teaspoons of garlic powder
- Two teaspoons of onion powder
- One teaspoon of lemon pepper
- A quarter teaspoon of black pepper
- Half teaspoon of sea salt

Instructions

- Preheat your air fryer toast oven to 400 degrees F.
- Line a baking sheet with baking paper and set it aside.
- In a food processor, pulse together cashews and pretzel sticks until coarsely ground.
- Combine garlic, onion, chili powder, lemon pepper, and salt in a small bowl.
- In a large bowl, combine half of the spice mixture and flour.
- Add almond milk to a separate bowl.

- In another bowl, combine cashew mixture, salt, pepper and olive oil; mix well.
- Sprinkle tofu slices with the remaining half of the spice mixture and coat each with the flour and then dip in almond milk; coat with the cashew mixture and bake for about 18 minutes or until golden brown.
- Serve the baked tofu with your favorite vegan salad.

Crispy Chicken Breast Sticks

Preparation Time-10 minutes | Cook Time-17 minutes | Servings-2 | Difficulty-Easy

Nutritional Facts- Calories-243 | Fats-4.8g |Carbohydrates-21g |Proteins-21.9g

Ingredients

- 3/4 cup of white flour
- One pound chicken breast, skinless, boneless, and cut into medium sticks
- One teaspoon of sweet paprika
- One cup of panko bread crumbs
- One whisked egg
- Salt and black pepper to the taste
- Two tablespoons of olive oil
- Zest from one lemon

Instructions

- In a bowl, mix paprika with flour, salt, pepper and lemon zest and stir.
- Put whisked egg in another bowl and the panko breadcrumbs in a third one.
- Dredge chicken pieces in flour, egg and panko and place them in your lined air fryer's basket, drizzle the oil over them, cook at 400 degrees F for 8 minutes, flip and cook for eight more minutes.
- Arrange them on a platter and serve them as a snack.
- Enjoy!

Crispy Fish Sticks

Preparation Time-10 minutes | Cook Time-12 minutes | Servings-2 | Difficulty-

Nutritional Facts- Calories-160 | Fats-1g|Carbohydrates-12g |Proteins-6g

Ingredients

- Four ounces of bread crumbs
- Four tablespoons of olive oil
- One whisked egg
- Four boneless, skinless, and cut into medium sticks white fish filets
- Salt and black pepper to the taste

Instructions

- In a bowl, mix bread crumbs with oil and stir well.
- Put egg in a second bowl, add salt and pepper and whisk well.
- Dip the fish stick in egg and then in bread crumb mix, place them in your air fryer's basket and cook at 360 degrees F for 12 minutes.
- Arrange fish sticks on a platter and serve as an appetizer.
- Enjoy.

Crispy Potatoes and Parsley

Preparation Time-10 minutes | Cook Time-10 minutes | Servings-2 | Difficulty-Easy

Nutritional Facts- Calories-153 | Fats-1g|Carbohydrates-16.8g |Proteins-4g

Ingredients

- One pound gold potatoes, cut into wedges
- Salt and black pepper to the taste
- Two tablespoons of olive
- Juice from half lemon
- A quarter cup of chopped parsley leaves

Instructions

- Rub potatoes with salt, pepper, lemon juice and olive oil, put them in your air fryer and cook at 350 degrees F for 10 minutes.
- Divide among plates, sprinkle parsley on top and serve.
- Enjoy!

Crunchy Fried Cabbage

Preparation Time-10 minutes | Cook Time-10 minutes | Servings-2 | Difficulty-

Nutritional Facts- Calories-105 | Fats-7.2g |Carbohydrates-10.2g |Proteins-2.1g

Ingredients

- Half cabbage head, sliced into 2-inch slices
- One tablespoon of olive oil
- Pepper
- Salt

Instructions

- Drizzle cabbage with olive oil and season with pepper and salt.
- Add cabbage slices into the air fryer basket and cook at 375 F for 5 minutes.
- Toss cabbage well and cook for 5 minutes more.
- Serve and enjoy.

Crunchy Salty Tortilla Chips

Preparation Time-5 minutes | Cook Time-10 minutes | Servings-2 | Difficulty-Easy

Nutritional Facts- Calories-155 | Fats-1.5g |Carbohydrates-6g |Proteins-25g

Ingredients

- Four six-inch corn tortillas, cut in half and slice into thirds
- One tablespoon of canola oil
- A quarter teaspoon of kosher salt
- Cooking spray

Instructions

- Spritz the air fry basket with cooking spray.
- On a clean work surface, brush the tortilla chips with canola oil, then transfer the chips to the air fry basket.
- Place the basket on the air fry position.
- Select Air Fry, set the temperature to 360 degrees F (182C) and set time to 10 minutes. Flip the chops and sprinkle with salt halfway through the cooking time.
- When cooked, the chips will be crunchy and lightly browned. Bring the chips to a plate lined with paper towels. Serve immediately.

Crunchy Zucchini Hash Browns

Preparation Time-30 minutes | Cook Time-15 minutes | Servings-2 | Difficulty-Moderate

Nutritional Facts- Calories-195 | Fats-6g |Carbohydrates-18g |Proteins-7.8g

Ingredients

- Four medium peeled and grated zucchinis
- One teaspoon of onion powder
- One teaspoon of garlic powder
- Two tablespoons of almond flour
- One to half teaspoon of chili flakes
- Salt and freshly ground pepper to taste
- Two teaspoons of olive oil

Instructions

- Put the grated zucchini in between layers of kitchen towel and squeeze to drain excess water. Pour one teaspoon of oil in a pan, preferably non-stick, over medium heat and sauté the potatoes for about 3 minutes.
- Transfer the zucchini to a shallow bowl and let cool. Sprinkle the zucchini with the remaining ingredients and mix until well combined.
- Transfer the zucchini mixture to a flat plate and pat it down to make one compact layer. Put it in the fridge and let it sit for 20 minutes.
- Set your air fryer toast oven to 360 degrees F.
- Meanwhile, take out the flattened zucchini and divide it into equal portions using a knife or cookie cutter.
- Lightly brush your air fryer toast oven's basket with the remaining teaspoon of olive oil.
- Gently place the zucchini pieces into the greased basket and fry for 12-15 minutes, flipping the hash browns halfway through.
- Enjoy hot!

Delicious Crab Cakes

Preparation Time-10 minutes | Cook Time-10 minutes | Servings-2 | Difficulty-Easy

Nutritional Facts- Calories-136 | Fats-12g |Carbohydrates-4.8g |Proteins-9.9g

Ingredients

- Four ounces of crab meat
- Two tablespoons of melted butter
- Two teaspoons of Dijon mustard
- One tablespoon of mayonnaise
- One egg, lightly beaten
- Half teaspoon of old bay seasoning
- One sliced green onion
- Two tablespoons of chopped parsley

- A quarter cup of almond flour
- A quarter teaspoon of pepper
- Half teaspoon of salt

Instructions

- Set all ingredients except butter in a mixing bowl and mix until well combined.
- Make four equal shapes of patties from the mixture and place them on a parchment-lined plate.
- Place plate in the fridge for 30 minutes.
- Spray air fryer basket with cooking spray.
- Brush melted butter on both sides of crab patties.
- Place crab patties in an air fryer basket and cook for 10 minutes at 350 F.
- Turn patties halfway through.
- Serve and enjoy.

Duck fingers

Preparation Time-10 minutes | Cook Time-25 minutes | Servings-2 | Difficulty-Easy

Nutritional Facts- Calories-156 | Fats-6.9g |Carbohydrates-7.8g |Proteins-19g

Ingredients

- One lb. of boneless duck (Cut into fingers)
- Two cups of dry breadcrumbs
- Two teaspoons of oregano
- Two teaspoons of red chili flakes

Marinade

- Two tablespoons of ginger-garlic paste
- Four tablespoons of lemon juice
- Two teaspoons of salt
- One teaspoon of pepper powder
- One teaspoon of red chili powder
- Six tablespoons of cornflour
- Four eggs

Instructions

- Mix all the ingredients for the marinade and put the duck fingers inside, and let it rest overnight.
- Mix the breadcrumbs, oregano and red chili flakes well and place the marinated fingers on this mixture. Cover it with plastic wrap and leave it till right before you serve to cook.

- Preheat the Air fryer at 160 degrees Fahrenheit for 5 minutes. Place the fingers in the fry basket and close it. Let them cook at the same temperature for another 15 minutes or so. Toss the fingers well so that they are cooked uniformly.

Egg White Chips

Preparation Time-5 minutes | Cook Time-10 minutes | Servings-2 | Difficulty-Easy

Nutritional Facts- Calories-180 | Fats-1g|Carbohydrates-12g |Proteins-6.9g

Ingredients

- One tablespoon of water
- Two tablespoons of shredded parmesan
- Four egg whites
- Salt and black pepper to the taste

Instructions

- In a bowl, mix egg whites with salt, pepper and water and whisk well.
- Spoon this into a muffin pan that fits your air fryer, sprinkle cheese on top, introduce it in your air fryer and cook at 350 degrees F for 8 minutes.
- Arrange egg-white chips on a platter and serve as a snack.
- Enjoy!

Everything Bagel Chips

Preparation Time-10 minutes | Cook Time-20 minutes | Servings-2 | Difficulty-Easy

Nutritional Facts- Calories-201 | Fats-7.8g |Carbohydrates-13.8g |Proteins-6g

Ingredients

- Two Pizza Crusts
- Olive oil spray
- Everything Bagel Seasoning
- Instructions
- Using a pizza cutter, cut the pizza crust into tiny chunks.
- Place each triangular chunk in the air fryer after spraying with olive oil spray and topping with Everything Bagel Seasoning.
- Bake for 10-15 minutes at 350°F, or until the chips are crisp to your liking.

- Chips with hummus, guacamole, or cheese spread are delicious!

Fish and Sweet Potato Chips

Preparation Time-20 minutes | Cook Time-25 minutes | Servings-2 | Difficulty-Moderate

Nutritional Facts- Calories-285 | Fats-15.9g |Carbohydrates-4g |Proteins-1g

Ingredients

- Four cups of sweet potatoes, sliced into strips
- One teaspoon of olive oil
- One beaten egg
- 2/3 cup of breadcrumbs
- One teaspoon of lemon zest
- Two fish fillets, sliced into strips
- Half cup of Greek yogurt
- One tablespoon of chopped shallots
- One tablespoon of chopped chives
- Two teaspoons of chopped dill

Instructions

- Toss sweet potatoes in oil.
- Cook at 360 F until crispy.
- Set aside.
- Dip fish fillet in egg.
- Dredge with breadcrumbs mixed with lemon zest.
- Air fry at 360 degrees F for 12 minutes.
- Mix yogurt and the remaining ingredients.
- Serve fish, sweet potato chips and sauce together.

Fish Nuggets

Preparation Time-10 minutes | Cook Time-15 minutes | Servings-2 | Difficulty-Easy

Nutritional Facts- Calories-332 | Fats-12g |Carbohydrates-16.8g |Proteins-15g

Ingredients

- Fourteen ounces of skinless and cut into medium pieces fish fillets
- Salt and black pepper to the taste
- Three tablespoons of flour
- One whisked egg
- Three tablespoons of water
- One and a half ounces of panko bread crumbs

- One tablespoon of garlic powder
- One tablespoon of smoked paprika
- Four tablespoons of homemade mayonnaise
- Lemon juice from half lemon
- One teaspoon of dried dill
- Cooking spray

Instructions

- In a bowl, mix flour with water and stir well.
- Add egg, salt and pepper and whisk well.
- In a second bowl, mix panko with garlic powder and paprika and stir well.
- Dip fish pieces in flour and egg mix and then in panko mix, place them in your air fryer's basket, spray them
- with cooking oil and cook at 400 degrees F for 12 minutes.
- Meanwhile, in a bowl, mix mayo with dill and lemon juice and whisk well.
- Arrange fish nuggets on a platter and serve with dill mayo on the side.
- Enjoy!

French Bread Pizza

Preparation Time-10 minutes | Cook Time-20 minutes | Servings-2 | Difficulty-Easy

Nutritional Facts- Calories-303 | Fats-6.9g |Carbohydrates-36.9g |Proteins-12.9g

Ingredients

- One teaspoon of dried oregano
- Half cup of fresh mushrooms
- One loaf of French bread
- A quarter cup of parmesan cheese
- One cup of mozzarella cheese
- Half green pepper
- 3/4 cup of spaghetti sauce

Instructions

- Put the spaghetti sauce on the French bread.
- Add green pepper, cheeses, mushroom, and oregano.
- Place it on the Air Fryer Grill pan.
- Set the Air Fryer Grill to the pizza function.
- Cook for 15 minutes at 370 degrees F.

French Fries with Seasoned Salt

Preparation Time-10 minutes | Cook Time-40 minutes | Servings-2 | Difficulty-Moderate

Nutritional Facts- Calories-235 | Fats-4.8g |Carbohydrates-23g |Proteins-4g

Ingredients

- Two teaspoons of chili powder
- Five sprays olive oil or avocado oil cooking spray
- One teaspoon of ground cumin
- One Russet potato
- Half teaspoon of garlic powder
- Two tablespoons of salt
- Half teaspoon of onion powder

Instructions

- Cut the potato into small strips about a quarter of an inch thick.
- Place the potato slices for about 30 minutes in a bowl of water to soak.
- Meanwhile, by combining the ingredients in a small bowl, prepare the seasoned salt. Just put it aside.
- Drain the slices of potato and use kitchen towels to dry properly.
- The potato slices should be put in a dry bowl. Spray with about five cooking oil sprays. Use your hands to coat them.
- To the potato slices, apply the preferred amount of Seasoned Salt and use your hands to toss to cover.
- Place the potato slices and spread them out as thinly as possible in the basket of your air fryer.
- Cook for 15 to 20 minutes at 390 degrees F (or your model's maximum temperature), flipping midway through until the fries are finely browned and crispy.
- Instantly serve.

French toast Casserole

Preparation Time-5 minutes | Cook Time-15 minutes | Servings-2 | Difficulty-Easy

Nutritional Facts- Calories-184 | Fats-10.8g |Carbohydrates-4.8g |Proteins-12g

Ingredients

- One large beaten egg

- Half cup of whole milk
- Half tablespoon of pure maple syrup
- Half teaspoon of vanilla extract
- A quarter teaspoon of cinnamon
- A quarter teaspoon of kosher salt
- One cup of stale bread cubes
- Half tablespoon of unsalted butter, at room temperature

Instructions

- In a medium bowl, merge together the eggs, milk, maple syrup, vanilla extract, cinnamon and salt. Stir in the bread cubes to coat well.
- Grease the bottom of a sheet pan with butter. Spread the bread mixture into the pan in an even layer.
- Slide the pan into the air fryer. Cook at the corresponding preset mode or Air Fry at 356 degrees Fahrenheit for 12 minutes.
- After about 10 minutes, remove the pan and check the casserole. The top should be browned, and the middle of the casserole just set. If more time is needed, return the pan to the air fryer and continue cooking.
- When cooking is complete, serve warm.

French Toast Sticks

Preparation Time-10 minutes | Cook Time-25 minutes | Servings-2 | Difficulty-Easy

Nutritional Facts- Calories-224 | Fats-9g |Carbohydrates-10.8g |Proteins-4g

Ingredients

- One-third cup of heavy cream
- Kosher salt
- Three tablespoons of granulated sugar
- A half teaspoon of pure vanilla extract
- Two large eggs
- One-third cup of whole milk
- Six thick slices Pullman or other white loaf or brioche, each slice cut into thirds
- A quarter teaspoon of ground cinnamon
- Maple syrup, for serving

Instructions

- In a big shallow baking dish, beat the cinnamon, eggs, cream, milk, sugar, vanilla and a pinch of salt. Insert the bread and turn a couple of times to coat.

- Arrange French toast in the air fryer basket, working in lots if necessary to prevent overcrowding the basket. Set the air fryer to 375°F and cook for about 8 minutes until golden, flipping halfway through. Drizzle with maple syrup and eat warm toast.

Fried Chicken and Waffles

Preparation Time-11 minutes | Cook Time-32 minutes | Servings-2 | Difficulty-Moderate

Nutritional Facts- Calories-461 | Fats-21.9g |Carbohydrates-37.8g |Proteins-27.9g

Ingredients

- One teaspoon of garlic powder
- Pepper
- Cooking oil
- Maple syrup (optional)
- Four whole chicken wings
- Chicken seasoning or rub
- Half cup of all-purpose flour
- Four frozen waffles

Instructions

- Season the chicken with garlic powder, chicken seasoning, and pepper to taste in a medium mixing bowl.
- Combine the chicken and flour in a sealable plastic bag. Shake to coat the chicken completely.
- Cooking oil should be sprayed into the air fryer basket.
- Transfer the chicken from the bag to the air fryer using tongs. It's fine to stack chicken wings on top of one another. Cooking oil should be sprayed over them. 5 minutes in a hot oven
- Shake the basket in the air fryer after unlocking it. Assume you'll be cooking the chicken. Continue shaking every 5 minutes until the chicken is fully cooked, about 20 minutes.
- Remove the fried chicken from the air fryer and place it on a plate to cool.
- Warm water should be used to clean the basket and the base. Return them to the air fryer.
- Preheat the air fryer to 370 degrees Fahrenheit.
- In the air fryer, place the frozen waffles. Do not create a pile. You may need to cook the waffles in

batches depending on the size of your air fryer. Cooking oil should be sprinkled on the waffles. 6 minutes in the oven

- Remove the cooked waffles from the air fryer if necessary, then repeat step 9 with the remaining waffles.
- Serve the waffles with the chicken and, if wanted, a drizzle of maple syrup.

Fried Pickles

Preparation Time-40 minutes | Cook Time-15 minutes | Servings-2 | Difficulty-Moderate

Nutritional Facts- Calories-160 | Fats-6g |Carbohydrates-7.8g |Proteins-17g

Ingredients

- A quarter cup of freshly grated Parmesan
- One teaspoon of garlic powder
- Half cup of bread crumbs
- Two cups of dill pickle slices
- One teaspoon of dried oregano
- One egg whisked with one tablespoon of water
- Ranch, for dipping

Instructions

- Pat pickle chips dry using paper towels. Stir the oregano, bread crumbs, parmesan and garlic powder in a medium bowl.
- Dredge pickle chips first in the egg and then bread crumb mixture. Working in batches, put in the air fryer basket in a single layer. Cook for 10 minutes at 400°F.

Serve warm with the ranch.

Friendly Bagels

Preparation Time-20 minutes | Cook Time-18 minutes | Servings-2 | Difficulty-Easy

Nutritional Facts- Calories-548 | Fats-21g |Carbohydrates-1.5g |Proteins-45.9g

Ingredients

- One cup of self-rising flour
- One cup of low Greek yogurt
- One egg

Instructions

- Mix together yogurt and flour until it becomes a ball of dough.

- Place a ball of dough on a flat surface and cover with flour.
- Separate into four balls.
- Roll each ball into a long rope
- Shape into a bagel form.
- Whisk egg.
- Coat each bagel with an egg wash and any toppings.
- Place in the air fryer or ninja basket
- Place on 350 degrees F for 10 minutes.

Garlic Bread

Preparation Time-10 minutes | Cook Time-15 minutes | Servings-2 | Difficulty-Easy

Nutritional Facts- Calories-151 | Fats-7.8g |Carbohydrates-18g |Proteins-4g

Ingredients

- Two stale French rolls
- Four tablespoons of Crushed or crumpled garlic
- One cup of mayonnaise
- Powdered grated Parmesan
- One tablespoon of olive oil

Instructions

- Preheat the air fryer to 200°C for 5 minutes.
- Mix mayonnaise with garlic and set aside.
- Cut the baguettes into slices, but without separating them completely.
- Fill the cavities of equals, then brush with olive oil and sprinkle with grated cheese.
- Put it in the basket of the air fryer. Cook for 10 minutes at 180°C. Serve.

Guacamole

Preparation Time-5 hours | Cook Time-15 minutes | Servings-2 | Difficulty-Hard

Nutritional Facts- Calories-167 | Fats-13.8g |Carbohydrates-1.5g |Proteins-1.5g

Ingredients

- Two teaspoons of cumin
- Eight tablespoons of almond flour
- Pepper and sea salt as per taste
- One egg
- Juice of one lime

- One-third cup of finely chopped fresh cilantro
- One egg white
- Three medium ripe avocados
- One-third cup of chopped onion
- One-third cup of almond flour
- One and a half cups of gluten-free panko
- Olive oil spray

Instructions

- Combine and crush the guacamole ingredients except for the flour(almond) In a bowl. Stir in the flour only after the guacamole is dense. To make it thick, add an extra tablespoon of flour to the batter. Place the bowl to solidify for around 2 hours in the refrigerator. (freezer)
- Line with nonstick foil or parchment paper the baking sheet. Using a spoon, take the guacamole out from the batch and give it the shape of a ball using your hands, and put it on the tray(baking). Repeat with the leftover guacamole very easily. Use nonstick foil to protect the tray and place it in the refrigerator (freezer) for around 5 to 6 hours or the whole night.
- Adjust your air fryer to 390 degrees F.
- Eggs are to be beaten altogether in a separate bowl.
- Work in batches. To make them 'sticky,' gently brush your prepared balls with olive oil, then dip them in the flour and then egg mixture and then the panko crumbs.
- Place the coated balls in the basket of the air fryer, spray with oil and let it cook for around 8 to 9 minutes or until golden brown on the outside. Take them out of the device if the balls start cracking. Let them cool slightly before savoring them because they become firmer.

Harvest Granola

Preparation Time-10 minutes | Cook Time-30 minutes | Servings-2 | Difficulty-Moderate

Nutritional Facts- Calories-105 | Fats-1g|Carbohydrates-4g |Proteins-18g

Ingredients

- One teaspoon of Canola Oil
- 1/3 cup of maple syrup
- Half cup of Dried Cranberries
- Half cup of pumpkin seeds

- One cup of rolled oats
- 2/3 cup of sliced almonds
- 3/2 teaspoons of salt

Instructions

- Bring together and mix the sunflower seeds, oats, pumpkin seeds, almonds and salt.
- Add the oil and syrup.
- Stir to combine.
- Place parchment onto three Air Fryer trays.
- Spray the granola mixture equally over the trays.
- Bake at 220 for 40 minutes, turning the trays midway over the cooking time.
- Add the cranberries and whisk to mix.
- Cool and serve.

Healthy Air Fried Chicken Tenders

Preparation Time-10 minutes | Cook Time-20 minutes | Servings-2 | Difficulty-Easy

Nutritional Facts- Calories-372 | Fats-10.8g |Carbohydrates-23g |Proteins-20g

Ingredients

- Twelve ounces of Chicken Breasts
- One Egg White
- 1/8 Cup of Flour
- Thirty-five grams Panko Bread Crumbs
- Pepper and salt

Instructions

- Trim the chicken breast and slice into tenders.
- With pepper and salt, season each side.
- Dip chicken tenders into egg whites. Then dip into panko bread crumbs and then into flour.
- Load and spray with olive spray into the air fryer basket.
- It has to be cooked for about ten minutes or until fully cooked at 350 degrees F.

Healthy Low Fat Air Fryer French Fries

Preparation Time-10 minutes | Cook Time-30 minutes | Servings-2 | Difficulty-

Nutritional Facts- Calories-272 | Fats-1g|Carbohydrates-26g |Proteins-12g

Ingredients

- Two tablespoons of parmesan cheese

- One tablespoon of olive oil plus more to brush wire basket
- Three medium russet potatoes
- Two tablespoons of finely chopped fresh parsley
- Salt

Instructions

- Potatoes are sliced into quarter" thick fries."
- To extract extra moisture, pat dry using a kitchen towel.
- Insert salt, parmesan cheese, fresh parsley and oil. To coat cheese, herbs, and oil evenly, toss or gently blend.
- Preheat the Air Fryer for 2-3 min at 360 degrees F. Rub some oil gently on the wire basket base.
- Then spread the seasoned fries uniformly on the mesh. Now cook for a total of 20 minutes.
- Using metal tongs, mix the fries gently after 10 minutes of frying.
- Continue to cook for another 5 minutes. Mix the fries again.
- Finally, cook for an extra 5 minutes.
- These fries are eaten warm with ketchup or your favorite sauce.

Home-Fried Potatoes

Preparation Time-8 minutes | Cook Time-30 minutes | Servings-2 | Difficulty-Easy

Nutritional Facts- Calories-279 | Fats-7.8g |Carbohydrates-15.9g |Proteins-6g

Ingredients

- One tablespoon of canola oil
- One teaspoon of paprika
- Pepper
- One and a half large russet potatoes
- One tablespoon of extra-virgin olive oil
- Salt
- One cup of chopped onion
- One cup of chopped green bell pepper
- One cup of chopped red bell pepper

Instructions

- Potatoes should be cut into 1/2-inch chunks. Allow the potatoes to soak for at least 30 minutes, preferably an hour, in a bowl of cold water.
- Dry the potatoes completely with paper towels

after drying. Return them to the dish that is now empty.

- Toss in the olive and canola oils, as well as the paprika, salt, and pepper to taste. Start by coating the potatoes completely.
- Place the potatoes in the air fryer to cook. Every 5 minutes, cook and reset the air fryer basket (a total of 4 times).
- In the air fryer basket, combine the onion, red, and green bell peppers. Fry for another 3 to 4 minutes, or until the potatoes are tender and the peppers are cooked through.
- Allow cooling before serving.

Hydrated Kale Chips

Preparation Time-5 minutes | Cook Time-10 minutes | Servings-2 | Difficulty-Easy

Nutritional Facts- Calories-103 | Fats-6.9g | Carbohydrates-7.8g | Proteins-17g

Ingredients

- Four cups of loosely packed stemmed kale
- Two teaspoons of ranch Seasoning
- Two tablespoons of olive oil
- One tablespoon of nutritional yeast
- A quarter teaspoon of salt

Instructions

- In a bowl, toss together kale pieces, oil, nutritional yeast, ranch seasoning, and salt until well coated.
- Transfer to a fryer basket and hydrate for 15 minutes, shaking halfway through cooking.
- Serve right away!

Hydrated Potato Wedges

Preparation Time-10 minutes | Cook Time-30 minutes | Servings-2 | Difficulty-Easy

Nutritional Facts- Calories-129 | Fats-5.28g | Carbohydrates-9.9g | Proteins-2.1g

Ingredients

- Two medium Russet potatoes, diced into wedges
- One and a half tablespoons of olive oil
- Half teaspoon of chili powder
- Half teaspoon of parsley
- Half teaspoon of paprika

- 1/8 teaspoon of black pepper
- Half teaspoon of sea salt

Instructions

- In a large bowl, mix potato wedges, olive oil, chili, parsley, paprika, salt and pepper until the potatoes are well coated.
- Transfer half of the potatoes to a fryer basket and hydrate for 20 minutes.
- Repeat with the remaining wedges. Serve hot with chilled orange juice.

Indian Potatoes

Preparation Time-10 minutes | Cook Time-15 minutes | Servings-2 | Difficulty-Easy

Nutritional Facts- Calories-241 | Fats-6.9g | Carbohydrates-15.9g | Proteins-17g

Ingredients

- One tablespoon of coriander seeds
- One tablespoon of cumin seeds
- Salt and black pepper to the taste
- Half teaspoon of turmeric powder
- Half teaspoon of red chili powder
- One teaspoon of pomegranate powder
- One tablespoon of chopped pickled mango
- Two teaspoons of dried fenugreek
- Four boiled, peeled and cubed potatoes
- Two tablespoons of olive oil

Instructions

- Heat up a pan that fits your air fryer with the oil over medium heat, add coriander and cumin seeds, stir and cook for 2 minutes.
- Add salt, pepper, turmeric, chili powder, pomegranate powder, mango, fenugreek and potatoes, toss, introduce in your air fryer and cook at 360 degrees F for 10 minutes.
- Divide among plates and serve hot.
- Enjoy!

Italian Eggplant Stew

Preparation Time-10 minutes | Cook Time-15 minutes | Servings-2 | Difficulty-Easy

Nutritional Facts- Calories-170 | Fats-12.9g | Carbohydrates-4.8g | Proteins-6.9g

Ingredients

- One chopped red onion
- Two chopped garlic cloves
- One bunch of chopped parsley
- Salt and black pepper to the taste
- One teaspoon of dried oregano
- Two eggplants, cut into medium chunks
- Two tablespoons of olive oil
- Two tablespoons of chopped capers
- One handful of pitted and sliced green olives
- Five chopped tomatoes
- Three tablespoons of herb vinegar

Instructions

- Heat up a pan that fits your air fryer with the oil over medium heat, add eggplant, oregano, salt and pepper, stir and cook for 5 minutes.
- Add garlic, onion, parsley, capers, olives, vinegar and tomatoes, stir, introduce in your air fryer and cook at 360 degrees F for 15 minutes.
- Divide into bowls and serve.
- Enjoy!

Jalapeno Balls

Preparation Time-10 minutes | Cook Time-5 minutes | Servings-2 | Difficulty-Easy

Nutritional Facts- Calories-172 | Fats-4g |Carbohydrates-12.9g |Proteins-6g

Ingredients

- Two cooked and crumbled bacon slices
- Two ounces of cream cheese
- A quarter teaspoon of onion powder
- Salt and black pepper to the taste
- One chopped jalapeno pepper
- Half teaspoon of dried parsley
- A quarter teaspoon of garlic powder

Instructions

- In a bowl, mix cream cheese with jalapeno pepper, onion and garlic powder, parsley, bacon, salt and pepper, and stir well.
- Shape small balls out of this mix, place them in your air fryer's basket, cook at 350 degrees F for 4 minutes, arrange on a platter and serve.
- Enjoy!

Kale chips

Preparation Time-10 minutes | Cook Time-10 minutes | Servings-2 | Difficulty-Easy

Nutritional Facts- Calories-100 | Fats-1.5g |Carbohydrates-13.8g |Proteins-4.8g

Ingredients

- Two teaspoons of olive oil
- One to two tablespoons of seasoning mix of your choice
- Four cups of loosely packed stemmed kale
- A pinch of salt

Instructions

- Lightly massage the kale in a medium-sized bowl of oil and salt. You're not going here for a kale salad. A touch of wilting is all right. Dump the coated kale into your air fryer's basket, then.
- Cook for 4-6 minutes at 370 ° F (do not preheat), shake after 2 minutes, check for thickening. Check-in for the last 2 minutes, every minute.
- Toss and eat quickly with the seasoning of choice.

Kale Salad Sushi Rolls with Sriracha Mayonnaise

Preparation Time-10 minutes | Cook Time-10 minutes | Servings-2 | Difficulty-Easy

Nutritional Facts- Calories-312 | Fats-23g |Carbohydrates-12.9g |Proteins-17g

Ingredients

Kale Salad

- One and a half cups of chopped kale
- One tablespoon of sesame seeds
- 1/3 teaspoon of soy sauce
- 1/3 teaspoon of toasted sesame oil
- Half teaspoon of rice vinegar
- A quarter teaspoon of ginger
- 1/8 teaspoon of garlic powder

Sushi Rolls

- Three sheets of sushi nori
- One batch of cauliflower rice
- Half sliced avocado

Sriracha Mayonnaise

- A quarter cup of Sriracha sauce

- A quarter cup of vegan mayonnaise

Coating

- Half cup of panko bread crumbs

Instructions

- In a medium bowl, merge all the ingredients for the salad together until well coated and set aside.
- Place a sheet of nori on a clean work surface and spread the cauliflower rice in an even layer on the nori. Scoop two to three tablespoons of kale salad on the rice and spread over. Place 1 or 2 avocado slices on top. Roll up the sushi, pressing gently to get a nice, tight roll. Repeat to make the remaining two rolls.
- In a bowl, stir together the Sriracha sauce and mayonnaise until smooth. Add bread crumbs to a separate bowl.
- Dredge the sushi rolls in Sriracha Mayonnaise, then roll in bread crumbs till well coated.
- Place the coated sushi rolls in the airflow racks.
- Slide the racks into the air fryer oven. Press the Power Button. Cook at 390F (199C) for 10 minutes.
- Flip the sushi rolls halfway through the cooking time.
- When cooking is complete, the sushi rolls will be golden brown and crispy.
- Bring to a platter and rest for 5 minutes before slicing each roll into eight pieces. Serve warm.

Lamb fries

Preparation Time-10 minutes | Cook Time-25 minutes | Servings-2 | Difficulty-Easy

Nutritional Facts- Calories-188 | Fats-9g |Carbohydrates-9g |Proteins-20g

Ingredients

- One lb. of boneless lamb cut into fingers
- Two cups of dry breadcrumbs
- Two teaspoons of oregano
- Two teaspoons of red chili flakes

Marinade

- Two tablespoons of ginger-garlic paste
- Four tablespoons of lemon juice
- Two teaspoons of salt
- One teaspoon of pepper powder

- One teaspoon of red chili powder
- Six tablespoons of cornflour
- Four eggs

Instructions

- Mix all the ingredients for the marinade and put the lamb fingers inside, and let it rest overnight.
- Mix the breadcrumbs, oregano and red chili flakes well and place the marinated fingers on this mixture. Cover it with plastic wrap and leave it till right before you serve to cook.
- Preheat the Air fryer at 160 degrees Fahrenheit for 5 minutes. Place the fingers in the fry basket and close it. Let them cook at the same temperature for another 15 minutes or so. Toss the fingers well so that they are cooked uniformly.

Lobster Kebab

Preparation Time-10 minutes | Cook Time-30 minutes | Servings-2 | Difficulty-Easy

Nutritional Facts- Calories-147 | Fats-6.9g |Carbohydrates-7.8g |Proteins-13.8g

Ingredients

- One lb. of shelled and cubed lobster
- Three chopped onions
- Five roughly chopped green chilies
- Two tablespoons of ginger paste
- One teaspoon of garlic paste
- One teaspoon of salt
- Three teaspoons of lemon juice
- Two teaspoons of garam masala
- Four tablespoons of chopped coriander
- Three tablespoons of cream
- Two tablespoons of coriander powder
- Four tablespoons of fresh mint chopped
- Three tablespoons of chopped capsicum
- Three eggs
- Two and a half tablespoons of white sesame seeds

Instructions

- Take all the ingredients mentioned under the first heading and mix them in a bowl. Grind them thoroughly to make a smooth paste.
- Take the eggs in a different bowl and beat them. Add a pinch of salt and leave them aside.

- Take a flat plate and in it mix the sesame seeds and breadcrumbs.
- Dip the lobster cubes in the egg and salt mixture and then in the mixture of breadcrumbs and sesame seeds. Leave these kebabs in the fridge for an hour or so to set.
- Preheat the Air fryer at 160 degrees Fahrenheit for around 5 minutes. Place the kebabs in the basket and let them cook for another 25 minutes at the same temperature. Turn the kebabs over in between the cooking process to get a uniform cook.
- Serve the kebabs with mint chutney.

Mexican Apple Snack

Preparation Time-10 minutes | Cook Time- 10 minutes | Servings-2 | Difficulty-Easy

Nutritional Facts- Calories-192 | Fats-4g |Carbohydrates-23g |Proteins-1.5g

Ingredients

- Two cored, peeled and cubed big apples
- Two teaspoons of lemon juice
- A quarter cup of chopped pecans
- Half cup of dark chocolate chips
- Half cup of clean caramel sauce

Instructions

- In a bowl, mix apples with lemon juice, stir and transfer to a pan that fits your air fryer.
- Add chocolate chips, pecans, drizzle the caramel sauce, toss, introduce in your air fryer and cook at 320 degrees F for 5 minutes.
- Toss gently, divide into small bowls and serve right away as a snack.
- Enjoy!

Mini Pizza

Preparation Time-10 minutes | Cook Time-30 minutes | Servings-2 | Difficulty-Easy

Nutritional Facts- Calories-273 | Fats-27g |Carbohydrates-23g |Proteins-21g

Ingredients

- One teaspoon of Italian herb seasoning
- A quarter cup of minced onion
- Three toasted and split muffins

- One and a half tablespoons of steak sauce
- One cup of mozzarella cheese
- A quarter cup of sliced green onion
- One can of tomato paste
- Half pound of ground beef
- One cup of parmesan cheese

Instructions

- Crumble meat in a bowl; add onion, tomato paste, Italian herb, and steak sauce.
- Stir well.
- Spread the mixture on muffins and transfer to the Air Fryer Grill pan.
- Set the Air Fryer Grill to the pizza function.
- Cook for about 20 minutes on both sides at 350F.
- Serve immediately with green onions and cheese.

Mini Spinach Quiches

Preparation Time-10 minutes | Cook Time-25 minutes | Servings-2 | Difficulty-Moderate

Nutritional Facts- Calories-329 | Fats-21.9g |Carbohydrates-23g |Proteins-7.8g

Ingredients

- One (9-inch) premade pie crust, thawed
- One egg
- A quarter cup of sharp shredded cheddar cheese
- A quarter cup of whole milk
- A quarter cup of heavy cream
- A quarter cup of frozen spinach, drained
- Salt and freshly ground black pepper, to taste

Instructions

- Arrange the circle into a muffin pan.
- With a fork, holes in the bottom of every pie shell and put aside.
- In a bowl, add the remaining ingredients and beat until well combined.
- Divide the mixture over each pie shell evenly.
- Turn the "Temperature Knob" of the Air Fryer Grill to line the temperature to 375 degrees F.
- Turn the "Function Knob" to settle on "Bake."
- Turn the "Timer Knob" to line the Time for 25 minutes.
- After preheating, arrange the muffin pan over the roasting rack.

- Insert the roasting rack at position 3 of the Air Fryer Grill.
- When the cooking time is over, remove the muffin pan and put it aside for about 5 minutes before serving.

Mushroom and Squash Toast

Preparation Time-10 minutes | Cook Time-15 minutes | Servings-2 | Difficulty-Easy

Nutritional Facts- Calories-136 | Fats-14g | Carbohydrates-4g | Proteins-10.2g

Ingredients

- One tablespoon of olive oil
- One red bell pepper, cut into strips
- One sliced green onion
- One cup of sliced button or cremini mushrooms
- One sliced small yellow squash
- Two tablespoons of softened butter
- Two slices of bread
- Half cup of soft goat cheese

Instructions

- Brush the crisper tray with olive oil.
- Place the crisper tray in the air fry position. Select Air Fry, set the temperature to 350 degrees F (177C) and set the time to 7 minutes.
- Put the red pepper, green onions, mushrooms, and squash inside the crisper tray and give them a stir. Air fry for 7 minutes or the vegetable is tender, shaking the crisper tray once throughout the cooking time.
- Remove the vegetables and set them aside.
- Spread the butter on the slices of bread and transfer to the crisper tray, butter-side up. Air fry for 3 minutes.
- Remove the toast from the grill and top with goat cheese and vegetables. Serve warm.

Mushroom Wonton

Preparation Time-10 minutes | Cook Time-25 minutes | Servings-2 | Difficulty-Easy

Nutritional Facts- Calories-132 | Fats-6g | Carbohydrates-12g | Proteins-6.9g

Ingredients

For dough

- One and a half cups of all-purpose flour
- Two teaspoons of salt or to taste
- Five tablespoons of water

For filling

- Two cups of cubed mushroom
- Two tablespoons of oil
- Two teaspoons of ginger-garlic paste
- Two teaspoons of soya sauce
- Two teaspoons of vinegar

Instructions

- Knead the dough and cover it with plastic wrap, and set it aside. Next, cook the ingredients for the filling and try to ensure that the mushroom is covered well with the sauce.
- Roll the dough and place the filling in the center. Now, wrap the dough to cover the filling and pinch the edges together.
- Preheat the Air fryer at 200° F for 5 minutes. Place the dumplings in the fry basket and close it. Let them cook at the same temperature for another 20 minutes.
- Recommended sides are chili sauce or ketchup.

Mushrooms Appetizer

Preparation Time-10 minutes | Cook Time-10 minutes | Servings-2 | Difficulty-Easy

Nutritional Facts- Calories-201 | Fats-15g | Carbohydrates-15g | Proteins-13.8g

Ingredients

- A quarter cup of mayonnaise
- One teaspoon of garlic powder
- One chopped small yellow onion
- Twenty-four ounces of white mushroom caps
- Salt and black pepper to the taste
- One teaspoon of curry powder
- Four ounces of soft cream cheese
- A quarter cup of sour cream
- Half cup of shredded Mexican cheese
- One cup of cooked, peeled, deveined and chopped shrimp

Instructions

- In a bowl, mix mayo with garlic powder, onion, curry powder, cream cheese, sour cream,

Mexican cheese, shrimp, salt and pepper to the taste and whisk well.

- Stuff mushrooms with this mix, place them in your air fryer's basket and cook at 300 degrees F for 10 minutes.
- Arrange on a platter and serve as an appetizer.

Mutton galette

Preparation Time-10 minutes | Cook Time-30 minutes | Servings-2 | Difficulty-Easy

Nutritional Facts- Calories-161 | Fats-7.8g |Carbohydrates-6.9g |Proteins-19g

Ingredients

- Two tablespoons of garam masala
- One lb. of minced mutton
- Three teaspoons of finely chopped ginger
- Two tablespoons of fresh coriander leaves
- Three finely chopped green chilies
- One and a half tablespoons of lemon juice
- Salt and pepper to taste

Instructions

- Mix the ingredients in a clean bowl.
- Mold this mixture into round and flat galettes.
- Wet the galettes slightly with water.
- Preheat the Air Fryer at 160 degrees Fahrenheit for 5 minutes. Place the galettes in the fry basket and let them cook for another 25 minutes at the same temperature. Keep rolling them over to get a uniform cook.
- Serve either with mint chutney or ketchup.

Nacho Coated Prawns

Preparation Time-30 minutes | Cook Time-10 minutes | Servings-2 | Difficulty-Easy

Nutritional Facts- Calories-190 | Fats-7.8g |Carbohydrates-21g |Proteins-13.8g

Ingredients

- Nine ounces of nacho chips
- One whisked egg
- Eighteen medium-sized prawns

Instructions

- Remove the shell and veins from the prawns, wash thoroughly and wipe dry.

- Grind the chips in a bowl until pieces are as that of breadcrumbs.
- Dip each prawn into the egg and then coat with the chip crumbs.
- Heat the air fryer to 356°F.
- Put the prawns into the air fryer and cook for 8 minutes. Serve with salsa or sour cream.

Onion Pakoda

Preparation Time-10 minutes | Cook Time-10 minutes | Servings-2 | Difficulty-Easy

Nutritional Facts- Calories-132 | Fats-12g |Carbohydrates-4g |Proteins-12.9g

Ingredients

- One cup of gram flour
- One tablespoon of coriander seeds of crushed
- One teaspoon of red chili powder
- A quarter teaspoon of turmeric powder
- Finely chopped coriander leaves(optional)
- Two onions medium-sized, peeled and thinly sliced
- One teaspoon of methi of kasoori
- 3/4 teaspoon of salt
- A quarter teaspoon of baking soda

Instructions

- Combine all of the ingredients in a large mixing basin and set aside for 5 minutes, covered. Due to the salt, the onions will release some moisture; use this to bind everything together into a dough, adding a few sprinkles of water as needed. If you make it too wet, it won't crisp up.
- By squeezing it into logs in your slightly oiled palm, you can make bite-sized pakodas.
- Turn the timer to 5 minutes to preheat the air fryer at 200 C, but the machine is ready when the indicator light goes out.
- Cover the basket with a sheet of parchment paper or lightly oiled aluminum foil, leaving some of the edges uncovered. This isn't required, but it makes cleaning a lot easier. Air fried the pakodas in a single layer for 5 minutes. After that, remove the basket, turn them around to the other side, or give it a shake, and cook for another 5 minutes, or until golden brown on all sides.

- Serve with green chutney, tamarind chutney, or ketchup right away. You can also create Pakoda Kadhi or Moar Kozhambu using these.

Parmesan Breaded Zucchini Chips

Preparation Time-15 minutes | Cook Time-20 minutes | Servings-2 | Difficulty-Easy

Nutritional Facts- Calories-201 | Fats-12.9g |Carbohydrates-1g|Proteins-6g

Ingredients

For the lemon aioli

- Half cup of mayonnaise
- Two tablespoons of olive oil
- Juice of one lemon
- One teaspoon of minced garlic
- Salt
- Pepper

For the zucchini chips

- Two medium zucchinis
- Two eggs
- 1/3 cup of bread crumbs
- 1/3 cup of grated Parmesan cheese
- Salt
- Pepper
- Cooking oil

Instructions

To make the zucchini chips

- Using a knife or mandolin, slice the zucchini into thin chips (approximately 1/8 inch thick).
- Beat the eggs in a small bowl. Combine the Parmesan cheese, bread crumbs, and salt & pepper to taste in a separate small bowl.
- Cooking oil should be sprayed into the air fryer basket.
- Dip the zucchini slices in the eggs one at a time, then in the bread crumb mixture. You can also use a spoon to sprinkle the bread crumbs on the zucchini slices.
- In the air fryer basket, arrange the zucchini chips but do not stack them.
- Fill the oven rack/basket with the mixture. Place the rack in the Air fryer oven's middle shelf. Cook in batches if possible. Cooking oil should be sprayed on the chips from a distance. Cook for 10 minutes before serving.
- Take the cooked zucchini chips from the air fryer and repeat with the rest of the zucchini.

To make the lemon aioli

- Combine the lemon juice, olive oil, mayonnaise, and garlic in a small bowl while the zucchini is cooking, seasoning with salt and pepper to taste. In a large mixing bowl, blend all of the ingredients until they are completely incorporated.
- Allow the zucchini to cool before serving with the aioli.

Patatas Bravas

Preparation Time-10 minutes | Cook Time-15 minutes | Servings-2 | Difficulty-Easy

Nutritional Facts- Calories-186 | Fats-6g |Carbohydrates-18g|Proteins-1.5g

Ingredients

- A pinch of sea salt & pepper
- Half teaspoon of cayenne (optional)
- One teaspoon of garlic powder
- One tablespoon of avocado oil
- Two red potatoes, cut into 1-inch chunks
- Pepper and sea salt to taste
- One tablespoon of smoked paprika
- Garlic aioli
- Dried chives

Instructions

- Bring a water pot to a boil. Insert the potatoes and let them boil for a period of 6 minutes. Use a strainer to extract the potatoes and put them on a towel (Kitchen) to pat them dry and let them cool. After the potatoes have cooled down to room temperature and are dry, add them with garlic powder, avocado oil, pepper and salt in a large bowl. The potatoes are then to be coated and then transfer ideally in batches to an air-fryer tray.
- Adjust the air fryer to 199C.
- Add this tray to your device and let it cook for around fifteen to sixteen minutes, shake the basket constantly every seven minutes. Also, brush the potatoes gently with oil(avocado) before frying to ensure a good crisp outer coating.

- Transfer the potatoes to a bowl and brush lightly with oil (avocado). Apply the seasonings and slightly shake the bowl in order to coat the potatoes, then enjoy with garlic aioli or any other condiment of your choice.

Pesto Crackers

Preparation Time-10 minutes | Cook Time- 20 minutes | Servings-2 | Difficulty-Easy

Nutritional Facts- Calories-194 | Fats-12g |Carbohydrates-4.8g |Proteins-7.8g

Ingredients

- Half teaspoon of baking powder
- Salt and black pepper to the taste
- One cup of flour
- A quarter teaspoon of basil, dried
- One minced garlic clove
- Two tablespoons of basil pesto
- Two tablespoons of butter

Instructions

- In a bowl, mix salt, pepper, baking powder, flour, garlic, cayenne, basil, pesto and butter and stir until you obtain a dough.
- Spread this dough on a lined baking sheet that fits your air fryer, introduce it in the fryer at 325 degrees F and bake for 17 minutes.
- Leave aside to cool down, cut crackers and serve them as a snack.
- Enjoy!

Philly Cheesesteaks

Preparation Time-20 minutes | Cook Time-20 minutes | Servings-2 | Difficulty-Easy

Nutritional Facts- Calories-122 | Fats-7.8g |Carbohydrates-14g |Proteins-4.2g

Ingredients

- Twelve ounces of thinly sliced boneless rib-eye steak
- Half teaspoon of Worcestershire sauce
- Half teaspoon of soy sauce
- Kosher salt and black pepper, to taste
- Half stemmed, deseeded, and thinly sliced green bell pepper
- Half thinly sliced small onion

- One tablespoon of vegetable oil
- Two soft hoagie rolls, split three-fourths of the way through
- One tablespoon of softened butter
- Two halved slices of provolone cheese

Instructions

- Combine the steak, Worcestershire sauce, soy sauce, salt, and ground black pepper in a large bowl. Toss to coat well. Set aside.
- Combine the bell pepper, onion, salt, ground black pepper, and vegetable oil in a separate bowl. Toss to coat the vegetables well.
- Pour the steak and vegetables into the air fryer basket.
- Slide the basket into the air fryer. Cook at the corresponding preset mode or Air Fry at 400F (205C) for 15 minutes.
- When cooked, the steak will be browned, and the vegetables will be tender. Transfer them to a plate. Set aside.
- Brush the hoagie rolls with butter and place them in the basket.
- Slide the basket in the air fryer and toast for 3 minutes. When done, the rolls should be lightly browned.
- Transfer the rolls to a clean work surface and divide the steak and vegetable mix in between the rolls. Spread with cheese. Put the stuffed rolls back in the basket.
- Cook for 2 minutes. Bring the basket back to the air fryer. When done, the cheese should be melted.
- Serve immediately.

Plantains

Preparation Time-10 minutes | Cook Time-13 minutes | Servings-2 | Difficulty-Easy

Nutritional Facts- Calories-130 | Fats-1g |Carbohydrates-20g |Proteins-12g

Ingredients

- One teaspoon of neutral oil
- One ripe plantain
- A pinch of salt

Instructions

- Cut the plantain, cutting parts that are around

1/2" thick.

- In a medium bowl, combine the plantain slices, oil, and salt together. Make sure all the pieces are covered in oil.
- Move to your air fryer basket and fry for 8-10 minutes at 400 ° F, shaking after 5 minutes. The plantains are finished when they are browned on the outside and soft on the inside. Depending on how ripe your plantains are, frying time can vary. Check-in at 8 minutes and, if necessary, add another minute or two to hit the nice, browned outside.

Polenta Bites

Preparation Time-10 minutes | Cook Time-20 minutes | Servings-2 | Difficulty-Easy

Nutritional Facts- Calories-231 | Fats-6.9g |Carbohydrates-12g |Proteins-4g

Ingredients

For the polenta

- One tablespoon of butter
- One cup of cornmeal
- One and a half cups of water
- Salt and black pepper to the taste

For the polenta bites

- Two tablespoons of powdered sugar
- Cooking spray

Instructions

- In a saucepan, combine water, cornmeal, butter, salt, and pepper; stir to combine; bring to a boil over medium heat; cook for 10 minutes; remove from heat; whisk once more; chill until cool.
- One tablespoon of polenta, shaped into a ball, placed on a work surface
- Repeat with the remaining polenta, then place all of the balls in the air fryer's cooking basket, spray with cooking spray, cover, and cook for 8 minutes at 380 degrees F.
- Serve polenta bits for breakfast by arranging them among plates and sprinkling sugar over them.
- Enjoy!

Popcorn

Preparation Time-10 minutes | Cook Time-10 minutes | Servings-2 | Difficulty-Easy

Nutritional Facts- Calories-30 | Fats-1g |Carbohydrates-4.8g |Proteins-0g

Ingredients

- Three tablespoons of dried corn kernels
- Two tablespoons of nutritional yeast dried chives
- Avocado oil spray or other oil like peanut oil, sunflower oil or coconut oil
- Pepper and sea salt to taste

Instructions

- Set the Air Fryer System to (199C).
- Add the kernels to the basket of the fryer and spray gently with a little oil. To avoid popped popcorn from escaping the basket and floating around in the air fryer, line the tray sides with aluminum foil if necessary.
- Insert the basket. Set 15 minutes time. Check it every 5 minutes to make sure that the kernels do not burn. Once they start popping, keep a close eye on them until the popping sound ceases, or until 15 minutes have passed.
- Immediately empty the basket and pour the contents into a large bowl. Spray with coconut or avocado oil gently.
- Enjoy warm or at room temperature.

Pork and Cabbage Gyoza

Preparation Time-10 minutes | Cook Time-10 minutes | Servings-2 | Difficulty-Easy

Nutritional Facts- Calories-230 | Fats-10.8g |Carbohydrates-1.5g |Proteins-27g

Ingredients

- Half pound of ground pork
- Half pound of thinly sliced and minced Napa cabbage
- Half cup of minced scallions
- One teaspoon of minced fresh chives
- One teaspoon of soy sauce
- One teaspoon of minced fresh ginger
- One tablespoon of minced garlic
- One teaspoon of granulated sugar
- Two teaspoons of kosher salt

- Twenty wonton or dumpling wrappers
- Cooking spray

Instructions

- Set the air fryer basket with cooking spray. Set aside.
- Make the filling: Combine all the ingredients, except for the wrappers, in a large bowl. Stir to mix well.
- Unfold a wrapper on a clean work surface, and then dab the edges with a little water. Scoop up Two teaspoons of the filling mixture in the center.
- Make the gyoza: Fold the wrapper over to filling and press the edges to seal. Pleat the edges if desired. Repeat with remaining wrappers and fillings.
- Arrange the gyozas in the basket and spritz with cooking spray.
- Slide the basket into the air fryer. Cook at the corresponding preset mode or Air Fry at 360F (182C) for 10 minutes.
- Flip the gyozas halfway through the cooking time.
- When cooked, the gyozas will be golden brown.
- Serve immediately.

Pork and Carrot Momos

Preparation Time-20 minutes | Cook Time-20 minutes | Servings-2 | Difficulty-Moderate

Nutritional Facts- Calories-290 | Fats-9.9g |Carbohydrates-1g|Proteins-40g

Ingredients

- Two tablespoons of olive oil
- One pound of ground pork
- One shredded carrot
- One chopped onion
- One teaspoon of soy sauce
- Sixteen wonton wrappers
- Salt and ground black pepper, to taste
- Cooking spray

Instructions

- Warm the olive oil in a nonstick skillet until shimmering.
- Add the ground pork, carrot, onion, soy sauce, salt, and ground black pepper and sauté for 10 minutes or until the pork is well browned and carrots are tender.

- Unfold the wrappers on a clean work surface, and then divide the cooked pork and vegetables on the wrappers. Set the edges around the filling to form momos. Nip the top to seal the momos.
- Arrange the momos in the air fryer basket and spritz with cooking spray.
- Slide the basket into the air fryer. Cook at the corresponding preset mode or Air Fry at 320 degrees F (160C) for 10 minutes.
- When cooking is complete, the wrappers will be lightly browned.
- Serve immediately.

Pork Rolls

Preparation Time-10 minutes | Cook Time-40 minutes | Servings-2 | Difficulty-Moderate

Nutritional Facts- Calories- 304| Fats-12g |Carbohydrates-15g |Proteins-23g

Ingredients

- One fifteen-ounce pork fillet
- Half teaspoon of chili powder
- One teaspoon of cinnamon powder
- One minced garlic clove
- Salt and black pepper to the taste
- Two tablespoons of olive oil
- One and a half teaspoons of ground cumin
- One chopped red onion
- Three tablespoons of chopped parsley

Instructions

- In a bowl, mix cinnamon with garlic, salt, pepper, chili powder, oil, onion, parsley and cumin and stir well.
- Put pork fillet on a cutting board, flatten it using a meat tenderizer. And use a meat tenderizer to flatten it.
- Spread onion mix on pork, roll tight, cut into medium rolls, place them in your preheated air fryer at 360 degrees F and cook them for 35 minutes.
- Arrange them on a platter and serve as an appetizer.
- Enjoy!

Pork Sliders

Preparation Time-10 minutes | Cook Time-15 minutes | Servings-2 | Difficulty-Easy

Nutritional Facts- Calories-122 | Fats-7.8g |Carbohydrates-14g |Proteins-4.2g

Ingredients

- Half pound of ground pork
- One tablespoon of Thai curry paste
- One tablespoon of fish sauce
- A quarter cup of thinly sliced scallions
- Two tablespoons of minced peeled fresh ginger
- One tablespoon of light brown sugar
- One teaspoon of ground black pepper
- Two to four slider buns split open lengthwise, warmed
- Cooking spray

Instructions

- Set the air fryer basket with cooking spray.
- Combine all the ingredients, except for the buns, in a large bowl. Stir to mix well.
- Divide and shape the mixture into six balls, then bash the balls into six 3-inch-diameter patties.
- Arrange the patties in the basket and spritz with cooking spray.
- Slide the basket into the air fryer. Cook at the corresponding preset mode or Air Fry at 375F (190C) for 14 minutes.
- Set the patties halfway through the cooking time.
- When cooked, the patties should be well browned.
- Assemble the buns with patties to make the sliders and serve immediately.

Pork Wontons

Preparation Time-10 minutes | Cook Time-25 minutes | Servings-2 | Difficulty-Easy

Nutritional Facts- Calories-151 | Fats-6.9g |Carbohydrates-12g |Proteins-15.9g

Ingredients

For dough

- One and a half cups of all-purpose flour
- Two teaspoons of salt
- Five tablespoons of water

For filling

- Two cups of minced pork
- Two tablespoons of oil
- Two teaspoons of ginger-garlic paste
- Two teaspoons of soya sauce
- Two teaspoons of vinegar

Instructions

- Knead the dough and cover it with plastic wrap, and set it aside. Next, cook the ingredients for the filling and try to ensure that the pork is covered well with the sauce.
- Roll the dough and place the filling in the center. Now, wrap the dough to cover the filling and pinch the edges together.
- Preheat the Air fryer at 200° F for 5 minutes. Place the wontons in the fry basket and close it. Let them cook at the same temperature for another 20 minutes.
- Recommended sides are chili sauce or ketchup.

Potato and Pea Samosas with Chutney

Preparation Time-30 minutes | Cook Time-22 minutes | Servings-2 | Difficulty-Moderate

Nutritional Facts- Calories-620 | Fats-30g |Carbohydrates-72g |Proteins-9.9g

Ingredients

Dough

- Two cups of all-purpose flour
- Four tablespoons of plain yogurt
- A quarter cup of cold unsalted butter
- Two teaspoons of kosher salt
- Half cup of ice water

Filling

- One tablespoon of vegetable oil
- Half diced onion
- One teaspoon of coriander
- One teaspoon of cumin
- One minced garlic clove
- One teaspoon of turmeric
- One teaspoon of kosher salt
- A quarter cup of peas, thawed if frozen
- Two cups of mashed potatoes
- Two tablespoons of yogurt

- Cooking spray

Chutney

- One cup of lightly packed mint leaves
- Two cups of lightly packed cilantro leaves
- Onc deseeded and minced green chili pepper
- Half cup of minced onion
- Juice of one lime
- One teaspoon of granulated sugar
- One teaspoon of kosher salt
- Two tablespoons of vegetable oil

Instructions

- Put the flour, yogurt, butter, and salt in a food processor. Pulse to combine until grainy. Pour in the water and pulse until a smooth and firm dough forms.
- Transfer the dough to a clean and lightly floured working surface. Knead the dough and shape it into a ball. Cut in half and flatten the halves into two discs. Wrap them in plastic and let them sit in the refrigerator until ready to use.
- Meanwhile, make the filling: Warmth the vegetable oil in a saucepan over medium heat.
- Attach the onion and sauté for 5 minutes or until lightly browned.
- Add the coriander, cumin, garlic, turmeric, and salt and sauté for 2 minutes or until fragrant.
- Add the peas, potatoes, and yogurt and stir to combine well. Turn off the heat and allow cooling.
- Meanwhile, combine the ingredients for the chutney in a food processor. Pulse to mix well until glossy. Set the chutney in a bowl and refrigerate until ready to use.
- Make the samosas: Remove the dough discs from the refrigerator and cut each disc into eight parts. Shape each part into a ball, and then roll the ball into a 6-inch circle. Divide the circle in half and roll each half into a cone.
- Scoop up two tablespoons of the filling into the cone; press the edges of the cone to seal and form into a triangle. Repeat with remaining dough and filling.
- Set the air fryer basket with cooking spray. Arrange the samosas in the basket and spritz with cooking spray.

- Slide the basket into the air fryer. Cook at the corresponding preset mode or Air Fry at 360F (182C) for 15 minutes.
- Flip the samosas halfway through the cooking time.
- When cooked, the samosas will be golden brown and crispy.
- Serve the samosas with the chutney.

Potato Spread

Preparation Time-10 minutes | Cook Time- 10 minutes | Servings-2 | Difficulty-Easy

Nutritional Facts- Calories-198 | Fats-1g|Carbohydrates-30g |Proteins- 10.8g

Ingredients

- Eight ounces canned garbanzo beans, drained
- One cup of peeled and chopped sweet potatoes
- A quarter cup of tahini
- Two tablespoons of lemon juice
- One tablespoon of olive oil
- Two minced garlic cloves
- Half teaspoon of ground cumin
- Two tablespoons of water
- A pinch of salt and white pepper

Instructions

- Put potatoes in your air fryer's basket, cook them at 360 degrees F for 15 minutes, cool them down, peel and put them in your food processor and pulse well.
- Add sesame paste, garlic, beans, lemon juice, cumin, water and oil and pulse really well.
- Add salt and pepper, pulse again, divide into bowls and serve.
- Enjoy!

Prawn galette

Preparation Time-10 minutes | Cook Time-30 minutes | Servings-2 | Difficulty-Easy

Nutritional Facts- Calories-147 | Fats-6.9g |Carbohydrates-7.8g |Proteins-13.8g

Ingredients

- Two tablespoons of garam masala
- One lb. of minced prawn
- Three teaspoons of finely chopped ginger

- Two tablespoons of fresh coriander leaves
- Three finely chopped green chilies
- Two tablespoons of lemon juice
- Salt and pepper to taste

Instructions

- Mix the ingredients in a clean bowl.
- Mold this mixture into round and flat galettes.
- Wet the galettes slightly with water.
- Preheat the Air Fryer at 160 degrees Fahrenheit for 5 minutes. Place the galettes in the fry basket and let them cook for another 25 minutes at the same temperature. Keep rolling them over to get a uniform cook.
- Serve either with mint chutney or ketchup.

Prawn Momos

Preparation Time-10 minutes | Cook Time-25 minutes | Servings-2 | Difficulty-Easy

Nutritional Facts- Calories-159 | Fats-1g|Carbohydrates-9g|Proteins-6.9g

Ingredients

For dough

- One and a half cups of all-purpose flour
- Two teaspoons of salt
- Five tablespoons of water

For filling

- Two cups of minced prawn
- Two tablespoons of oil
- Two teaspoons of ginger-garlic paste
- Two teaspoons of soya sauce
- Two teaspoons of vinegar

Instructions

- Knead the dough and cover it with plastic wrap, and set it aside. Next, cook the ingredients for the filling and try to ensure that the prawn is covered well with the sauce.
- Roll the dough and cut it into a square. Place the filling in the center. Now, wrap the dough to cover the filling and pinch the edges together.
- Preheat the Air fryer at 200° F for 5 minutes. Place the wontons in the fry basket and close it. Let them cook at the same temperature for another 20 minutes.
- Recommended sides are chili sauce or ketchup.

Pumpkin Muffins

Preparation Time-10 minutes | Cook Time-20 minutes | Servings-2 | Difficulty-

Nutritional Facts- Calories-60 | Fats-17g|Carbohydrates-1.5g|Proteins-1.5g

Ingredients

- A quarter cup of butter
- 3/4 cup of pumpkin puree
- Two tablespoons of flaxseed meal
- A quarter cup of flour
- Half cup of sugar
- Half teaspoon of nutmeg, ground
- One teaspoon of cinnamon powder
- Half teaspoon of baking soda
- One egg
- Half teaspoon of baking powder

Instructions

- In a bowl, mix butter with pumpkin puree and egg and blend well.
- Add flaxseed meal, flour, sugar, baking soda, baking powder, nutmeg and cinnamon and stir well.
- Spoon this into a muffin pan that fits your fryer, introduce it in the fryer at 350 degrees F and bake for 15 minutes.
- Serve muffins cold as a snack.
- Enjoy!

Radish Hash Browns

Preparation Time-10 minutes | Cook Time-15 minutes | Servings-2 | Difficulty-Easy

Nutritional Facts- Calories-70 | Fats-4g |Carbohydrates-6.9g|Proteins-1.2g

Ingredients

- Half lb. radishes washed and cut off roots
- One tablespoon of olive oil
- Half teaspoon of paprika
- Half teaspoon of onion powder
- Half teaspoon of garlic powder
- One medium onion
- A quarter teaspoon of pepper
- 3/4 teaspoon of sea salt

Instructions

- Using a mandolin slicer, thinly slice the onion and radishes.
- Toss sliced radishes and onions with olive oil in a large mixing basin.
- Cook for 8 minutes at 360°F in an air fryer basket with onion and radish pieces. Shake the basket twice more.
- Toss the radish and onion slices with the seasonings in a mixing bowl.
- In an air fryer basket, cook radish and onion slices for 5 minutes at 400 degrees F. Halfway through, give the basket a good shake.
- Serve and have fun.

Rice, Shrimp, and Spinach Frittata

Preparation Time-15 minutes | Cook Time-16 minutes | Servings-2 | Difficulty-Easy

Nutritional Facts- Calories-192 | Fats-9.9g |Carbohydrates-15g |Proteins-12.9g

Ingredients

- Two eggs
- Pinch salt
- A quarter cup of cooked rice
- A quarter cup of chopped cooked shrimp
- A quarter cup of baby spinach
- A quarter cup of grated Monterey Jack cheese
- Nonstick cooking spray

Instructions

- Set a baking pan with nonstick cooking spray.
- Pour the eggs and salt in a small bowl until frothy.
- Set the cooked rice, shrimp, and baby spinach in the baking pan. Set in the whisked eggs and scatter the cheese on top.
- Bring the pan into the air fryer oven. Press the Power Button. Cook at 320F (160C) for 16 minutes.
- When cooking is processed, the frittata should be golden and puffy.
- Set the frittata to cool for 5 minutes before slicing to serve.

Risotto Croquettes with Tomato Sauce

Preparation Time-One hour and 40 minutes | Cook Time-54 minutes | Servings-2 | Difficulty-Hard

Nutritional Facts- Calories-384 | Fats-23g |Carbohydrates-10.5g |Proteins-34.2g

Ingredients

Risotto Croquettes

- Two tablespoons of unsalted butter
- One small yellow onion, minced
- Half cup of Arborio rice
- Two and a half cups of chicken stock
- Half cup of dry white wine
- Two eggs
- Zest of one lemon
- Half cup of grated Parmesan cheese
- One ounce of fresh Mozzarella cheese
- A quarter cup of peas
- Two tablespoons of water
- Half cup of all-purpose flour
- One cup of panko bread crumbs
- Kosher salt and black pepper, to taste
- Cooking spray

Tomato Sauce

- Two tablespoons of extra-virgin olive oil
- Two minced cloves of garlic
- A quarter teaspoon of red pepper flakes
- One can of crushed tomatoes
- Two teaspoons of granulated sugar
- Kosher salt and black pepper, to taste

Instructions

- Melt the butter in a pot over medium heat, then add the onion and salt to taste. Set for 5 minutes or until the onion is translucent.
- Add the rice and stir to coat well. Cook for 3 minutes or until the rice is lightly browned. Pour in the chicken stock and wine.
- Bring to a boil. Then cook for 20 minutes or until the rice is tender and liquid is almost absorbed.
- Make the risotto: When the rice is cooked, break the egg into the pot. Add the lemon zest and Parmesan cheese. Sprinkle with salt and ground black pepper. Stir to mix well.
- Pour the risotto into a baking sheet, then level with a spatula to spread the risotto evenly. Wrap

the baking sheet in plastic and refrigerate for 1 an hour.

- Meanwhile, heat the olive oil in a saucepan over medium heat until shimmering.
- Add the garlic and sprinkle with red pepper flakes. Sauté for a minute or until fragrant.
- Add the crushed tomatoes and sprinkle with sugar. Stir to mix well. Bring to a boil. Set the heat to low and simmer for 15 minutes or until slightly thickened. Sprinkle with salt and pepper to taste. Set aside until ready to serve.
- Remove the risotto from the refrigerator. Scoop the risotto into twelve 2-inch balls, and then flatten the balls with your hands.
- Arrange an about 1/2-inch piece of Mozzarella and five peas in the center of each flattened ball, and then wrap them back into balls.
- Bring the balls to a baking sheet lined with parchment paper, then refrigerate for 15 minutes or until firm.
- Whisk the remaining two eggs with two tablespoons of water in a bowl. Pour the flour into a second bowl and pour the panko into a third bowl.
- Dredge the risotto balls in the bowl of flour first, then into the eggs, and then into the panko. Shake the excess off.
- Transfer the balls to the air fry basket and spritz with cooking spray.
- Place the basket on the bake position.
- Select Bake, set temperature to 400F (205C) and set time to 10 minutes. Flip the balls halfway through the cooking time.
- When cooking is complete, the balls should be golden brown.
- Serve the risotto balls with tomato sauce.

Salmon Fritters

Preparation Time-10 minutes | Cook Time-35 minutes | Servings-2 | Difficulty-Easy

Nutritional Facts- Calories-147 | Fats-6.9g |Carbohydrates-7.8g |Proteins-13.8g

Ingredients

- Two tablespoons of garam masala
- One lb. of fileted Salmon
- Three teaspoons of finely chopped ginger
- Two tablespoons of fresh coriander leaves
- Three finely chopped green chilies
- Two tablespoons of lemon juice
- Salt and pepper to taste

Instructions

- Mix the ingredients in a clean bowl.
- Mold this mixture into round and flat galettes.
- Wet the galettes slightly with water.
- Preheat the Air Fryer at 160 degrees Fahrenheit for 5 minutes. Place the galettes in the fry basket and let them cook for another 25 minutes at the same temperature. Keep rolling them over to get a uniform cook.
- Serve either with mint chutney or ketchup.

Sausage and Cream Cheese Biscuits

Preparation Time-5 minutes | Cook Time-15 minutes | Servings-2 | Difficulty-Easy

Nutritional Facts- Calories-224 | Fats-12.9g |Carbohydrates-20g |Proteins-9.9g

Ingredients

- Six ounces of chicken breakfast sausage
- Three ounces of biscuit dough
- 1/8 cup of cream cheese

Instructions

- Make two tiny patties out of the sausage.
- In the air fryer, place the sausage patties. 5 minutes in the oven
- Activate the air fryer. Turn the patties over. Cook for a further 5 minutes.
- Take the cooked sausages out of the air fryer and set them aside.
- Make two biscuits using the biscuit dough.
- In the air fryer, place the biscuits. 3 minutes in the oven
- Activate the air fryer. Turn the biscuits over. Cook for a further 2 minutes.
- Take the baked biscuits out of the air fryer and set them aside.
- Each biscuit should be split in two. One spoonful of cream cheese should be spread on the bottom of each biscuit. Serve with the second half of the biscuit and a sausage patty on top.

Scrambled Eggs Wonton Cup

Preparation Time-10 minutes | Cook Time-25 minutes | Servings-2 | Difficulty-Easy

Nutritional Facts- Calories-130 | Fats-6.9g |Carbohydrates-7.8g |Proteins-9g

Ingredients

- Four Wonton wrappers
- Four eggs
- One and a half Breakfast sausages
- One large pepper
- Two mushrooms
- One and a half onions
- Butter
- Salt and pepper to taste

Instructions

- Preheat the Air Fryer Grill to 177 C or 350 F.
- Make the scrambled eggs.
- Fold the wrappers brushed with butter into the muffin pan
- Mix the ingredients in a bowl and put them in the wrappers.
- Bake for 10 minutes.

Seafood Appetizer

Preparation Time-10 minutes | Cook Time-25 minutes | Servings-2 | Difficulty-Easy

Nutritional Facts- Calories-169 | Fats-7.8g |Carbohydrates-6.9g |Proteins-6.9g

Ingredients

- Half cup of chopped yellow onion
- One cup of chopped green bell pepper
- One cup of chopped celery
- One cup of peeled and deveined baby shrimp
- One cup of flaked crabmeat
- One cup of homemade mayonnaise
- One teaspoon of Worcestershire sauce
- Salt and black pepper to the taste
- Two tablespoons of bread crumbs
- One tablespoon of butter
- One teaspoon of sweet paprika

Instructions

- In a bowl, mix shrimp with crab meat, bell pepper, onion, mayo, celery, salt and pepper and stir.
- Add Worcestershire sauce, stir again and pour everything into a baking dish that fits your air fryer.
- Sprinkle bread crumbs and add butter, introduce in your air fryer and cook at 320 degrees F for 25 minutes, shaking halfway.
- Divide into a bowl and serve with paprika sprinkled on top as an appetizer.
- Enjoy!

Seafood Pizza

Preparation Time-15 minutes | Cook Time-20 minutes | Servings-2 | Difficulty-Easy

Nutritional Facts- Calories-235 | Fats-9g |Carbohydrates-30g |Proteins-17g

Ingredients

- One pizza base
- Grated pizza cheese (mozzarella cheese preferably) for topping
- Some pizza topping sauce
- Cooking oil for brushing and topping purposes

For toppings

- Two chopped Onions
- Two cups of mixed seafood
- Two chopped capsicums
- Two deseeded and chopped tomatoes
- One tablespoon of mushrooms/corns
- Two teaspoons of pizza seasoning
- Some small cottage cheese cubes (optional)

Instructions

- Put the pizza base in a pre-heated Air fryer for around 5 minutes. (Preheated to 340 Fahrenheit).
- Take out the base. Pour some pizza sauce on top of the base at the center. Using a spoon, spread the sauce over the base, making sure that you leave some gap around the circumference. Grate some mozzarella cheese and sprinkle it over the sauce layer.
- Take all the vegetables and the seafood and mix them in a bowl. Add some oil and seasoning. Also, add some salt and pepper according to taste. Mix them properly. Put this topping over the layer of cheese on the pizza. Now sprinkle some more

grated cheese and pizza seasoning on top of this layer.

- Preheat the Air Fryer at 250 degrees Fahrenheit for around 5 minutes. Open the fry basket and place the pizza inside.
- Close the basket and keep the fryer at 170 degrees for another 10 minutes. If you feel that it is undercooked, you may put it at the same temperature for another 2 minutes or so.

Sheet Pan Shakshuka

Preparation Time-5 minutes | Cook Time-25 minutes | Servings-2 | Difficulty-Easy

Nutritional Facts- Calories-219 | Fats-10.8g | Carbohydrates-20g | Proteins-9.9g

Ingredients

- Two large eggs
- One chopped Anaheim chili
- One tablespoon of vegetable oil
- Half cup of chopped onion
- One teaspoon of ground cumin
- Two minced garlic cloves
- Half cup of feta cheese
- Half teaspoon of paprika
- Half of the tomatoes
- Salt and pepper

Instructions

- Sauté the chili and onions in oil until tender.
- Pour in the remaining ingredients apart from eggs and cook until thick.
- Make two pockets to pour in the eggs.
- Bake for 10 minutes at 191 C or 375 F in the Air Fryer Grill.
- Top it off with feta.

Shrimp and Chestnut Rolls

Preparation Time-10 minutes | Cook Time-15 minutes | Servings-2 | Difficulty-

Nutritional Facts- Calories-157 | Fats-4g | Carbohydrates-12g | Proteins-4g

Ingredients

- Half pound already cooked and chopped shrimp
- Eight ounces of chopped water chestnuts
- Half pounds of chopped shiitake mushrooms

- Two cups of chopped cabbage
- Two tablespoons of olive oil
- One minced garlic clove
- One teaspoon of grated ginger
- Three chopped scallions
- Salt and black pepper to the taste
- One tablespoon of water
- One egg yolk
- Six spring roll wrappers

Instructions

- Heat up a pan with the oil over medium-high heat, add cabbage, shrimp, chestnuts, mushrooms, garlic, ginger, scallions, salt and pepper, stir and cook for 2 minutes.
- In a bowl, mix egg with water and stir well.
- Arrange roll wrappers on a working surface, divide shrimp and veggie mix on them, seal edges with egg wash, place them all in your air fryer's basket, cook at 360 degrees F for 15 minutes, transfer to a platter and serve as an appetizer.
- Enjoy!

Shrimp and Sesame Seed Toasts

Preparation Time-15 minutes | Cook Time-10 minutes | Servings-2 | Difficulty-Easy

Nutritional Facts- Calories-523 | Fats-12g | Carbohydrates-34g | Proteins-41g

Ingredients

- A quarter-pound of peeled and deveined raw shrimp
- One beaten egg
- Two chopped scallions plus more for garnish
- Two tablespoons of chopped fresh cilantro
- Two teaspoons of grated fresh ginger
- One teaspoon of sriracha sauce
- One teaspoon of soy sauce
- Half teaspoon of toasted sesame oil
- Four slices of thinly sliced white sandwich bread
- A quarter cup of sesame seeds
- Cooking spray
- Thai chili sauce, for serving

Instructions

- In a food processor, attach the shrimp, egg, scallions, cilantro, ginger, sriracha sauce, soy sauce and sesame oil, and pulse until chopped finely. Transfer the shrimp mixture to a bowl.

- On a clean work surface, cut the crusts off the sandwich bread. Using a brush, generously brush one side of each slice of bread with shrimp mixture.
- Put the sesame seeds on a plate. Press bread slices, shrimp side down, into sesame seeds to coat evenly. Cut each slice diagonally into quarters.
- Set the air fryer basket with cooking spray. Spread the coated slices in a single layer in the air fryer basket.
- Slide the basket into the air fryer. Cook at the corresponding preset mode or Air Fry at 400F (205C) for 8 minutes.
- Flip the bread slices halfway through.
- When cooking is processed, it should be golden and crispy. Detach from the air fryer to a plate and let cool for 5 minutes. Top with the chopped scallions and serve warm with Thai chili sauce.

Shrimp Muffins

Preparation Time-10 minutes | Cook Time-30 minutes | Servings-2 | Difficulty-Moderate

Nutritional Facts- Calories-60 | Fats-1.5g |Carbohydrates-4g |Proteins-4g

Ingredients

- Half of the spaghetti squash, peeled and halved
- One tablespoon of mayonnaise
- Half cup of mozzarella, shredded
- Four ounces of shrimp, peeled, cooked and chopped
- One cup of panko
- One teaspoon of parsley flakes
- One minced garlic clove
- Salt and black pepper to the taste
- Cooking spray

Instructions

- Put squash halves in your air fryer, cook at 350 degrees F for 16 minutes, leave aside to cool down and scrape flesh into a bowl.
- Add salt, pepper, parsley flakes, panko, shrimp, mayo and mozzarella and stir well.
- Spray a muffin tray that fits your air fryer with cooking spray and divide squash and shrimp mix in each cup.

- Introduce in the fryer and cook at 360 degrees F for 10 minutes.
- Arrange muffins on a platter and serve as a snack.
- Enjoy!

Simple Roasted Okra

Preparation Time-10 minutes | Cook Time-15 minutes | Servings-2 | Difficulty-Easy

Nutritional Facts- Calories-176 | Fats-17g |Carbohydrates-6g |Proteins-2.4g

Ingredients

- One lb. of trimmed and sliced okra
- Two teaspoons of olive oil
- Pepper
- Salt

Instructions

- Preheat the air fryer to 350 F.
- Mix together okra, oil, pepper, and salt.
- Add okra into the air fryer basket and cook for 10 minutes. Toss halfway through.
- Toss well and cook for 2 minutes more.
- Serve and enjoy.

Simple Stuffed Tomatoes

Preparation Time-10 minutes | Cook Time-15 minutes | Servings-2 | Difficulty-Easy

Nutritional Facts- Calories-143 | Fats-4g |Carbohydrates-9.9g |Proteins-4g

Ingredients

- Two pulp scooped and chopped tomatoes
- Salt and black pepper to the taste
- Half chopped yellow onion
- One tablespoon of butter
- One tablespoon of chopped celery
- Half cup of chopped mushrooms
- One tablespoon of bread crumbs
- Half cup of cottage cheese
- A quarter teaspoon of caraway seeds
- One tablespoon of chopped parsley

Instructions

- Heat up a pan with the butter over medium heat, melt it, add onion and celery, stir and cook for 3 minutes.

- Add tomato pulp and mushrooms, stir and cook for 1 minute more.
- Add salt, pepper, crumbled bread, cheese, caraway seeds and parsley, stir, cook for 4 minutes more and take off the heat.
- Stuff tomatoes with this mix, place them in your air fryer and cook at 350 degrees F for 8 minutes.
- Divide stuffed tomatoes among plates and serve.
- Enjoy!

Smoked Ham and Venison Sausage

Preparation Time-10 minutes | Cook Time-20 minutes | Servings-2 | Difficulty-Easy

Nutritional Facts- Calories-112 | Fats-7.8g |Carbohydrates-4g |Proteins-9.9g

Ingredients

- One teaspoon of dried sage
- Cayenne
- One teaspoon of thyme
- One and a half lb. of venison
- One teaspoon of salt
- Half lb. of smoked ham
- One teaspoon of ground pepper
- Half lb. of bacon

Instructions

- In a bowl, mix venison, thyme, sage, ground pepper, salt, and cayenne.
- Cut the meats into pieces.
- Mix all ingredients.
- Shape platter out of it.
- Place the platter on the Air Fryer Grill pan.
- Set the Air Fryer Grill to the broil function.
- Cook for 15 minutes at 400 F.

Spicy Brussels Sprouts

Preparation Time-10 minutes | Cook Time-15 minutes | Servings-2 | Difficulty-Easy

Nutritional Facts- Calories-82 | Fats-4g |Carbohydrates-10.8g |Proteins-4g

Ingredients

- Half lb. of trimmed and halved Brussels sprouts
- One tablespoon of chopped chives
- A quarter teaspoon of cayenne

- Half teaspoon of chili powder
- Two tablespoons of olive oil

Instructions

- Add all ingredients into the large bowl and toss well.
- Spread Brussels sprouts in the air fryer basket and cook at 370 F for 14 minutes. Shake basket halfway through.

Spicy Cabbage

Preparation Time-10 minutes | Cook Time-8 minutes | Servings-2 | Difficulty-Easy

Nutritional Facts- Calories-32 | Fats-0g |Carbohydrates-6g |Proteins-1.5g

Ingredients

- One grated carrot
- Half teaspoon of cayenne pepper
- A quarter cup of apple cider vinegar
- Half cabbage
- One teaspoon of red pepper flakes
- One tablespoon of sesame seed oil
- A quarter cup of apple juice

Instructions

- Put carrot, cayenne, cabbage, and oil on the Air Fryer Grill pan.
- Add vinegar, pepper flakes, and apple juice.
- Set the Air Fryer Grill to the air fry function.
- Cook for 8 minutes at 350 degrees F.
- Serve immediately.
- If desired, serve with maple syrup.

Spicy Chicken Ginger Soup

Preparation Time-10 minutes | Cook Time-Three hours | Servings-2 | Difficulty-Hard

Nutritional Facts- Calories-589 | Fats-27.9g |Carbohydrates-45.9g |Proteins-40g

Ingredients

- One lb. of cooked and diced chicken
- Fourteen ounces can of coconut milk
- One tablespoon of garlic powder
- One cup of uncooked rice
- Two tablespoons of fresh chopped basil
- One tablespoon of ground ginger

- One tablespoon of green curry paste
- Two teaspoons of thyme
- Four cups of chicken stock

Instructions

- Place the inner pot in the grill air fryer combo base.
- Add all ingredients into the inner pot and mix well.
- Cover the inner pot with a glass lid.
- Select slow cook mode, then press the temperature button and set the time for 3 hours. Press start.
- When the timer reaches 0, then press the cancel button.
- Serve and enjoy.

Spinach & Ricotta Cups

Preparation Time-10 minutes | Cook Time-10 minutes | Servings-2 | Difficulty-Easy

Nutritional Facts- Calories-138 | Fats-12g |Carbohydrates-1.5g |Proteins-7.8g

Ingredients

- Two large eggs
- Two tablespoons of heavy cream
- Two tablespoons of frozen spinach, thawed
- Four teaspoons of crumbled ricotta cheese
- Salt and freshly ground black pepper, to taste

Instructions

- Grease 2 ramekins.
- In each prepared ramekin, crack one egg.
- Divide the cream spinach, cheese, salt, and black pepper in each ramekin and gently stir to mix without breaking the yolks.
- Turn the "Temperature Knob" of the Air Fryer Grill to line the temperature to 330 degrees F.
- Turn the "Function Knob" to settle on "Air Fry."
- Turn the "Timer Knob" to line the Time for 10 minutes.
- After preheating, arrange the ramekins pan over the roasting rack.
- Insert the roasting rack at position 2 of the Air Fryer Grill.

- When the cooking time is over, remove the ramekins and place them onto a wire rack to chill for five minutes before serving.

Squab fingers

Preparation Time-10 minutes | Cook Time-30 minutes | Servings-2 | Difficulty-Easy

Nutritional Facts- Calories-150 | Fats-6.9g |Carbohydrates-6g |Proteins-15g

Ingredients

- Half lb. of squab fingers
- Two cups of dry breadcrumbs
- One cup of oil for frying

Marinade

- One and a half tablespoons of ginger-garlic paste
- Three tablespoons of lemon juice
- Two teaspoons of salt
- One teaspoon of pepper powder
- One teaspoon of red chili flakes or to taste
- Three eggs
- Five tablespoons of cornflour
- Two teaspoons of tomato ketchup

Instructions

- Make the marinade and transfer the fingers into the marinade. Leave them on a plate to dry for fifteen minutes.
- Now cover the fingers with the crumbs and set them aside to dry for fifteen minutes.
- Preheat the Air Fryer at 160 degrees Fahrenheit for 5 minutes or so. Keep the fish in the fry basket now and close it properly. Let the fingers cook at the same temperature for another 25 minutes. In between the cooking process, toss the fish once in a while to avoid burning the food.
- Serve either with tomato ketchup or chili sauce. Mint chutney also works well with the fish.

Sriracha Roasted Potatoes

Preparation Time-10 minutes | Cook Time- 30 minutes | Servings-2 | Difficulty-Easy

Nutritional Facts- Calories-147 | Fats-4.8g |Carbohydrates-25g |Proteins-4g

Ingredients

- Two diced potatoes
- Two teaspoons of sriracha
- A quarter teaspoon of garlic powder
- Salt & pepper
- Olive oil
- Chopped fresh parsley

Instructions

- Combine the potatoes with the remaining ingredients.
- Preheat the Air Fryer Grill at 230 degrees C or 450 degrees F.
- Line the pan with olive oil and spread the coated potatoes. Sprinkle parsley.
- Bake for 30 minutes.

Sriracha-Honey Chicken Wings

Preparation Time-10 minutes | Cook Time-40 minutes | Servings-2 | Difficulty-Moderate

Nutritional Facts- Calories-197 | Fats-9g |Carbohydrates-19g |Proteins-21g

Ingredients

- Two tablespoons of sriracha sauce
- One and a half tablespoons of soy sauce
- One tablespoon of butter
- Juice of half lime
- One pound chicken wings
- A quarter cup of honey
- Cilantro, chives, or scallions for garnish

Instructions

- The air fryer is preheated to 360 degrees F. To make sure the wings are sufficiently browned, put the chicken wings into the air fryer basket and cook for thirty minutes, turning the chicken around every 7 minutes with tongs.
- Insert the sauce ingredients into a small saucepan as the wings are frying, and bring to a boil for about three minutes.
- Toss them in a bowl with the sauce when the wings are cooked until thoroughly covered. Then sprinkle with the garnish. Serve immediately.

Stuffed Zucchini Caps

Preparation Time-10 minutes | Cook Time-30 minutes | Servings-2 | Difficulty-Moderate

Nutritional Facts- Calories-283 | Fats-4g |Carbohydrates-16.8g |Proteins-24g

Ingredients

- Half cup of carrot
- A quarter teaspoon of ground fennel seed
- One oregano sprig
- A quarter cup of red bell pepper
- A quarter cup of plain breadcrumbs
- Three tablespoons of butter
- Two medium zucchinis
- One pinch of freshly ground black pepper
- A quarter teaspoon of Sea Salt
- Two sweet sausages
- A quarter cup of shredded mozzarella
- A quarter cup of Onion

Instructions

- Take away the sausages from their casings.
- Position the sausages on an Air Flow Rack. Place the rack on the center shelf of the Power Air Fryer.
- Press the Power Button (370F for 15 minutes).
- Take out the sausages and slice them into small bits.
- Expose the interior of the zucchinis, leaving a layer in the bottom.
- Slice the pulp of the zucchinis.
- Melt the butter in a sauté pan on medium-high heat and sauté the onion, fennel seed, zucchini pulp, red pepper, carrot, and sausage bits until soft.
- Include the oregano, breadcrumbs, ground black pepper, and sea salt cook for 2 minutes over medium heat.
- Include the mozzarella in the prepared mixture and mix wholly.
- Serve the cooked blend into each zucchini cap.
- Place the stuffed zucchinis on two Racks. Position the Racks on the bottom and center shelves of the appliance.
- Press the Power Button and then the Baking Button (350F) and reduce the cooking time to 15 minutes.

Sweet and Spicy Peanuts

Preparation Time-5 minutes | Cook Time-5 minutes | Servings-2 | Difficulty-Easy

Nutritional Facts- Calories-122 | Fats-7.8g |Carbohydrates-14g |Proteins-4.2g

Ingredients

- Two cups of shelled raw peanuts
- One tablespoon of hot red pepper sauce
- Two tablespoons of granulated white sugar

Instructions

Put the peanuts in a large bowl, then drizzle with hot red pepper sauce and sprinkle with sugar. Toss to coat well.

- Pour the peanuts into the air fry basket.
- Place the basket on the air fry position.
- Select Air Fry, set the temperature to 400F (205C) and set time to 5 minutes. Set the peanuts halfway through the cooking time.
- When cooking is complete, the peanuts will be crispy and browned. Remove from the air fryer grill.
- Serve immediately.

Sweet Baby Carrots

Preparation Time-15 minutes | Cook Time-10 minutes | Servings-2 | Difficulty-Easy

Nutritional Facts- Calories-77 | Fats-1g|Carbohydrates-13.8g |Proteins-4g

Ingredients

- One tablespoon of brown sugar
- Two cups of baby carrots
- Two tablespoons of melted butter
- Black pepper and salt

Instructions

- Mix butter, sugar, pepper, carrot, and salt in a bowl.
- Transfer the mix to the Air Fryer Grill pan.
- Set the Air Fryer Grill to the air fry function.
- Cook for 10 minutes at 350 degrees F.
- Serve immediately.
- If desired, serve with maple syrup.

Sweet Bacon Snack

Preparation Time-10 minutes | Cook Time-30 minutes | Servings-2 | Difficulty-Easy

Nutritional Facts- Calories-159 | Fats-6.9g |Carbohydrates-12g |Proteins-9g

Ingredients

- Half teaspoon of cinnamon powder
- Eight bacon slices
- Half tablespoon of avocado oil
- One and a half ounces of dark chocolate
- One teaspoon of maple extract

Instructions

- Arrange bacon slices in your air fryer's basket, sprinkle cinnamon mix over them and cook them at 300 degrees F for 30 minutes.
- Heat up a pot with the oil over medium heat, add chocolate and stir until it melts.
- Add maple extract, stir, take off the heat and leave aside to cool down a bit.
- Take bacon strips out of the oven, leave them to cool down, dip each in chocolate mix, place them on parchment paper and leave them to cool down completely.
- Serve cold as a snack.

Sweet Popcorn

Preparation Time-10 minutes | Cook Time- 10 minutes | Servings-2 | Difficulty-Easy

Nutritional Facts- Calories-80 | Fats-1.5g |Carbohydrates-6.9g |Proteins-1.5g

Ingredients

- Two tablespoons of corn kernels
- Two tablespoons of butter
- Two ounces of brown sugar

Instructions

- Put corn kernels in your air fryer's pan, cook at 400 degrees F for 6 minutes, transfer them to a tray, spread and leave aside for now.
- Heat up a pan over low heat, add butter, melt it, add sugar and stir until it dissolves.
- Add popcorn, toss to coat, take off the heat and spread on the tray again.
- Cool down, divide into bowls and serve as a snack.

- Enjoy.

Sweet Potato Chips

Preparation Time-One hour | Cook Time-15 minutes | Servings-2 | Difficulty-Moderate

Nutritional Facts- Calories-233 | Fats-4g |Carbohydrates-25g |Proteins-1.5g

Ingredients

- A quarter cup of Olive Oil
- Pepper and salt to taste
- Two thinly sliced medium-sized Sweet Potatoes
- One teaspoon of ground Cinnamon optional

Instructions

- Cut rather finely the sweet potatoes. And use a food processor or mandolin.
- Soak the sweet potato slices in cold water for 30 minutes.
- Drain and pat the slices thoroughly to dry. Repeat several times until it's fully dry.
- Add the cinnamon, salt, olive oil, and pepper to sweet potato slices ensuring that each slice is covered with oil.
- The air-fry basket is lightly greased.
- Air fry the sweet potatoes at 390 degrees F for 15 min in batches, giving the basket a strong shake for cooking every 7 to 8 minutes. Suppose it is still not crisp; fry for an extra 5 minutes.
- Serve warm with ketchup.

Toasted Seasoned Nuts

Preparation Time-10 minutes | Cook Time-50 minutes | Servings-2 | Difficulty-Hard

Nutritional Facts- Calories-198 | Fats-6.9g |Carbohydrates-16.8g |Proteins-15.9g

Ingredients

- A quarter teaspoon of ground garlic cloves
- Half pound of cashews
- Four tablespoons of sugar
- Eight ounces of pecan halves
- One whisked egg white
- One teaspoon of salt
- Half teaspoon of cinnamon
- A quarter teaspoon of mixed spice
- A quarter teaspoon of cayenne pepper

- One cup of almonds

Instructions

- Mix the sugar, garlic, mixed spice, pepper, salt, cinnamon and egg together in a bowl.
- Heat your air fryer to 300°F.
- Put the cashews, almonds and pecan, into the egg mixture and toss.
- Coat the fryer basket with oil using a brush and pour half the nut mixture on it. Toast for 25 minutes until crunchy,
- stirring the nuts at intervals. Do the same with the second batch of nuts.
- Store in a sealed jar if not eaten immediately.

Tomato-Corn Frittata with Avocado Dressing

Preparation Time-10 minutes | Cook Time- 20 minutes| Servings-2 | Difficulty-Easy

Nutritional Facts- Calories-279 | Fats-7.8g |Carbohydrates-34.8g |Proteins-6g

Ingredients

- Half cup of cherry tomatoes
- Kosher salt and black pepper, to taste
- Six large eggs, lightly beaten
- Half cup of fresh corn kernels
- A quarter cup of milk
- One tablespoon of finely chopped fresh dill
- Half cup of shredded Monterey Jack cheese

Avocado Dressing

- One ripe avocado pitted and peeled
- Two tablespoons of fresh lime juice
- A quarter cup of olive oil
- One scallion, finely chopped
- Eight fresh basil leaves, finely chopped

Instructions

- Bring the tomato halves in a colander and lightly season with salt. Set aside to drain well. Set the tomatoes into a large bowl and fold in the eggs, corn, milk, and dill. Set with salt and pepper and stir until mixed.
- Whisk the egg mixture into a baking pan.
- Bring the pan into the air fryer oven. Press the Power Button. Cook at 300F (150C) for 15 minutes.

- When done, detach from the air fryer oven. Scatter the cheese on top.
- Press the Power Button. Cook at 315F (157C) for 5 minutes. Bring the pan back to the air fryer oven.
- When cooking is processed, the frittata will be puffy and set.
- Meanwhile, set the avocado dressing: Press the avocado with the lime juice in a medium bowl until smooth. Merge in the olive oil, scallion, and basil and stir until well incorporated.
- Set the frittata to cool for 5 minutes and serve alongside the avocado dressing.

Tortilla Chips

Preparation Time-10 minutes | Cook Time-10 minutes | Servings-2 | Difficulty-Easy

Nutritional Facts- Calories-212 | Fats-9.9g | Carbohydrates-12g | Proteins-7.8g

Ingredients

- One tablespoon of olive oil
- One tablespoon of McCormick Spice Blend
- Twelve corn tortillas
- Two teaspoons of kosher salt
- Guacamole, for serving

Instructions

- Preheat the fryer to 350 degrees Fahrenheit.
- Brush both sides of the tortillas with olive oil.
- Then season the tortillas with salt and the Delicious Jazzy Spice Mix.
- Any tortilla can be cut into six wedges.
- Working in batches, add the tortilla wedges to the air fryer in a single layer and 'fried' for about 5 minutes, or until crisp and golden brown.
- Serve with guacamole on the side.
- Enjoy.

Tuna Cakes

Preparation Time-10 minutes | Cook Time-10 minutes | Servings-2 | Difficulty-Easy

Nutritional Facts- Calories-159 | Fats-1g | Carbohydrates-9g | Proteins-6.9g

Ingredients

- Six ounces of drained and flaked canned tuna

- Two eggs
- Half teaspoon of dried dill
- One teaspoon of dried parsley
- A quarter cup of chopped red onion
- One teaspoon of garlic powder
- Salt and black pepper to the taste
- Cooking spray

Instructions

- In a bowl, mix tuna with salt, pepper, dill, parsley, onion, garlic powder and eggs, stir well and shape medium cakes out of this mix.
- Place tuna cakes in your air fryer's basket, spray them with cooking oil and cook at 350 degrees F for 10 minutes, flipping them halfway.
- Arrange them on a platter and serve as an appetizer.
- Enjoy!

Twice Baked Potatoes

Preparation Time-10 minutes | Cook Time-2 hours | Servings-2 | Difficulty-Hard

Nutritional Facts- Calories-140 | Fats-6.9g | Carbohydrates-15.9g | Proteins-4g

Ingredients

- Kosher salt
- Half cup of butter softened
- Half cup of milk
- Half cup of sour cream
- One and a half cups of shredded Cheddar, divided
- Two green onions, thinly sliced, plus more for garnish
- Three large russet potatoes scrubbed clean
- One tablespoon of extra-virgin olive oil
- Freshly ground black pepper

Instructions

- Using paper towels, completely dry the potatoes. Poke the potatoes all over with a fork, then brush them with oil and season with salt. Place the potatoes in an air fryer basket in batches and cook for 40 minutes at 400 degrees F. Place it on a large baking sheet to cool until it is safe to handle.
- Cut a tiny layer from the top of each potato by cutting lengthwise. Leave a 12" margin around each potato after scooping it out. Put the insides

of it in a large mixing basin. Keep the potato tops and roast them on the tray as a snack!

- Add the sour cream, butter, and milk to the bowl with the potatoes and mash until the butter is melted and the potatoes are virtually smooth but still have some lumps. Insert Stir together one cup of green onions and the cheese until well mixed. Season with pepper and salt.

- Return the baked potatoes to the air fryer basket and cover them with the potato mixture. Add the remaining half cup of cheddar cheese on top. Cook at 400°F for 5 minutes, or until the cheese is melted and the outside is crispy.

- Garnish with additional green onions before serving.

Vegan Beignets

Preparation Time-One hour | Cook Time-One hour | Servings-2 to 4 | Difficulty-Hard

Nutritional Facts- Calories-151 | Fats-9g |Carbohydrates-9.9g |Proteins-17g

Ingredients

- One cup of Whole Earth Sweetener Baking Blend

Proofing

Three tablespoons of powdered baking blend

- Three cups of unbleached white flour plus extra to sprinkle on the cutting board
- One cup of Full-fat coconut milk from a can

Dough

- Two tablespoons of melted coconut oil
- One teaspoon of organic corn starch
- One and a half teaspoons of active baking yeast
- Two tablespoons of aquafaba drained water from a can of chickpeas
- Two teaspoons of vanilla

Instructions

- Insert into your mixer the corn starch and Whole Earth Baking Blend and process until smooth and powdery.

- Heat the coconut milk until it is warm yet cold enough that without burning yourself, you can dip your finger in it. With the yeast and sugar, add it to the mixer. Let the yeast sit for 10 minutes before it starts to foam.

- Mix in the aquafaba, coconut oil, and vanilla with the paddle attachment. Then, add a cup of flour at a time.

- If you have one, turn to your dough hook once the flour is added in and the dough comes from the sides of the mixer.

- For about 3 minutes, knead the dough in your mixer. The dough would be wetter in contrast to the dough you make when you are making a loaf of bread, but without it sitting on your side, you must be able to scrape out the dough & form a ball.

- In a mixing bowl, put the dough and cover it with a clean dish towel and let it rise for 1 hour.

- Sprinkle some flour on a large cutting board and pat the dough out into a 1/3-inch-thick rectangle. Slice into 24 squares and leave for 30 minutes to proof before cooking them.

- Cook in batches of 3 to 6 at a time.

- Preheat the oven to 350 degrees F. Place the beignets on a parchment paper-lined baking sheet.

- Bake until golden brown or for about 15 minutes, flipping after every 3 minutes. Sprinkle with the powdered baking mix you made in the beginning and eat it liberally.

Vegetable Egg Cups

Preparation Time-10 minutes | Cook Time-20 minutes | Servings-2 | Difficulty-Easy

Nutritional Facts- Calories-194 | Fats-11.4g |Carbohydrates-6.9g |Proteins-12g

Ingredients

- Two eggs
- One tablespoon of chopped cilantro
- Two tablespoons of half and half
- Half cup of shredded cheddar cheese
- One cup of vegetables, diced
- Pepper
- Salt

Instructions

- Set aside four ramekins that have been sprayed with cooking spray.

- Whisk eggs with half and half, cilantro, veggies, pepper, a half cup of cheese, and salt in a mixing bowl.

- Fill the four ramekins with the egg mixture.
- Put ramekins in air fryer basket and bake for 12 minutes at 300°F.
- Cook for another 2 minutes at 400 degrees F on top of the remaining half cup of cheese.
- Serve and have fun.

Vegetable Supreme Pan Pizza

Preparation Time-10 minutes | Cook Time-30 minutes | Servings-2 | Difficulty-Easy

Nutritional Facts- Calories-245 | Fats-15g |Carbohydrates-15g |Proteins-24g

Ingredients

- Eight slices of White Onion
- Twelve slices of Tomato
- Two tablespoons of olive oil
- 3/2 cups of shredded mozzarella
- Eight cremini mushrooms
- Half green pepper
- Four tablespoons of Pesto
- One Pizza Dough
- One cup of spinach

Instructions

- Roll the pizza dough halves until each one reaches the size of the Air Flow racks.
- Lightly grease both sides of each dough with olive oil.
- Place each pizza on a rack. Place the racks on the upper and lower shelves of the electric fryer.
- Press the power button then the French fries button (400 F) and decrease the cooking time to 13 minutes.
- After 5 minutes, flip the dough onto the top shelf and turn the racks.
- After 4 minutes, turn the dough onto the top shelf.
- Take out both racks and drizzle the pizzas with the toppings.
- Place the racks on the upper and lower shelves of the electric fryer.
- Press the power button then the French fries button (400 F) and decrease the cooking time to 7 minutes.
- After 4 minutes, rotate the pizzas.

- Once the pizzas are done, let them rest for 4 minutes before cutting.

Vegetarian Pizza

Preparation Time-15 minutes | Cook Time-10 minutes | Servings-2 | Difficulty-Easy

Nutritional Facts- Calories-260 | Fats-12.9g |Carbohydrates-1.5g |Proteins-34g

Ingredients

Two pizza crusts
One tablespoon of olive oil
A quarter cup of tomato sauce
One cup of mushrooms
Half cup of sliced black olives
One minced clove of garlic
Half teaspoon of oregano
Salt and pepper to taste
One cup of shredded mozzarella

Instructions

- Brush pizza crust with oil.
- Spread tomato sauce on top.
- Arrange mushrooms and olives on top.
- Sprinkle with garlic and oregano.
- Season with salt and pepper.
- Top with mozzarella cheese.
- Place inside the air fryer.
- Set it to bake.
- Cook at 400 F for 10 minutes.

Venison Loaf

Preparation Time-10 minutes | Cook Time-One hour and 20 minutes | Servings-2 | Difficulty-Hard

Nutritional Facts- Calories-211 | Fats-4g |Carbohydrates-13g |Proteins-9g

Ingredients

- Chopped onion
- Half lb. of sausage
- One cup of milk
- Two eggs
- Four ounces of barbecue sauce
- Two cups of cracker crumbs
- Tomato sauce
- Half lb. of ground venison

Instructions

- Mix cracker crumbs, milk, ground venison, and barbecue sauce in a bowl.
- Add sausage, eggs, and onion.
- Place the mixture on the Air Fryer Grill pan.
- Set the Air Fryer Grill to the air fry function.
- Bake for 1 hour at 350 degrees F.
- Serve immediately or allow cooling before serving.

Chapter 5-Air Fried Sides Recipes

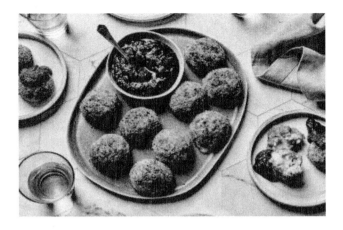

Arancini

Preparation Time-10 minutes | Cook Time-30 minutes | Servings-2 to 4 | Difficulty-Moderate

Nutritional Facts- Calories-218 | Fats-9g |Carbohydrates-12g |Proteins-26g

Ingredients

- 2/3 cup of raw white Arborio rice
- Two teaspoons of butter
- Half teaspoon of salt
- One and 1/3 cups of water
- Two well beaten large eggs
- One and a quarter cup of seasoned Italian-style dried bread crumbs
- Ten 1/3-inch semi-firm Mozzarella cubes
- Cooking spray

Instructions

- Pour the rice, butter, salt, and water into a pot. Stir to mix well and bring a boil over medium-high heat. Keep stirring.
- Reduce the heat to low and cover the pot. Simmer for 20 minutes or until the rice is tender.
- Turn off the heat and let sit, covered, for 10 minutes, then open the lid and fluffy the rice with a fork. Allow cooling for ten more minutes.
- Pour the beaten eggs into a bowl, and then pour the bread crumbs into a separate bowl.
- Scoop two tablespoons of the cooked rice up and form it into a ball, then press the Mozzarella into the ball and wrap.
- Dredge the ball in the eggs first, and then shake the excess off the dunk the ball in the bread

crumbs. Roll to coat evenly. Repeat to make ten balls in total with the remaining rice.

- Transfer the balls to the airflow racks and spritz with cooking spray.
- Slide the racks into the air fryer oven. Press the Power Button. Cook at 375F (190C) for 10 minutes.
- When cooking is complete, the balls should be lightly browned and crispy.
- Remove the balls from the air fryer oven and allow them to cool before serving.

Artichokes and Tarragon Sauce

Preparation Time-10 minutes | Cook Time-20 minutes | Servings-2 | Difficulty-Easy

Nutritional Facts- Calories-215 | Fats-1g|Carbohydrates-27.9g |Proteins-6g

Ingredients

- Four trimmed artichokes
- Two tablespoons of chopped tarragon
- Two tablespoons of chicken stock
- Lemon zest from two lemons
- Two tablespoons of lemon juice
- One chopped celery stalk
- Half cup of olive oil
- Salt to the taste

Instructions

- In your food processor, mix tarragon, chicken stock, lemon zest, lemon juice, celery, salt and olive oil and pulse very well.
- In a bowl, mix artichokes with tarragon and lemon sauce, toss well, transfer them to your air fryer's basket and cook at 380 degrees F for 18 minutes.
- Divide artichokes among plates, drizzle the rest of the sauce all over and serve as a side dish.

Asparagus with Almonds

Preparation Time-10 minutes | Cook Time-10 minutes | Servings-2 | Difficulty-Easy

Nutritional Facts- Calories-122 | Fats-11.1g |Carbohydrates-4.8g |Proteins-4g

Ingredients

- Twelve asparagus spears

- 1/3 cup of sliced almonds
- Two tablespoons of olive oil
- Two tablespoons of balsamic vinegar
- Pepper
- Salt

Instructions

- Drizzle asparagus spears with oil and vinegar.
- Arrange asparagus spears into the air fryer basket and season with pepper and salt.
- Sprinkle sliced almond over asparagus spears.
- Cook asparagus at 350 F for 5 minutes. Shake basket halfway through.
- Serve and enjoy.

Avocado Fries

Preparation Time-10 minutes | Cook Time-10 minutes | Servings-2 | Difficulty-Easy

Nutritional Facts- Calories-131 | Fats-9g |Carbohydrates-15.9g |Proteins-4g

Ingredients

- One pitted, peeled, and sliced avocado
- Salt and black pepper to the taste
- Half cup of panko bread crumbs
- One tablespoon of lemon juice
- One whisked egg
- One tablespoon of olive oil

Instructions

- In a bowl, mix panko with salt and pepper and stir.
- In another bowl, mix the egg with a pinch of salt and whisk.
- In a third bowl, mix avocado fries with lemon juice and oil and toss.
- Dip fries in egg, then in panko, place them in your air fryer's basket and cook at 390 degrees F for 10 minutes, shaking halfway.
- Divide among plates and serve as a side dish.

Baked Grits

Preparation Time-5 minutes | Cook Time-35 minutes | Servings-2 | Difficulty-Moderate

Nutritional Facts- Calories-189 | Fats-10.8g |Carbohydrates-4.8g |Proteins-12g

Ingredients

- One cup of grits or polenta (not instant or quick cook)
- Two cups of milk
- Two cups of chicken or vegetable stock
- Two tablespoons of unsalted butter, divided into four pieces
- One teaspoon of kosher salt or a half teaspoon of fine salt

Instructions

- Add the grits to the baking pan. Stir in the milk, stock, butter, and salt.
- Place the pan on the bake position. Choose Bake, set the temperature to 325°F (163°C), and set the time for 1 hour and 5 minutes.
- After 15 minutes, detach the pan from the air fryer grill and stir the polenta. Return the pan to the air fryer grill and continue cooking.
- After 30 minutes, remove the pan again and stir the polenta again. Return the pan to the air fryer grill and continue cooking for 15 to 20 minutes or until the polenta is soft and creamy and the liquid is absorbed.
- When done, remove the pan from the air fryer grill.
- Serve immediately.

Baked White Rice

Preparation Time-5 minutes | Cook Time-35 minutes | Servings-2 | Difficulty-Moderate

Nutritional Facts- Calories-522 | Fats-12g |Carbohydrates-34g |Proteins-39g

Ingredients

- One cup of washed and drained long-grain white rice
- Two cups of water
- One tablespoon of melted unsalted butter or One tablespoon of extra-virgin olive oil
- One teaspoon of kosher salt or a half teaspoon of fine salt

Instructions

- Add the butter and rice to the baking pan and stir to coat. Pour in the water and sprinkle with the salt. Stir until the salt is dissolved.

- Place the pan on the bake position. Set Bake, set the temperature to 325°F (163°C) and set the time for 35 minutes.
- After 20 minutes, remove the pan from the air fryer grill. Stir the rice. Transfer the pan back to the air fryer grill and continue cooking for 10 to 15 minutes or until the rice is mostly cooked through and the water is absorbed.
- When done, remove the pan from the air fryer grill and cover it with aluminum foil. Let stand for 10 minutes. Using a fork, gently fluff the rice.
- Serve immediately.

Balsamic Artichokes

Preparation Time-11 minutes | Cook Time-8 minutes | Servings-2 | Difficulty-Easy

Nutritional Facts- Calories-533 | Fats-28.9g |Carbohydrates-65g |Proteins-13.8g

Ingredients

- Two teaspoons of balsamic vinegar
- Black pepper and salt
- A quarter cup of olive oil
- One teaspoon of oregano
- Four big trimmed artichokes
- Two tablespoons of lemon juice
- Two cloves of garlic

Instructions

- Sprinkle the artichokes with pepper and salt.
- Brush oil over the artichokes and add lemon juice.
- Place the artichokes on the Air Fryer Grill.
- Set the Air Fryer Grill at Air fryer/Grill, Timer at 7 minutes at 360 degrees F.
- Mix garlic, lemon juice, pepper, vinegar, oil in a bowl.
- Add oregano and salt.
- Mix well.
- Serve the artichokes with balsamic vinaigrette.

Balsamic Mushrooms

Preparation Time-11 minutes | Cook Time-8 minutes | Servings-2 | Difficulty-Easy

Nutritional Facts- Calories-123 | Fats-1g|Carbohydrates-6g |Proteins-7.8g

Ingredients

- Eight ounces of mushrooms
- One teaspoon of fresh chopped parsley
- Two teaspoons of balsamic vinegar
- Half teaspoon of granulated garlic
- One teaspoon of olive oil
- Pepper
- Salt

Instructions

- Toss mushrooms with garlic, oil, pepper, and salt.
- Add mushrooms into the air fryer basket and cook at 375 F for 8 minutes. Toss halfway through.
- Toss mushrooms with parsley and balsamic vinegar.
- Serve and enjoy.

Barley Risotto

Preparation Time-10 minutes | Cook Time-30 minutes | Servings-2 | Difficulty-Moderate

Nutritional Facts- Calories-124 | Fats-4g |Carbohydrates-10.8g |Proteins-4g

Ingredients

- Five cups of veggie stock
- Three tablespoons of olive oil
- Two chopped yellow onions
- Two minced cloves of garlic
- 3/4 pound of barley
- Three ounces of sliced mushrooms
- Two ounces of skim milk
- One teaspoon of dried thyme
- One teaspoon of dried tarragon
- Salt and black pepper to the taste
- Two pounds of peeled and chopped sweet potato

Instructions

- Put stock in a pot, add barley, stir, bring to a boil over medium heat and cook for 15 minutes.
- Heat up your air fryer at 350 degrees F, add oil and heat it up.
- Add barley, onions, garlic, mushrooms, milk, salt, pepper, tarragon and sweet potato, stir and cook for 15 minutes more.
- Divide among plates and serve as a side dish.

Beer Risotto

Preparation Time-10 minutes | Cook Time-30 minutes | Servings-2 | Difficulty-Moderate

Nutritional Facts- Calories-143 | Fats-4g |Carbohydrates-10.8g |Proteins-17g

Ingredients

- Two tablespoons of olive oil
- Two chopped yellow onions
- One cup of sliced mushrooms
- One teaspoon of dried basil
- One teaspoon of dried oregano
- One and a half cups of rice
- Two cups of beer
- Two cups of chicken stock
- One tablespoon of butter
- Half cup of grated parmesan

Instructions

- In a dish that fits your air fryer, mix oil with onions, mushrooms, basil and oregano and stir.
- Add rice, beer, butter, stock and butter, stir again, place in your air fryer's basket and cook at 350 degrees F for 30 minutes.
- Divide among plates and serve with grated parmesan on top as a side dish.
- Enjoy!

Beet Salad with Parsley Dressing

Preparation Time-15 minutes | Cook Time-15 minutes | Servings-2 | Difficulty-Easy

Nutritional Facts- Calories-185 | Fats-15.9g |Carbohydrates-10.8g |Proteins-7.8g

Ingredients

- Black pepper and salt
- One clove of garlic
- Two tablespoons of balsamic vinegar
- Four beets
- Two tablespoons of capers
- One bunch of chopped parsley
- One tablespoon of olive oil

Instructions

- Place beets on the Air Fryer Grill pan.
- Set the Air Fryer Grill to the air fry function.

- Set Timer and temperature to 15 minutes and 360 degrees F.
- In another bowl, mix pepper, garlic, capers, salt, and olive oil. Mix well
- Remove the beets from the Air Fryer Grill and place them on a flat surface.
- Peel and put it in the salad bowl
- Serve with vinegar.

Beets and Arugula Salad

Preparation Time-10 minutes | Cook Time-10 minutes | Servings-2 | Difficulty-Easy

Nutritional Facts- Calories-121 | Fats-1.5g |Carbohydrates-13.8g |Proteins-4g

Ingredients

- One and a half pounds of peeled and quartered beets
- A drizzle of olive oil
- Two teaspoons of grated orange zest
- Two tablespoons of cider vinegar
- Half cup of orange juice
- Two tablespoons of brown sugar
- Two chopped scallions
- Two teaspoons of mustard
- Two cups of arugula

Instructions

- Rub beets with the oil and orange juice, place them in your air fryer and cook at 350 degrees F for 10 minutes.
- Transfer beet quarters to a bowl, add scallions, arugula and orange zest and toss.
- In a separate bowl, mix sugar with mustard and vinegar, whisk well, add to salad, toss and serve.

Beets and Blue Cheese Salad

Preparation Time-10 minutes | Cook Time-15 minutes | Servings-2 | Difficulty-Easy

Nutritional Facts- Calories-105 | Fats-4.8g |Carbohydrates-13.8g |Proteins-4.8g

Ingredients

- Six peeled and quartered beets
- Salt and black pepper to the taste
- A quarter cup of crumbled blue cheese
- One tablespoon of olive oil

Instructions

- Put beets in your air fryer, cook them at 350 degrees F for 14 minutes and transfer them to a bowl.
- Add blue cheese, salt, pepper and oil, toss and serve.

Blistered Tomatoes

Preparation Time-6 minutes | Cook Time-10 minutes | Servings-2 | Difficulty-

Nutritional Facts- Calories-283 | Fats-4g |Carbohydrates-16.8g |Proteins-26g

Ingredients

- Two pounds of cherry tomatoes
- Two tablespoons of olive oil
- Two teaspoons of balsamic vinegar
- Half teaspoon of salt
- Half teaspoon of ground black pepper

Instructions

- Toss the cherry tomatoes with olive oil in a large bowl to coat well. Pour the tomatoes into a baking pan.
- Bring the pan into the air fryer oven. Press the Power Button. Cook at 400 degrees F (205C) for 10 minutes.
- Set the tomatoes halfway through the cooking time.
- When cooking is complete, the tomatoes will be blistered and lightly wilted.
- Transfer the blistered tomatoes to a large bowl and toss with balsamic vinegar, salt, and black pepper before serving.

Bratwurst and Pickle Kabobs

Preparation Time-10 minutes | Cook Time-30 minutes | Servings-2 | Difficulty-Moderate

Nutritional Facts- Calories-286 | Fats-4.8g |Carbohydrates-19g |Proteins-23g

Ingredients

- Twenty pretzel nuggets, thawed
- Four diced dill pickles
- Four wholly cooked and sliced bratwurst
- A quarter cup of pretzel salt
- Spicy Mustard for serving

Instructions

- Alternate between placing five bratwurst medallions and four pickle medallions on a skewer in your Air Fryer Oven.
- Make four extra skewers with meat and pickles.
- Using a skewer, skewer four pretzel nuggets.
- Spray with water and sprinkle with pretzel salt.
- Prepare four more pretzel skewers.
- Attach the skewers, swapping out pretzel and pork skewers as needed.
- Preheat oven to 350°F and bake for 10 minutes.
- Serve with spicy mustard on the side.

Breaded Dill Pickles with Buttermilk Dressing

Preparation Time-45 minutes | Cook Time-10 minutes | Servings-2 | Difficulty-Moderate

Nutritional Facts- Calories-515 | Fats-1g |Carbohydrates-1.5g |Proteins-45g

Ingredients

Buttermilk Dressing

- A quarter cup of buttermilk
- A quarter cup of chopped scallions
- 1/3 cup of mayonnaise
- Half cup of sour cream
- Half teaspoon of cayenne pepper
- Half teaspoon of onion powder
- Half teaspoon of garlic powder
- One tablespoon of chopped chives
- Two tablespoons of chopped fresh dill
- Kosher salt and black pepper, to taste

Fried Dill Pickles

- 1/3 cup of all-purpose flour
- One (Two pounds) jar kosher dill pickles, cut into four spears, drained
- Two and a half cups panko bread crumbs
- Two eggs, beaten with Two tablespoons of water
- Kosher salt and black pepper, to taste
- Cooking spray

Instructions

- Merge the ingredients for the dressing in a bowl. Stir to mix well.
- Wrap the bowl in plastic and refrigerate for 30

minutes or until ready to serve.

- Pour the flour into a bowl and sprinkle with salt and ground black pepper. Stir to mix well. Put the bread crumbs in a separate bowl. Set the beaten eggs in a third bowl.
- Dredge the pickle spears in the flour, then into the eggs, and then into the panko to coat well. Shake the excess off.
- Arrange the pickle spears in a single layer in the air fry basket and spritz with cooking spray.
- Place the basket on the air fry position.
- Select Air Fry, set the temperature to 400 degrees F (205C) and set time to 8 minutes. Flip the pickle spears halfway through the cooking time.
- When cooking is complete, remove the pan from the air fryer grill.
- Serve the pickle spears with buttermilk dressing.

Broccoli Salad

Preparation Time-15 minutes | Cook Time-10 minutes | Servings-2 | Difficulty-Easy

Nutritional Facts- Calories-199 | Fats-13.8g |Carbohydrates-16.8g |Proteins-7.8g

Ingredients

- Six cloves of garlic
- One head of broccoli
- Black pepper and salt
- One tablespoon of Chinese rice wine vinegar
- One tablespoon of peanut oil

Instructions

- Mix oil, salt, broccoli, and pepper.
- Place the mixture on the Air Fryer Grill pan.
- Set the Air Fryer Grill to the air fry function.
- Cook for 9 minutes at 350 degrees F.
- Place the broccoli in the salad bowl and add peanuts oil, rice vinegar, and garlic.
- Serve immediately.

Brussels Sprout with Tomatoes Mix

Preparation Time-10 minutes | Cook Time-10 minutes | Servings-2 | Difficulty-Easy

Nutritional Facts- Calories-57 | Fats-1g |Carbohydrates-12g |Proteins-4.8g

Ingredients

- Six halved cherry tomatoes
- One tablespoon of olive oil
- One pound of Brussel sprouts
- Black pepper and salt
- A quarter cup of chopped green onions

Instructions

- Sprinkle pepper and salt on the Brussels sprout.
- Place it on the Air Fryer Grill pan.
- Set the Air Fryer Grill to the air fry function.
- Cook for 10 minutes at 350 degrees F.
- Place the cooked sprout in a bowl, add pepper, green onion, salt, olive oil, and cherry tomatoes.
- Mix well and serve immediately

Brussels Sprouts and Pomegranate Seeds Side Dish

Preparation Time-5 minutes | Cook Time-10 minutes | Servings-2 | Difficulty-Easy

Nutritional Facts- Calories-156 | Fats-4.8g |Carbohydrates-19g |Proteins-4g

Ingredients

- One pound of trimmed and halved Brussels sprouts
- Salt and black pepper to the taste
- One cup of pomegranate seeds
- A quarter cup of toasted pine nuts
- One tablespoon of olive oil
- Two tablespoons of veggie stock

Instructions

- In a heat-proof dish that fits your air fryer, mix Brussels sprouts with salt, pepper, pomegranate seeds, pine nuts, oil and stock, stir, place in your air fryer's basket and cook at 390 degrees F for 10 minutes.
- Divide among plates and serve as a side dish.

Cajun Onion Wedges

Preparation Time-10 minutes | Cook Time-15 minutes | Servings-2 | Difficulty-Easy

Nutritional Facts- Calories-200 | Fats-4.8g |Carbohydrates-15.9g |Proteins-6.9g

Ingredients

- Two big white onions, cut into wedges
- Salt and black pepper to the taste
- Two eggs
- A quarter cup of milk
- 1/3 cup of panko
- A drizzle of olive oil
- One and a half teaspoons of paprika
- One teaspoon of garlic powder
- Half teaspoon of Cajun seasoning

Instructions

- In a bowl, mix panko with Cajun seasoning and oil and stir.
- In another bowl, mix egg with milk, salt and pepper and stir.
- Sprinkle onion wedges with paprika and garlic powder, dip them in egg mix, then in bread crumbs mix, place in your air fryer's basket, cook at 360 degrees F for 10 minutes, flip and cook for 5 minutes more.
- Divide among plates and serve as a side dish.

Carrots and Rhubarb

Preparation Time-10 minutes | Cook Time-40 minutes | Servings-2 | Difficulty-Moderate

Nutritional Facts- Calories-172 | Fats-1.5g |Carbohydrates-9.9g |Proteins-4g

Ingredients

- One pound baby carrots
- Two teaspoons of walnut oil
- One pound of roughly chopped rhubarb
- One orange, peeled, cut into medium segments and zest grated
- Half cup of halved walnuts,
- Half teaspoon of stevia

Instructions

- Put the oil in your air fryer, add carrots, toss and fry them at 380 degrees F for 20 minutes.
- Add rhubarb, orange zest, stevia and walnuts, toss and cook for 20 minutes more.
- Add orange segments, toss and serve as a side dish.

Cauliflower and Broccoli Delight

Preparation Time-10 minutes | Cook Time-10 minutes | Servings-2 | Difficulty-Easy

Nutritional Facts- Calories-289 | Fats-4.8g |Carbohydrates-27.9g |Proteins-4g

Ingredients

- Two florets separated and steamed cauliflower heads
- One floret separated and steamed broccoli head
- Zest from one orange
- Juice from one orange
- A pinch of hot pepper flakes
- Four anchovies
- One tablespoon of chopped capers
- Salt and black pepper to the taste
- Four tablespoons of olive oil

Instructions

- In a bowl, mix the orange zest with orange juice, pepper flakes, anchovies, capers salt, pepper and olive oil and whisk well.
- Add broccoli and cauliflower, toss well, transfer them to your air fryer's basket and cook at 400 degrees F for 7 minutes.
- Divide among plates and serve as a side dish with some of the orange vinaigrette drizzled on top.

Cauliflower Cakes

Preparation Time-10 minutes | Cook Time-10 minutes | Servings-2 | Difficulty-Easy

Nutritional Facts- Calories-125 | Fats-1.5g |Carbohydrates-13.8g |Proteins-4g

Ingredients

- Three and a half cups of cauliflower rice
- Two eggs
- A quarter cup of white flour
- Half cup of grated parmesan
- Salt and black pepper to the taste
- Cooking spray

Instructions

- In a bowl, mix cauliflower rice with salt and pepper, stir and squeeze excess water.
- Transfer cauliflower to another bowl, add eggs,

salt, pepper, flour and parmesan, stir really well and shape your cakes.

- Grease your air fryer with cooking spray, heat it up at 400 degrees, add cauliflower cakes and cook them for 10 minutes, flipping them halfway.
- Divide cakes among plates and serve as a side dish.

Cauliflower Rice

Preparation Time-10 minutes | Cook Time-40 minutes | Servings-2 | Difficulty-Moderate

Nutritional Facts- Calories-142 | Fats-1g|Carbohydrates-9.9g |Proteins-4g

Ingredients

- One tablespoon of peanut oil
- One tablespoon of sesame oil
- Four tablespoons of soy sauce
- Three minced garlic cloves
- One tablespoon of grated ginger
- Juice from half lemon
- One riced cauliflower head
- Nine ounces of drained water chestnuts
- 3/4 cup of peas
- Fifteen ounces of chopped mushrooms
- One whisked egg

Instructions

- In your air fryer, mix cauliflower rice with peanut oil, sesame oil, soy sauce, garlic, ginger and lemon juice, stir, cover and cook at 350 degrees F for 20 minutes.
- Add chestnuts, peas, mushrooms and egg, toss and cook at 360 degrees F for 20 minutes more.
- Divide among plates and serve.

Cheddar Biscuits

Preparation Time-10 minutes | Cook Time-20 minutes | Servings-2 | Difficulty-Easy

Nutritional Facts- Calories-221 | Fats-1g|Carbohydrates-20g |Proteins-4g

Ingredients

- Two and 1/3 cup of self-rising flour
- Half cup plus one tablespoon of melted butter
- Two tablespoons of sugar
- Half cup of grated cheddar cheese

- One and 1/3 cup of buttermilk
- One cup of flour

Instructions

- In a bowl, mix self-rising flour with Half a cup of butter, sugar, cheddar cheese and buttermilk and stir until you obtain a dough.
- Spread One cup of flour on a working surface, roll dough, flatten it, cut eight circles with a cookie cutter and coat them with flour.
- Line your air fryer's basket with tin foil, add biscuits, brush them with melted butter and cook them at 380 degrees F for 20 minutes.
- Divide among plates and serve as an aside.

Cheesy Artichokes

Preparation Time-15 minutes | Cook Time-6 minutes | Servings-2 | Difficulty-Easy

Nutritional Facts- Calories-379 | Fats-19g |Carbohydrates-39g |Proteins-7.8g

Ingredients

- One teaspoon of onion powder
- Half cup of chicken stock
- Fourteen ounces of artichoke hearts
- Eight ounces of mozzarella
- Half cup of mayonnaise
- Eight ounces of cream cheese
- Ten ounces of spinach
- Three cloves of garlic
- Sixteen ounces of grated parmesan cheese
- Half cup of sour cream

Instructions

- Mix cream cheese, onion powder, chicken stock, and artichokes in a bowl.
- Add sour cream, mayonnaise, spinach to the bowl.
- Transfer the mixture to the Air Fryer Grill pan
- Set the Air Fryer Grill to Air fryer/Grill.
- Set Timer to 6 minutes at 350 degrees F.
- Serve immediately.

Cheesy Wafer

Preparation Time-5 minutes | Cook Time-5 minutes | Servings-2 | Difficulty-Easy

Nutritional Facts- Calories-184 | Fats-10.8g |Carbohydrates-4.8g |Proteins-12g

Ingredients

- One cup of shredded aged Manchego cheese
- One teaspoon of all-purpose flour
- Half teaspoon of cumin seeds
- A quarter teaspoon of cracked black pepper

Instructions

- Line the air fry basket with parchment paper.
- Merge the cheese and flour in a bowl. Stir to mix well. Spread the mixture in the basket into a 4-inch round.
- Combine the cumin and black pepper in a small bowl. Stir to mix well. Sprinkle the cumin mixture over the cheese round.
- Place the basket on the air fry position.
- Select Air Fry, set the temperature to 375 degrees F (190C) and set time to 5 minutes.
- When cooked, the cheese will be lightly browned and frothy.
- Use tongs to transfer the cheese wafer onto a plate and slice to serve.

Chicken and Spinach Salad

Preparation Time-10 minutes | Cook Time-15 minutes | Servings-2 | Difficulty-Easy

Nutritional Facts- Calories-178 | Fats-12.9g |Carbohydrates-12g |Proteins-20g

Ingredients

- Two teaspoons of dried parsley
- Two skinless and boneless chicken breasts
- Half teaspoon of onion powder
- Two teaspoons of sweet paprika
- Half cup of lemon juice
- Salt and black pepper to the taste
- Five cups of baby spinach
- Eight sliced strawberries
- One sliced small red onion
- Two tablespoons of balsamic vinegar
- One pitted, peeled and chopped avocado
- A quarter cup of olive oil
- One tablespoon of chopped tarragon

Instructions

- Put chicken in a bowl, add lemon juice, parsley, onion powder and paprika and toss.
- Transfer chicken to your air fryer and cook at 360 degrees F for 12 minutes.
- In a bowl, mix spinach, onion, strawberries and avocado and toss.
- In another bowl, mix oil with vinegar, salt, pepper and tarragon, whisk well, add to the salad and toss.
- Divide chicken among plates, add spinach salad on the side and serve.
- Enjoy!

Chile Relleno Boats

Preparation Time-10 minutes | Cook Time-15 minutes | Servings-2 | Difficulty-Easy

Nutritional Facts- Calories-291 | Fats-9g |Carbohydrates-9g |Proteins-20g

Ingredients

- One large poblano pepper
- Half cup of cauliflower rice
- Fiesta blend seasoning
- A quarter cup of reduced-fat shredded cheddar or Mexican blend cheese
- Canned green chilis
- Green onions
- One small onion sliced and sauteed
- One ounce of fat-free cream cheese
- One packet Sloppy joe mix
- Sliced roasted red peppers
- Jalapeno slices
- Cilantro
- A quarter cup of salsa
- A quarter cup of fat-free sour cream

Instructions

- Cut the poblano pepper in half lengthwise and remove the seeds.
- To taste, combine cauliflower rice, sauteed onion, cream cheese, and fiesta blend.
- Adding a squeeze of lime juice to the fiesta blend seasoning will make it even better.

- Spread the pepper on top.
- Prepare the sloppy joe mix, reducing the amount of water if desired for a thicker consistency.
- Using a spatula, spread the cream cheese mixture over the top.
- Lastly, top with shredded cheese.
- As desired, add the remaining toppings.
- Bake for 10 minutes in the air fryer until the cheese is melted and gently browned.
- If desired, top with salsa and sour cream.

Coconut Cream Potatoes

Preparation Time-10 minutes | Cook Time-20 minutes | Servings-2 | Difficulty-Easy

Nutritional Facts- Calories-188 | Fats-4.8g |Carbohydrates-15.9g |Proteins-16.8g

Ingredients

- Two whisked eggs
- Salt and black pepper to the taste
- One tablespoon of grated cheddar cheese
- One tablespoon of flour
- Two sliced potatoes
- Four ounces of coconut cream

Instructions

- Place potato slices in your air fryer's basket and cook at 360 degrees F for 10 minutes.
- Meanwhile, in a bowl, mix eggs with coconut cream, salt, pepper and flour.
- Arrange potatoes in your air fryer's pan, add coconut cream mix over them, sprinkle cheese, return to the air fryer's basket and cook at 400 degrees F for 10 minutes more.
- Divide among plates and serve as a side dish.
- Enjoy!

Colored Veggie Rice

Preparation Time-10 minutes | Cook Time-25 minutes | Servings-2 | Difficulty-Easy

Nutritional Facts- Calories-283 | Fats-4.8g |Carbohydrates-34g |Proteins-15g

Ingredients

- Two cups of basmati rice
- One cup of mixed carrots, peas, corn and green beans

- Two cups of water
- Half teaspoon of green chili, minced
- Half teaspoon of grated ginger
- Three minced garlic cloves
- Two tablespoons of butter
- One teaspoon of cinnamon powder
- One tablespoon of cumin seeds
- Two bay leaves
- Three whole cloves
- Five black peppercorns
- Two whole cardamoms
- One tablespoon of sugar
- Salt to the taste

Instructions

- Put the water in a heatproof dish that fits your air fryer, add rice, mixed veggies, green chili, grated ginger, garlic cloves, cinnamon, cloves, butter, cumin seeds, bay leaves, cardamoms, black peppercorns, salt and sugar, stir, put in your air fryer's basket and cook at 370 degrees F for 25 minutes.
- Divide among plates and serve as a side dish.
- Enjoy!

Corn with Lime and Cheese

Preparation Time-10 minutes | Cook Time-15 minutes | Servings-2 | Difficulty-Easy

Nutritional Facts- Calories-200 | Fats-6g |Carbohydrates-12.9g |Proteins-6g

Ingredients

- Two corns on the cob, husks removed
- A drizzle of olive oil
- Half cup of grated feta cheese
- Two teaspoons of sweet paprika
- Juice from two limes

Instructions

- Rub corn with oil and paprika, place in your air fryer and cook at 400 degrees F for 15 minutes, flipping once.
- Divide corn among plates, sprinkle cheese on top, drizzle lime juice and serve as a side dish.
- Enjoy!

Creamy Air Fried Potato Side Dish

Preparation Time-10 minutes | Cook Time-One hour and 20 minutes | Servings-2 | Difficulty-Hard

Nutritional Facts- Calories-172 | Fats-4.8g |Carbohydrates-15.9g |Proteins-4g

Ingredients

- One big potato
- Two cooked and chopped bacon strips
- One teaspoon of olive oil
- 1/3 cup of shredded cheddar cheese
- One tablespoon of chopped green onions
- Salt and black pepper to the taste
- One tablespoon of butter
- Two tablespoons of heavy cream

Instructions

- Rub potato with oil, season with salt and pepper, place in the preheated air fryer and cook at 400 degrees F for 30 minutes.
- Flip potato, cook for 30 minutes more, transfer to a cutting board, cool it down, slice in half lengthwise and scoop pulp in a bowl.
- Add bacon, cheese, butter, heavy cream, green onions, salt and pepper, stir well and stuff potato skins with this mix.
- Return potatoes to your air fryer and cook them at 400 degrees F for 20 minutes.
- Divide among plates and serve as a side dish.
- Enjoy!

Creamy Cabbage

Preparation Time-10 minutes | Cook Time-20 minutes | Servings-2 | Difficulty-Easy

Nutritional Facts- Calories-208 | Fats-9.9g |Carbohydrates-19g |Proteins-6g

Ingredients

- One chopped green cabbage head
- One chopped yellow onion
- Salt and black pepper to the taste
- Four chopped bacon slices
- One cup of whipped cream
- Two tablespoons of cornstarch

Instructions

- Put cabbage, bacon and onion in your air fryer.
- In a bowl, mix cornstarch with cream, salt and pepper, stir and add over cabbage.
- Toss, cook at 400 degrees F for 20 minutes, divide among plates and serve as a side dish.
- Enjoy!

Creamy Endives

Preparation Time-10 minutes | Cook Time-10 minutes | Servings-2 | Difficulty-

Nutritional Facts- Calories-122 | Fats-1g|Carbohydrates-9g |Proteins-4.8g

Ingredients

- Six trimmed and halved endives
- One teaspoon of garlic powder
- Half cup of Greek yogurt
- Half teaspoon of curry powder
- Salt and black pepper to the taste
- Three tablespoons of lemon juice

Instructions

- In a bowl, mix endives with garlic powder, yogurt, curry powder, salt, pepper and lemon juice, toss, leave aside for 10 minutes and transfer to your preheated air fryer at 350 degrees F.
- Cook endives for 10 minutes, divide them among plates and serve as a side dish.
- Enjoy!

Creamy Roasted Peppers Side Dish

Preparation Time-10 minutes | Cook Time-10 minutes | Servings-2 | Difficulty-Easy

Nutritional Facts- Calories-181 | Fats-1g|Carbohydrates-4.8g |Proteins-6g

Ingredients

- One tablespoon of lemon juice
- One red bell pepper
- One green bell pepper
- One yellow bell pepper
- One lettuce head
- One ounce of rocket leaves
- Salt and black pepper to the taste
- Three tablespoons of Greek yogurt
- Two tablespoons of olive oil

Instructions

- Place bell peppers in your air fryer's basket, cook at 400 degrees F for 10 minutes, transfer to a bowl, leave aside for 10 minutes, peel them, discard seeds, cut them into strips, transfer to a larger bowl, add rocket leaves and lettuce strips and toss.
- In a bowl, mix oil with lemon juice, yogurt, salt and pepper and whisk well.
- Add this over bell peppers mix, toss to coat, divide among plates and serve as a side salad.
- Enjoy!

Crispy Brussels Sprouts and Potatoes

Preparation Time-10 minutes | Cook Time-10 minutes | Servings-2 | Difficulty-Easy

Nutritional Facts- Calories-162 | Fats-4g |Carbohydrates-16.8g |Proteins-7.8g

Ingredients

- One and a half pounds of washed and trimmed Brussels sprouts
- One cup of chopped new potatoes
- One and a half tablespoons of bread crumbs
- Salt and black pepper to the taste
- One and a half tablespoons of butter

Instructions

- Put Brussels sprouts and potatoes in your air fryer's pan, add bread crumbs, salt, pepper and butter, toss well and cook at 400 degrees F for 8 minutes.
- Divide among plates and serve as a side dish.
- Enjoy!

Crispy Kale Chips with Soy Sauce

Preparation Time-5 minutes | Cook Time-5 minutes | Servings-2 | Difficulty-Easy

Nutritional Facts- Calories-171 | Fats-4.8g |Carbohydrates-4.8g |Proteins-25g

Ingredients

- Four medium kale leaves, about One ounce each, stems removed, tear the leaves in thirds
- Two teaspoons of soy sauce
- Two teaspoons of olive oil

Instructions

- Toss the kale leaves with olive oil and soy sauce in a large bowl to coat well. Place the leaves in the baking pan.
- Slide the pan into the air fryer grill.
- Select Air Fry, set the temperature to 400 degrees F (205C) and set time to 5 minutes. Flip the leaves with tongs gently halfway through.
- When cooked, the kale leaves should be crispy. Remove the pan from the air fryer grill.
- Serve immediately.

Crunchy Potato Chips

Preparation Time-20 minutes | Cook Time-15 minutes | Servings-2 | Difficulty-Easy

Nutritional Facts- Calories-287 | Fats-4g |Carbohydrates-19g |Proteins-6g

Ingredients

- Two large sliced russet potatoes
- Sea salt and ground black pepper, to taste
- Cooking spray

Lemony Cream Dip

- Half cup of sour cream
- A quarter teaspoon of lemon juice
- Two minced scallions
- One tablespoon of olive oil
- A quarter teaspoon of salt
- Freshly ground black pepper, to taste

Instructions

- Soak the potato slices in water for 10 minutes, and then pat dry with paper towels.
- Transfer the potato slices to the air fry basket. Spritz the slices with cooking spray.
- Place the basket on the air fry position.
- Select Air Fry, set the temperature to 300 degrees F (150C) and set time to 15 minutes. Stir the potato slices three times during cooking. Sprinkle with salt and ground black pepper at the last minute.
- Meanwhile, combine the ingredients for the dip in a small bowl. Stir to mix well.
- When cooking is complete, the potato slices will be crispy and golden brown. Remove the basket from the air fryer grill.

- Serve the potato chips immediately with the dip.

Easy Roasted Carrots

Preparation Time-10 minutes | Cook Time-20 minutes | Servings-2 | Difficulty-Easy

Nutritional Facts- Calories-62 | Fats-1.5g |Carbohydrates-12g |Proteins-1.5g

Ingredients

- Sixteen ounces of peeled carrots
- One teaspoon of olive oil
- Pepper
- Salt

Instructions

- Preheat the air fryer to 360 F.
- Toss carrots with oil and season with pepper and salt.
- Add carrots into the air fryer basket and cook for 15-18 minutes. Shake basket 3-4 Times.
- Serve and enjoy.

Easy Soy Garlic Mushrooms

Preparation Time-10 minutes | Cook Time-15 minutes | Servings-2 | Difficulty-Easy

Nutritional Facts- Calories-91 | Fats-7.8g |Carbohydrates-6.9g |Proteins-4g

Ingredients

- Eight ounces of cleaned mushrooms
- One tablespoon of chopped fresh parsley
- One teaspoon of soy sauce
- Half teaspoon of garlic powder
- One tablespoon of olive oil
- Pepper
- Salt

Instructions

- Toss mushrooms with soy sauce, garlic powder, oil, pepper, and salt.
- Add mushrooms into the air fryer basket and cook at 380 F for 10-12 minutes.
- Garnish with parsley and serve.

Eggplant Fries

Preparation Time-10 minutes | Cook Time-10 minutes | Servings-2 | Difficulty-Easy

Nutritional Facts- Calories-162 | Fats-6g |Carbohydrates-12g |Proteins-6.9g

Ingredients

- Cooking spray
- One peeled and cut into fries eggplant
- Two tablespoons of milk
- One whisked egg
- Two cups of panko bread crumbs
- Half cup of shredded Italian cheese
- A pinch of salt and black pepper to the taste

Instructions

- In a bowl, mix egg with milk, salt and pepper and whisk well.
- In another bowl, mix panko with cheese and stir.
- Dip eggplant fries in egg mix, then coat in panko mix, place them in your air fryer greased with cooking spray and cook at 400 degrees F for 5 minutes.
- Divide among plates and serve as a side dish.
- Enjoy!

Eggplant Side Dish

Preparation Time-10 minutes | Cook Time-10 minutes | Servings-2 | Difficulty-Easy

Nutritional Facts- Calories-200 | Fats-6.9g |Carbohydrates-12g |Proteins-6g

Ingredients

- Eight baby eggplants, scooped in the center and pulp reserved
- Salt and black pepper to the taste
- A pinch of dried oregano
- One chopped green bell pepper
- One tablespoon of tomato paste
- One bunch of chopped coriander
- Half teaspoon of garlic powder
- One tablespoon of olive oil
- One chopped yellow onion
- One chopped tomato

Instructions

- Heat up a pan with the oil over medium heat, add

onion, stir and cook for 1 minute.

- Add salt, pepper, eggplant pulp, oregano, green bell pepper, tomato paste, garlic powder, coriander and tomato; stir, cook for 1-2 minutes more, take off the heat and cool down.
- Stuff eggplants with this mix, place them in your air fryer's basket and cook at 360 degrees F for 8 minutes.
- Divide eggplants among plates and serve them as a side dish.
- Enjoy!

Fast Teriyaki Shrimp Skewers

Preparation Time-10 minutes | Cook Time-8 minutes | Servings-2 | Difficulty-Easy

Nutritional Facts- Calories-290 | Fats-9.9g |Carbohydrates-1g|Proteins-40g

Ingredients

- One and a half tablespoons of mirin
- One and a half teaspoons of ginger juice
- One and a half tablespoons of soy sauce
- Twelve large peeled and deveined shrimp
- One large egg
- 1/3 cup of panko bread crumbs
- Cooking spray

Instructions

- Combine the mirin, soy sauce, and ginger juice in a large bowl. Stir to mix well.
- Dunk the shrimp in the bowl of mirin mixture, then wrap the bowl in plastic and refrigerate for 1 hour to marinate.
- Spritz the air fry basket with cooking spray.
- Run twelve 4-inch skewers through each shrimp.
- Whisk the egg in the bowl of the marinade to combine well. Pour the bread crumbs on a plate.
- Dredge the shrimp skewers in the egg mixture, then shake the excess off and roll over the bread crumbs to coat well.
- Arrange the shrimp skewers in the air fry basket and spritz with cooking spray.
- Place the basket on the air fry position.
- Select Air Fry, set the temperature to 400 degrees F (205C) and set time to 6 minutes. Flip the shrimp skewers halfway through the cooking time.

- When done, the shrimp will be opaque and firm.
- Serve immediately.

Flavored Cauliflower Side Dish

Preparation Time-10 minutes | Cook Time-10 minutes | Servings-2 | Difficulty-Easy

Nutritional Facts- Calories-77 | Fats-1.5g |Carbohydrates-12g |Proteins-17g

Ingredients

- Twelve steamed cauliflower florets
- Salt and black pepper to the taste
- A quarter teaspoon of turmeric powder
- One and a half teaspoons of red chili powder
- One tablespoon of grated ginger
- Two teaspoons of lemon juice
- Three tablespoons of white flour
- Two tablespoons of water
- Cooking spray
- Half teaspoon of cornflour

Instructions

- In a bowl, mix chili powder with turmeric powder, ginger paste, salt, pepper, lemon juice, white flour, cornflour and water, stir, add cauliflower, toss well and transfer them to your air fryer's basket.
- Coat them with cooking spray, cook them at 400 degrees F for 10 minutes, divide among plates and serve as a side dish.
- Enjoy!

Fried Pickles

Preparation Time-10 minutes | Cook Time-20 minutes | Servings-2 | Difficulty-Easy

Nutritional Facts- Calories-212 | Fats-9.9g |Carbohydrates-7.8g |Proteins-21.9g

Ingredients

- One package of Pancake mix
- One egg white
- One teaspoon of garlic powder
- One teaspoon of baking powder
- Two tablespoons of water
- One small jar of dill pickle chips

Instructions

- Using a paper towel, pat the pickle chips dry.
- In a large mixing bowl, combine the garlic powder, Pancake mix, and baking powder.
- Combine all of the ingredients, including the egg white and water, in a mixing bowl.
- Dill pickle chips are dipped in batter.
- Bake pickle chips for 8-10 minutes at 400 degrees F in an Air fryer.
- Alternatively, arrange pickles on a baking sheet and bake for 8 minutes on each side at 450 degrees F.
- Allow cooling before eating your fried pickles!

Fried Red Cabbage

Preparation Time-10 minutes | Cook Time-15 minutes | Servings-2 | Difficulty-Easy

Nutritional Facts- Calories-173 | Fats-6.9g |Carbohydrates-12.9g |Proteins-4.8g

Ingredients

- Four minced garlic cloves
- Half cup of chopped yellow onion
- One tablespoon of olive oil
- Six cups of chopped red cabbage
- One cup of veggie stock
- One tablespoon of apple cider vinegar
- One cup of applesauce
- Salt and black pepper to the taste

Instructions

- In a heat-proof dish that fits your air fryer, mix cabbage with onion, garlic, oil,
- stock, vinegar, applesauce, salt and pepper, toss really well, place the dish in your air fryer's basket and cook at 380 degrees F for 15 minutes.
- Divide among plates and serve as a side dish.
- Enjoy!

Fried Tomatoes

Preparation Time-10 minutes | Cook Time-5 minutes | Servings-2 | Difficulty-Easy

Nutritional Facts- Calories-133 | Fats-4.8g |Carbohydrates-9g |Proteins-4.8g

Ingredients

- Two sliced green tomatoes

- Salt and black pepper to the taste
- Half cup of flour
- One cup of buttermilk
- One cup of panko bread crumbs
- Half tablespoon of Creole seasoning
- Cooking spray

Instructions

- Season tomato slices with salt and pepper.
- Put flour in a bowl, buttermilk in another and panko crumbs and Creole seasoning in a third one.
- Dredge tomato slices in flour, then in buttermilk and panko bread crumbs, place them in your air fryer's basket greased with cooking spray and cook them at 400 degrees F for 5 minutes.
- Divide among plates and serve as a side dish.
- Enjoy!

Garlic Beet Wedges

Preparation Time-10 minutes | Cook Time-15 minutes | Servings-2 | Difficulty-Easy

Nutritional Facts- Calories-182 | Fats-6.9g |Carbohydrates-10.8g |Proteins-1.5g

Ingredients

- Four washed, peeled and wedge-cut beets
- One tablespoon of olive oil
- Salt and black to the taste
- Two minced cloves of garlic
- One teaspoon of lemon juice

Instructions

- In a bowl, mix beets with oil, salt, pepper, garlic and lemon juice, toss well, transfer
- to your air fryer's basket and cook them at 400 degrees F for 15 minutes.
- Divide beets wedges among plates and serve as a side dish.
- Enjoy!

Garlic Green Beans

Preparation Time-10 minutes | Cook Time-10 minutes | Servings-2 | Difficulty-Easy

Nutritional Facts- Calories-69 | Fats-4g |Carbohydrates-9g |Proteins-17g

Ingredients

- One lb. of trimmed fresh green beans
- One teaspoon of garlic powder
- One tablespoon of olive oil
- Pepper
- Salt

Instructions

- Drizzle green beans with oil and season with garlic powder, pepper, and salt.
- Place green beans into the air fryer basket and cook at 370 F for 8 minutes. Toss halfway through.
- Serve and enjoy.

Garlic Potatoes

Preparation Time-10 minutes | Cook Time-20 minutes | Servings-2 | Difficulty-Easy

Nutritional Facts- Calories-162 | Fats-4.8g | Carbohydrates-7.8g | Proteins-4.8g

Ingredients

- Two tablespoons of chopped parsley
- Five minced garlic cloves
- Half teaspoon of dried basil
- Half teaspoon of dried oregano
- Three pounds of halved red potatoes
- One teaspoon of dried thyme
- Two tablespoons of olive oil
- Salt and black pepper to the taste
- Two tablespoons of butter
- 1/3 cup of grated parmesan

Instructions

- In a bowl, mix potato halves with parsley, garlic, basil, oregano, thyme, salt, pepper, oil and butter, toss really well and transfer to your air fryer's basket.
- Cover and cook at 400 degrees F for 20 minutes, flipping them once.
- Sprinkle parmesan on top, divide potatoes among plates and serve as a side dish.
- Enjoy!

Garlic Tomatoes

Preparation Time-10 minutes | Cook Time-15 minutes | Servings-2 | Difficulty-Easy

Nutritional Facts- Calories-92 | Fats-0g | Carbohydrates-1.5g | Proteins-6g

Ingredients

- Four crushed garlic cloves
- One pound of mixed cherry tomatoes
- Three chopped thyme springs
- Salt and black pepper to the taste
- A quarter cup of olive oil

Instructions

- In a bowl, mix tomatoes with salt, black pepper, garlic, olive oil and thyme, toss to coat, introduce in your air fryer and cook at 360 degrees F for 15 minutes.
- Divide the tomatoes, mix among plates and serve.
- Enjoy!

Garlicky Zucchini and Squash

Preparation Time-10 minutes | Cook Time-10 minutes | Servings-2 | Difficulty-Easy

Nutritional Facts- Calories-325 | Fats-16.2g | Carbohydrates-24g | Proteins-40.5g

Ingredients

- Two large peeled and spiralized zucchini
- Two large yellow summer squashes
- One tablespoon of olive oil, divided
- Half teaspoon of kosher salt
- One garlic clove
- Two tablespoons of fresh chopped basil
- Cooking spray

Instructions

- Spritz the air fry basket with cooking spray.
- Combine the zucchini and summer squash with One teaspoon of salt and olive oil in a large bowl. Toss to coat well.
- Bring the zucchini and summer squash to the air fry basket and add the garlic.
- Place the basket on the air fry position.
- Select Air Fry, set the temperature to 360 degrees F (182C) and set time to 10 minutes. Stir the

zucchini and summer squash halfway through the cooking time.

- When cooked, the zucchini and summer squash will be tender and fragrant. Transfer the cooked zucchini and summer squash onto a plate and set aside.

- Remove the garlic from the air fryer grill and allow it to cool for 5 minutes. Mince the garlic and combine it with the remaining olive oil in a small bowl. Stir to mix well.

- Drizzle the spiralized zucchini and summer squash with garlic oil and sprinkle with basil. Toss to serve.

Glazed Beets

Preparation Time-10 minutes | Cook Time-40 minutes | Servings-2 | Difficulty-Moderate

Nutritional Facts- Calories-121 | Fats-4g |Carbohydrates-1g|Proteins-4g

Ingredients

- Three pounds of trimmed small beets
- Four tablespoons of maple syrup
- One tablespoon of duck fat

Instructions

- Heat up your air fryer at 360 degrees F, add duck fat and heat it up.
- Add beets and maple syrup, toss and cook for 40 minutes.
- Divide among plates and serve as a side dish.
- Enjoy!

Golden Garlicky Olive Stromboli

Preparation Time-25 minutes | Cook Time-25 minutes | Servings-2 | Difficulty-Moderate

Nutritional Facts- Calories-147 | Fats-4.8g |Carbohydrates-10.8g |Proteins-15.9g

Ingredients

- Four large unpeeled cloves of garlic
- Three tablespoons of grated Parmesan cheese
- Half cup of packed fresh basil leaves
- Half cup of marinated pitted green and black olives
- A quarter teaspoon of crushed red pepper
- Half pound of pizza dough, at room temperature

- Four ounces of sliced provolone cheese
- Cooking spray

Instructions

- Spritz the air fry basket with cooking spray. Put the unpeeled garlic in the air fry basket.
- Place the basket on the air fry position.
- Select Air Fry, set the temperature to 370 degrees F (188C) and set the time to 10 minutes.
- When cooked, the garlic will be softened completely. Remove from the air fryer grill and allow to cool until you can handle it.
- Peel the garlic and set it into a food processor with two tablespoons of basil, crushed red pepper, Parmesan, and olives. Pulse to mix well. Set aside.
- Arrange the pizza dough on a clean work surface, and then roll it out with a rolling pin into a rectangle. Cut the rectangle in half.
- Sprinkle half of the garlic mixture over each rectangle half, and leave 1/2-inch edges to uncover. Top them with the provolone cheese.
- Brush one long side of each rectangle half with water, and then roll them up. Spritz the air fry basket with cooking spray. Transfer the rolls to the air fry basket. Spritz with cooking spray and scatter with remaining Parmesan.
- Place the basket on the air fry position.
- Select Air Fry and set the time to 15 minutes. Set the rolls halfway through the cooking time. When done, the rolls should be golden brown.
- Remove the rolls from the air fryer grill and allow them to cool for a few minutes before serving.

Greek Beef Meatballs Salad

Preparation Time-10 minutes | Cook Time-10 minutes | Servings-2 | Difficulty-Easy

Nutritional Facts- Calories-200 | Fats-4.8g |Carbohydrates-12.9g |Proteins-27g

Ingredients

- A quarter cup of milk
- Sixteen ounces of ground beef
- One grated yellow onion
- Five cubed bread slices
- One whisked egg
- A quarter cup of chopped parsley
- Salt and black pepper to the taste

- Two minced cloves of garlic
- A quarter cup of chopped mint
- Two and a half teaspoons of dried oregano
- One tablespoon of olive oil
- Cooking spray
- Seven ounces of halved cherry tomatoes
- One cup of baby spinach
- One and a half tablespoons of lemon juice
- Seven ounces of Greek yogurt

Instructions

- Put torn bread in a bowl, add milk, soak for a few minutes, squeeze and transfer to another bowl.
- Add beef, salt, egg, pepper, , mint, oregano, garlic, parsley, and onion; stir and shape medium meatballs out of this mix.
- Spray them with cooking spray, place them in your air fryer and cook at 370 degrees F for 10 minutes.
- In a salad bowl, mix spinach with cucumber and tomato.
- Add meatballs, the oil, some salt, pepper, lemon juice and yogurt, toss and serve.
- Enjoy!

Greek Veggie Side Dish

Preparation Time-10 minutes | Cook Time-45 minutes | Servings-2 | Difficulty-Moderate

Nutritional Facts- Calories-210 | Fats-1.5g |Carbohydrates-10.8g |Proteins-6g

Ingredients

- One sliced eggplant
- One sliced zucchini
- Two chopped red bell peppers
- Two minced cloves of garlic
- Three tablespoons of olive oil
- One bay leaf
- One chopped thyme spring
- Two chopped onions
- Four tomatoes, cut into quarters
- Salt and black pepper to the taste

Instructions

- In your air fryer's pan, mix eggplant slices with zucchini ones, bell peppers, garlic, oil, bay leaf,

thyme, onions, tomatoes, salt and pepper, toss and cook them at 300 degrees F for 35 minutes.
- Divide among plates and serve as a side dish.
- Enjoy!

Green Beans Side Dish

Preparation Time-10 minutes | Cook Time-25 minutes | Servings-2 | Difficulty-Easy

Nutritional Facts- Calories-161 | Fats-4g |Carbohydrates-10.8g |Proteins-4g

Ingredients

- One and a half pounds of trimmed green beans, steamed for 2 minutes
- Salt and black pepper to the taste
- Half pound of chopped shallots
- A quarter cup of toasted almonds
- Two tablespoons of olive oil

Instructions

- In your air fryer's basket, mix green beans with salt, pepper, shallots, almonds and oil, toss well and cook at 400 degrees F for 25 minutes.
- Divide among plates and serve as a side dish.
- Enjoy!

Hasselback Potatoes

Preparation Time-10 minutes | Cook Time-20 minutes | Servings-2 | Difficulty-Easy

Nutritional Facts- Calories-172 | Fats-6.9g |Carbohydrates-9g |Proteins-6g

Ingredients

- Two peeled and thinly sliced potatoes
- Two tablespoons of olive oil
- One teaspoon of minced garlic
- Salt and black pepper to the taste
- Half teaspoon of dried oregano
- Half teaspoon of dried basil
- Half teaspoon of sweet paprika

Instructions

- In a bowl, mix oil with garlic, salt, pepper, oregano, basil and paprika and whisk really well.
- Rub potatoes with this mix, place them in your air fryer's basket and fry them at 360 degrees F for 20 minutes.

- Divide them among plates and serve as a side dish.
- Enjoy!

Herbed Tomatoes

Preparation Time-10 minutes | Cook Time-15 minutes | Servings-2 | Difficulty-Easy

Nutritional Facts- Calories-112 | Fats-1.5g |Carbohydrates-6.9g |Proteins-4g

Ingredients

- Four big halved tomatoes
- Salt and black pepper to the taste
- One tablespoon of olive oil
- Two minced cloves of garlic
- Half teaspoon of chopped thyme

Instructions

- In your air fryer, mix tomatoes with salt, pepper, oil, garlic and thyme, toss and cook at 390 degrees F for 15 minutes.
- Divide among plates and serve them as a side dish.
- Enjoy!

Indian Turnips Salad

Preparation Time-10 minutes | Cook Time-12 minutes | Servings-2 | Difficulty-Easy

Nutritional Facts- Calories-101 | Fats-1g|Carbohydrates-12g |Proteins-4g

Ingredients

- Twenty ounces of peeled and chopped turnips
- One teaspoon of minced garlic
- One teaspoon of grated ginger
- Two chopped yellow onions
- Two chopped tomatoes
- One teaspoon of ground cumin
- One teaspoon of ground coriander
- Two chopped green chilies
- Half teaspoon of turmeric powder
- Two tablespoons of butter
- Salt and black pepper to the taste
- A handful of chopped coriander leaves

Instructions

- Heat up a pan that fits your air fryer with the butter, melt it, add green chilies, garlic and ginger, stir and cook for 1 minute.
- Add onions, salt, pepper, tomatoes, turmeric, ground cumin, coriander and turnips, stir, introduce in your air fryer and cook at 350 degrees F for 10 minutes.
- Divide among plates, sprinkle fresh coriander on top and serve.
- Enjoy!

Leeks

Preparation Time-10 minutes | Cook Time-10 minutes | Servings-2 | Difficulty-Easy

Nutritional Facts- Calories-102 | Fats-4g |Carbohydrates-7.8g |Proteins-1.5g

Ingredients

- Four washed and halved leeks
- Salt and black pepper to the taste
- One tablespoon of melted butter
- One tablespoon of lemon juice

Instructions

- Rub leeks with melted butter, season with salt and pepper, put in your air fryer and cook at 350 degrees F for 7 minutes.
- Arrange on a platter, drizzle lemon juice all over and serve.
- Enjoy!

Lemony Artichokes

Preparation Time-10 minutes | Cook Time-15 minutes | Servings-2 | Difficulty-Easy

Nutritional Facts- Calories-121 | Fats-1g|Carbohydrates-9g |Proteins-4g

Ingredients

- Two medium trimmed and halved artichokes
- Cooking spray
- Two tablespoons of lemon juice
- Salt and black pepper to the taste

Instructions

- Grease your air fryer with cooking spray, add artichokes, drizzle lemon juice and sprinkle salt and black pepper and cook them at 380 degrees F for 15 minutes.

- Divide them among plates and serve as a side dish.
- Enjoy!

Lemony Corn and Bell Pepper

Preparation Time-10 minutes | Cook Time-10 minutes | Servings-2 | Difficulty-Easy

Nutritional Facts- Calories-264 | Fats-4g |Carbohydrates-24g |Proteins-31.8g

Ingredients

Corn

- One and a half cups of thawed frozen corn kernels
- One cup of mixed diced bell peppers
- One diced jalapeño
- One cup of diced yellow onion
- Half teaspoon of ancho chili powder
- One tablespoon of fresh lemon juice
- One teaspoon of ground cumin
- Half teaspoon of kosher salt
- Cooking spray

For Serving

- A quarter cup of feta cheese
- A quarter cup of chopped fresh cilantro
- One tablespoon of fresh lemon juice

Instructions

- Spritz the air fry basket with cooking spray.
- Combine the ingredients for the corn in a large bowl. Stir to mix well.
- Pour the mixture into the air fry basket.
- Place the basket on the air fry position.
- Select Air Fry, set the temperature to 375 degrees F (190C) and set time to 10 minutes. Stir the mixture halfway through the cooking time.
- When done, the corn and bell peppers should be soft.
- Transfer them onto a large plate, and then spread with feta cheese and cilantro. Drizzle with lemon juice and serve.

Lemony-Garlicky Asparagus

Preparation Time-5 minutes | Cook Time-10 minutes | Servings-2 | Difficulty-Easy

Nutritional Facts- Calories-211 | Fats-10.8g |Carbohydrates-21g |Proteins-6g

Ingredients

- Ten spears asparagus, snap the ends off
- One tablespoon of lemon juice
- Two teaspoons of minced garlic
- Half teaspoon of salt
- A quarter teaspoon of ground black pepper
- Cooking spray

Instructions

- Line the air fry basket with parchment paper.
- Put the asparagus spears in a large bowl. Drizzle with a sprinkle with minced garlic,
- lemon juice and salt, and ground black pepper. Toss to coat well.
- Transfer the asparagus to the air fry basket and spritz it with cooking spray.
- Place the basket on the air fry position.
- Select Air Fry, set the temperature to 400 degrees F (205C) and set time to 10 minutes. Flip the asparagus halfway through cooking.
- When cooked, the asparagus should be wilted and soft. Remove the basket from the air fryer grill.
- Serve immediately.

Lentils Fritters

Preparation Time-10 minutes | Cook Time-10 minutes | Servings-2 | Difficulty-Easy

Nutritional Facts- Calories-143 | Fats-1g|Carbohydrates-12g |Proteins-4g

Ingredients

- One cup of yellow lentils, soaked in water for 1 hour and drained
- One chopped hot chili pepper
- One-inch grated ginger piece
- Half teaspoon of turmeric powder
- One teaspoon of garam masala
- One teaspoon of baking powder
- Salt and black pepper to the taste
- Two teaspoons of olive oil

- 1/3 cup of water
- Half cup of chopped cilantro
- One and a half cups of chopped spinach
- Four minced garlic cloves
- 3⁄4 cup of chopped red onion
- Mint chutney for serving

Instructions

- In your blender, mix lentils with chili pepper, ginger, turmeric, garam masala, baking powder, salt, pepper, olive oil, water, cilantro, spinach, onion and garlic, blend well and shape medium balls out of this mix.
- Place them all in your preheated air fryer at 400 degrees F and cook for 10 minutes.
- Serve your veggie fritters with a side salad for lunch.
- Enjoy!

Lunch Chicken Salad

Preparation Time-10 minutes | Cook Time-20 minutes | Servings-2 | Difficulty-Easy

Nutritional Facts- Calories-372 | Fats-6g |Carbohydrates-9.9g |Proteins-6g

Ingredients

- Two hulled ears of corn
- One pound of boneless chicken tenders
- Olive oil as needed
- Salt and black pepper to the taste
- One teaspoon of sweet paprika
- One tablespoon of brown sugar
- Half teaspoon of garlic powder
- Half iceberg lettuce head, cut into medium strips
- Half romaine lettuce head, cut into medium strips
- One cup of canned black beans, drained
- One cup of shredded cheddar cheese
- Three tablespoons of chopped cilantro
- Four chopped green onions
- Twelve sliced cherry tomatoes
- A quarter cup of ranch dressing
- Three tablespoons of BBQ sauce

Instructions

- Put corn in your air fryer, drizzle some oil, toss, cook at 400 degrees F for 10 minutes, transfer to a plate and leave aside for now.

- Put chicken in your air fryer's basket, add salt, pepper, brown sugar, paprika and garlic powder, toss, drizzle some more oil, cook at 400 degrees F for 10 minutes, flipping them halfway, transfer tenders to a cutting board and chop them.
- Cur kernels off the cob, transfer corn to a bowl, add chicken, iceberg lettuce, romaine lettuce, black beans, cheese, cilantro, tomatoes, onions, BBQ sauce and ranch dressing, toss well and serve for lunch.
- Enjoy!

Lunch Potato Salad

Preparation Time-10 minutes | Cook Time-25 minutes | Servings-2 | Difficulty-Easy

Nutritional Facts- Calories-211 | Fats-6.9g |Carbohydrates-12g |Proteins-4.8g

Ingredients

- Two pounds of halved red potatoes
- Two tablespoons of olive oil
- Salt and black pepper to the taste
- Two chopped green onions
- One chopped red bell pepper
- 1/3 cup of lemon juice
- Three tablespoons of mustard

Instructions

- On your air fryer's basket, mix potatoes with half of the olive oil, salt and pepper and cook at 350 degrees F for 25 minutes, shaking the fryer once.
- In a bowl, mix onions with bell pepper and roasted potatoes and toss.
- In a small bowl, mix lemon juice with the rest of the oil and mustard and whisk really well.
- Add this to potato salad, toss well and serve for lunch.
- Enjoy!

Mediterranean Vegetables

Preparation Time-10 minutes | Cook Time-15 minutes | Servings-2 | Difficulty-Easy

Nutritional Facts- Calories-63 | Fats-1.2g |Carbohydrates-13.8g |Proteins-2.7g

Ingredients

- Six halved cherry tomatoes

- One diced eggplant
- One diced zucchini
- One diced green bell pepper
- One teaspoon of thyme
- One teaspoon of oregano
- Pepper
- Salt

Instructions

- In a bowl, toss eggplant, zucchini, bell pepper, thyme, oregano, pepper, and salt.
- Add vegetable mixture into the air fryer basket and cook at 360 F for 12 minutes.
- Add cherry tomatoes and shake basket well and cook for 3 minutes more.
- Serve and enjoy.

Mushroom Cakes

Preparation Time-10 minutes | Cook Time-10 minutes | Servings-2 | Difficulty-Easy

Nutritional Facts- Calories-192 | Fats-1g | Carbohydrates-18g | Proteins-6.9g

Ingredients

- Four ounces of chopped mushrooms
- One chopped yellow onion
- Salt and black pepper to the taste
- Half teaspoon of ground nutmeg
- Two tablespoons of olive oil
- One tablespoon of butter
- One and a half tablespoons of flour
- One tablespoon of bread crumbs
- Fourteen ounces of milk

Instructions

- Heat up a pan with the butter over medium-high heat, add onion and mushrooms, stir, cook for 3 minutes, add flour, stir well again and take off the heat.
- Add milk gradually, salt, pepper and nutmeg, stir and leave aside to cool down completely.
- In a bowl, mix oil with bread crumbs and whisk.
- Take spoonfuls of the mushroom filling, add to breadcrumbs mix, coat well, shape patties out of this mix,
- place them in your air fryer's basket and cook at 400 degrees F for 8 minutes.

- Divide among plates and serve as a side for a steak.
- Enjoy!

Mushroom Side Dish

Preparation Time-10 minutes | Cook Time-10 minutes | Servings-2 | Difficulty-Easy

Nutritional Facts- Calories-241 | Fats-7.8g | Carbohydrates-13.8g | Proteins-6g

Ingredients

Ten stems removed button mushrooms
- One tablespoon of Italian seasoning
- Salt and black pepper to the taste
- Two tablespoons of grated cheddar cheese
- One tablespoon of olive oil
- Two tablespoons of grated mozzarella
- One tablespoon of chopped dill

Instructions

- In a bowl, mix mushrooms with Italian seasoning, salt, pepper, oil and dill and rub well.
- Arrange mushrooms in your air fryer's basket, sprinkle mozzarella and cheddar in each and cook them at 360 degrees F for 8 minutes.
- Divide them among plates and serve them as a side dish.
- Enjoy!

Mushrooms and Sour Cream

Preparation Time-10 minutes | Cook Time-10 minutes | Servings-2 | Difficulty-Easy

Nutritional Facts- Calories-211 | Fats-4g | Carbohydrates-15g | Proteins-4g

Ingredients

- Two chopped bacon strips
- One chopped yellow onion
- One chopped green bell pepper
- Twenty-four stems removed mushrooms
- One grated carrot
- Half cup of sour cream
- One cup of grated cheddar cheese
- Salt and black pepper to the taste

Instructions

- Heat up a pan over medium-high heat, add

bacon, onion, bell pepper and carrot, stir and cook for 1 minute.

- Add salt, pepper and sour cream, stir, cook for 1 minute more, take off the heat and cool down.
- Stuff mushrooms with this mix, sprinkle cheese on top and cook at 360 degrees F for 8 minutes.
- Divide among plates and serve as a side dish.
- Enjoy!

Mutton Momos

Preparation Time-5 minutes | Cook Time-30 minutes | Servings-2 | Difficulty-Easy

Nutritional Facts- Calories-471 | Fats-13.8g |Carbohydrates-21g |Proteins-30g

Ingredients

For dough

- One and a half cups of all-purpose flour
- Five tablespoons of water
- Half teaspoon of salt

For filling

- Two teaspoons of vinegar
- Two tablespoons of coriander leaves
- One teaspoon of. ground cumin
- One chopped onion
- Two teaspoons of soy-sauce
- Two cups of minced mutton
- Two teaspoons of ginger-garlic paste
- Two tablespoons of oil

Instructions

- In a bowl, add the dough ingredients and mix. Knead the dough and cover with a plastic wrap, set aside.
- Preheat the air fryer to 200F.
- For the filling, add all the ingredients to a bowl and mix thoroughly. Roll out the dough and cut it into small squares. Place the dough's middle fillings, wrap the dough to cover the fillings, and pinch the edges together.
- Transfer to the air fryer and close the lid. Set time to 20 minutes.
- Serve and enjoy with sauce or ketchup.

Okra and Corn Salad

Preparation Time-10 minutes | Cook Time-15 minutes | Servings-2 | Difficulty-Easy

Nutritional Facts- Calories-164 | Fats-4.8g |Carbohydrates-21g |Proteins-4g

Ingredients

- One pound of trimmed okra
- Six chopped scallions
- Three chopped green bell peppers
- Black pepper and salt as per taste
- Two tablespoons of olive oil
- One teaspoon of sugar
- Twenty-eight ounces of chopped canned tomatoes
- One cup of con

Instructions

- Heat the oil in a pan large enough to fit your air fryer over medium-high heat, then add the bell peppers and scallions, stir, and cook for 5 minutes.
- Stir in the tomatoes, okra, pepper, salt, sugar, and corn, then transfer to your air fryer and cook for 7 minutes at 360 degrees F.
- Serve the okra mixture warm among plates.
- Enjoy!

Okra Chips

Preparation Time-5 minutes | Cook Time-16 minutes | Servings-2 | Difficulty-Easy

Nutritional Facts- Calories-321 | Fats-19g |Carbohydrates-4g |Proteins-12g

Ingredients

- Two pounds of fresh okra pods
- Two tablespoons of canola oil
- One teaspoon of coarse sea salt

Instructions

- Stir the salt and oil in a bowl to mix well. Add the okra and toss to coat well. Place the okra in the air fry basket.
- Place the basket on the air fry position.
- Select Air Fry, set the temperature to 400 degrees F (205C) and set time to 16 minutes. Flip the okra at least three times during cooking.

- When cooked, the okra should be lightly browned. Remove from the air fryer grill.
- Serve immediately.

Old Bay Shrimp and Corn Bake

Preparation Time-10 minutes | Cook Time-18 minutes | Servings-2 | Difficulty-Easy

Nutritional Facts- Calories-283 | Fats-4.8g |Carbohydrates-16.8g |Proteins-24g

Ingredients

- One ear corn, husk and silk detach
- Eight ounces of unpeeled red potatoes
- Two teaspoons of Old Bay Seasoning, divided
- Two teaspoons of vegetable oil, divided
- A quarter teaspoon of ground black pepper
- Eight ounces of deveined large shrimps
- Six ounces of Andouille or chorizo sausage
- Two minced cloves of garlic
- One tablespoon of chopped fresh parsley

Instructions

- Put the corn rounds and potatoes in a large bowl. Sprinkle with One teaspoon of Old Bay seasoning and drizzle with vegetable oil. Toss to coat well.
- Transfer the corn rounds and potatoes onto a baking pan.
- Place the pan on the bake position.
- Select Bake, set temperature to 400F (205C) and set time to 18 minutes.
- After 6 minutes, remove the pan from the air fryer grill. Stir the corn rounds and potatoes. Return the pan to the air fryer grill and continue cooking.
- Meanwhile, cut slits into the shrimps but be careful not to cut them through. Combine the remaining Old Bay seasoning, remaining vegetable oil, shrimps, and sausage in the large bowl. Toss to coat well.
- After 6 minutes, remove the pan from the air fryer grill. Add the shrimp and sausage to the pan. Return the pan to the air fryer grill and continue cooking for 6 minutes. Stir the shrimp mixture halfway through the cooking time.
- When done, the shrimps should be opaque. Remove the pan from the air fryer grill.
- Transfer the dish to a plate and spread with parsley before serving.

Panko Crusted Calf's Liver Strips

Preparation Time-15 minutes | Cook Time-5 minutes | Servings-2 | Difficulty-Easy

Nutritional Facts- Calories-244 | Fats-12g |Carbohydrates-2g |Proteins-12g

Ingredients

- One pound of sliced calf's liver
- Two eggs
- Two tablespoons of milk
- Half cup of whole wheat flour
- Two cups of panko breadcrumbs
- Salt and ground black pepper, to taste
- Cooking spray

Instructions

- Spritz the airflow racks with cooking spray.
- Rub the calf's liver strips with salt and ground black pepper on a clean work surface.
- Whisk the eggs with milk in a large bowl. Pour the flour into a shallow dish. Pour the panko into a separate shallow dish.
- Dunk the liver strips in the flour, then in the egg mixture. Shake the excess off and roll the strips over the panko to coat well.
- Arrange the liver strips in the racks and spritz with cooking spray.
- Slide the racks into the air fryer oven. Press the Power Button. Cook at 390F (199C) for 5 minutes.
- Flip the strips halfway through.
- When cooking is processed, the strips should be browned.
- Serve immediately.

Panko-Crusted Shrimp

Preparation Time-15 minutes | Cook Time-10 minutes | Servings-2 | Difficulty-Easy

Nutritional Facts- Calories-283 | Fats-4g |Carbohydrates-16.8g |Proteins-26g

Ingredients

- One tablespoon of Sriracha sauce
- One teaspoon of Worcestershire sauce
- Two tablespoons of sweet chili sauce
- 1/3 cup of mayonnaise
- One beaten egg

- One cup of panko bread crumbs
- One pound of raw shelled and deveined, rinsed and drained shrimp
- Lime wedges, for serving
- Cooking spray

Instructions

- Spritz the air fry basket with cooking spray.
- Combine the Sriracha sauce, Worcestershire sauce, chili sauce, and mayo in a bowl. Stir to mix well. Reserve 1/3 cup of the mixture as the dipping sauce.
- Combine the remaining sauce mixture with the beaten egg. Stir to mix well. Put the panko in a separate bowl.
- Dredge the shrimp in the sauce mixture first, then into the panko. Roll the shrimp to coat well. Shake the excess off.
- Place the shrimp in the air fry basket, then spritz with cooking spray.
- Place the basket on the air fry position.
- Select Air Fry, set the temperature to 360°F (182°C) and set the time to 10 minutes. Flip the shrimp halfway through the cooking time.
- When cooking is processed, the shrimp should be opaque.
- Remove the shrimp from the air fryer grill and serve with reserve sauce mixture and squeeze the lime wedges over.

Parmesan Mushrooms

Preparation Time-10 minutes | Cook Time-15 minutes | Servings-2 | Difficulty-Easy

Nutritional Facts- Calories-124 | Fats-4g |Carbohydrates-10.8g |Proteins-17g

Ingredients

- Nine button mushroom caps
- Three crumbled cream cracker slices
- One egg white
- Two tablespoons of grated parmesan
- One teaspoon of Italian seasoning
- A pinch of salt and black pepper
- One tablespoon of melted butter

Instructions

- In a bowl, mix crackers with egg white, parmesan, Italian seasoning, butter, salt and

pepper, stir well and stuff mushrooms with this mix.
- Arrange mushrooms in your air fryer's basket and cook them at 360 degrees F for 15 minutes.
- Divide among plates and serve as a side dish.
- Enjoy!

Pasta Salad

Preparation Time-12 minutes | Cook Time-17 minutes | Servings-2 | Difficulty-Easy

Nutritional Facts- Calories-201 | Fats-4.8g |Carbohydrates-18g |Proteins-6.9g

Ingredients

- One sliced and roughly chopped zucchini
- One roughly chopped orange bell pepper
- One roughly chopped green bell pepper
- One roughly chopped red onion
- Four ounces of brown halved mushrooms
- Salt and black pepper to the taste
- One teaspoon of Italian seasoning
- One pound of already cooked penne rigate
- One cup of halved cherry tomatoes
- Half cup of pitted and halved kalamata olive
- A quarter cup of olive oil
- Three tablespoons of balsamic vinegar
- Two tablespoons of chopped basil

Instructions

- Combine zucchini, orange bell pepper, Italian seasoning, mushrooms, green bell pepper, salt, red onion, pepper, and oil in a mixing bowl; toss well, then transfer to an air fryer preheated to 380 degrees F and cook for 12 minutes.
- Toss the spaghetti with the cooked vegetables, vinegar, olives, cherry tomatoes, and basil in a large salad bowl and serve.

Pork Belly Bites

Preparation Time-15 minutes | Cook Time-20 minutes | Servings-2 | Difficulty-Easy

Nutritional Facts- Calories-156 | Fats-4g |Carbohydrates-6g |Proteins-24g

Ingredients

- One lb. of diced pork belly
- Salt and pepper to taste

- Half teaspoon of garlic powder
- One teaspoon of Worcestershire sauce

Instructions

- Select the grill setting in your air fryer.
- Preheat it to 400 degrees F.
- Flavor pork with salt, pepper, garlic powder and Worcestershire sauce.
- Add to the air fryer.
- Cook at 400 degrees F for 20 minutes, flipping twice.

Potato Casserole

Preparation Time-15 minutes | Cook Time-40 minutes | Servings-2 | Difficulty-Moderate

Nutritional Facts- Calories-162 | Fats-4.8g |Carbohydrates-19g |Proteins-4g

Ingredients

- Three pounds of scrubbed sweet potatoes
- A quarter cup of milk
- Half teaspoon of ground nutmeg
- Two tablespoons of white flour
- A quarter teaspoon of ground allspice
- Salt to the taste

For the topping

- Half cup of almond flour
- Half cup of soaked, drained and ground walnuts
- A quarter cup of soaked, drained and ground pecans
- A quarter cup of shredded coconut
- One tablespoon of chia seeds
- A quarter cup of sugar
- One teaspoon of cinnamon powder
- Five tablespoons of butter

Instructions

- Place potatoes in your air fryer's basket, prick them with a fork and cook at 360 degrees F for 30 minutes.
- Meanwhile, in a bowl, mix almond flour with pecans, walnuts, A quarter cup of coconut, A quarter cup of sugar, chia seeds, one teaspoon of cinnamon and the butter and stir everything.

- Transfer potatoes to a cutting board, cool them, peel and place them in a baking dish that fits your air fryer.
- Add milk, flour, salt, nutmeg and allspice and stir
- Add the crumble mix you've made earlier on top, place the dish in your air fryer's basket and cook at 400 degrees F for 8 minutes.
- Divide among plates and serve as a side dish.

Potato Wedges

Preparation Time-10 minutes | Cook Time-25 minutes | Servings-2 | Difficulty-Easy

Nutritional Facts- Calories-171 | Fats-7.8g |Carbohydrates-15.9g |Proteins-6.9g

Ingredients

- Two potatoes, cut into wedges
- One tablespoon of olive oil
- Salt and black pepper to the taste
- Three tablespoons of sour cream
- Two tablespoons of sweet chili sauce

Instructions

- In a bowl, mix potato wedges with oil, salt and pepper, toss well, add to air fryer's basket and cook at 360 degrees F for 25 minutes, flipping them once.
- Divide potato wedges among plates, drizzle sour cream and chili sauce all over and serve them as a side dish.

Potatoes Patties

Preparation Time-10 minutes | Cook Time-10 minutes | Servings-2 | Difficulty-Easy

Nutritional Facts- Calories-141 | Fats-4.8g |Carbohydrates-16.8g |Proteins-4.8g

Ingredients

- Four cubed, boiled and mashed potatoes
- One cup of grated parmesan
- Salt and black pepper to the taste
- A pinch of nutmeg
- Two egg yolks
- Two tablespoons of white flour
- Three tablespoons of chopped chives

For the breading

- A quarter cup of white flour
- Three tablespoons of vegetable oil
- Two whisked eggs
- A quarter cup of bread crumbs

Instructions

- In a bowl, mix mashed potatoes with egg yolks, salt, pepper, nutmeg, parmesan, chives and two tablespoons of flour, stir well, shape medium cakes and place them on a plate.
- In another bowl, mix vegetable oil with bread crumbs and stir.
- Put whisked eggs in a third bowl and a quarter cup of flour in a fourth one.
- Dip cakes in flour, then in eggs and in breadcrumbs at the end, place them in your air fryer's basket, cook them at 390 degrees F for 8 minutes, divide among plates and serve as a side dish.
- Enjoy!

Pumpkin Rice

Preparation Time-5 minutes | Cook Time-30 minutes | Servings-2 | Difficulty-Easy

Nutritional Facts- Calories-261 | Fats-6g |Carbohydrates-28.9g |Proteins-4g

Ingredients

- Two tablespoons of olive oil
- One chopped small yellow onion
- Two minced cloves of garlic
- Twelve ounces of white rice
- Four cups of chicken stock
- Six ounces of pumpkin puree
- Half teaspoon of nutmeg
- One teaspoon of chopped thyme
- Half teaspoon of grated ginger
- Half teaspoon of cinnamon powder
- Half teaspoon of allspice
- Four ounces of heavy cream

Instructions

- In a dish that fits your air fryer, mix oil with onion, garlic, rice, stock, pumpkin puree, nutmeg, thyme, ginger, cinnamon, allspice and

cream, stir well, place in your air fryer's basket and cook at 360 degrees F for 30 minutes.
- Divide among plates and serve as a side dish.

Rice and Sausage Side Dish

Preparation Time-10 minutes | Cook Time-20 minutes | Servings-2 | Difficulty-Easy

Nutritional Facts- Calories-240 | Fats-12g |Carbohydrates-25g |Proteins-13.8g

Ingredients

Two cups of boiled white rice
- One tablespoon of butter
- Salt and black pepper to the taste
- Four minced garlic cloves
- One chopped pork sausage
- Two tablespoons of chopped carrot
- Three tablespoons of grated cheddar cheese
- Two tablespoons of shredded mozzarella cheese

Instructions

- Heat up your air fryer at 350 degrees F, add butter, melt it, add garlic, stir and brown for 2 minutes.
- Add sausage, salt, pepper, carrots and rice, stir and cook at 350 degrees F for 10 minutes.
- Add cheddar and mozzarella, toss, divide among plates and serve as a side dish.

Roasted Eggplant

Preparation Time-10 minutes | Cook Time-20 minutes | Servings-2 | Difficulty-Easy

Nutritional Facts- Calories-173 | Fats-4.8g |Carbohydrates-12g |Proteins-4g

Ingredients

- One and a half pounds of cubed eggplant
- One tablespoon of olive oil
- One teaspoon of garlic powder
- One teaspoon of onion powder
- One teaspoon of sumac
- Two teaspoons of za'atar
- Juice from half lemon
- Two bay leaves

Instructions

- In your air fryer, mix eggplant cubes with oil, garlic powder, onion powder, sumac, za'atar, lemon juice and bay leaves, toss and cook at 370 degrees F for 20 minutes.
- Divide among plates and serve as a side dish.

Roasted Parsnips

Preparation Time-10 minutes | Cook Time-40 minutes | Servings-2 | Difficulty-Moderate

Nutritional Facts- Calories-124 | Fats-1g | Carbohydrates-10.8g | Proteins-4g

Ingredients

- Two pounds of peeled parsnips, cut into medium chunks
- Two tablespoons of maple syrup
- One tablespoon of dried parsley flakes
- One tablespoon of olive oil

Instructions

- Preheat your air fryer at 360 degrees F, add oil and heat it up as well.
- Add parsnips, parsley flakes and maple syrup, toss and cook them for 40 minutes.
- Divide among plates and serve as a side dish.

Roasted Peppers

Preparation Time-10 minutes | Cook Time-20 minutes | Servings-2 | Difficulty-Easy

Nutritional Facts- Calories-145 | Fats-4g | Carbohydrates-12g | Proteins-4g

Ingredients

- One tablespoon of sweet paprika
- One tablespoon of olive oil
- Two red bell peppers, cut into medium strips
- Two yellow bell peppers, cut into medium strips
- Two green bell peppers, cut into medium strips
- One chopped yellow onion
- Salt and black pepper to the taste

Instructions

- In your air fryer, mix red bell peppers with green and yellow ones.
- Add paprika, oil, onion, salt and pepper, toss and cook at 350 degrees F for 20 minutes.

- Divide among plates and serve as a side dish.

Roasted Pumpkin

Preparation Time-10 minutes | Cook Time-12 minutes | Servings-2 | Difficulty-Easy

Nutritional Facts- Calories-201 | Fats-6g | Carbohydrates-10.8g | Proteins-17g

Ingredients

- One and a half-pound of deseeded, sliced and roughly chopped pumpkin
- Three minced garlic cloves
- One tablespoon of olive oil
- A pinch of sea salt
- A pinch of brown sugar
- A pinch of nutmeg, ground
- A pinch of cinnamon powder

Instructions

- In your air fryer's basket, mix pumpkin with garlic, oil, salt, brown sugar, cinnamon and nutmeg, toss well, cover and cook at 370 degrees F for 12 minutes.
- Divide among plates and serve as a side dish.
- Enjoy!

Sausage Rolls

Preparation Time-10 minutes | Cook Time-10 minutes | Servings-2 | Difficulty-Easy

Nutritional Facts- Calories- 292 | Fats-13.8g | Carbohydrates-1.5g | Proteins-37.8g

Ingredients

- One can refrigerated crescent roll dough
- One small package of mini smoked sausages patted dry
- Two tablespoons of melted butter
- Two teaspoons of sesame seeds
- One teaspoon of onion powder

Instructions

- Place the crescent roll dough on a clean work surface and separate it into eight pieces. Cut each piece in half, and you will have 16 triangles.
- Make the pigs in the blanket: Arrange each sausage on each dough triangle, and then roll the sausages up.

- Brush the pigs with melted butter and place the pigs in the blanket in the air fry basket. Sprinkle with sesame seeds and onion powder.
- Place the basket on the bake position.
- Select Bake, set temperature to 330F (166C) and set time to 8 minutes. Flip the pigs halfway through the cooking time.
- When cooking is complete, the pigs should be fluffy and golden brown.
- Serve immediately.

Scallops and Spring Veggies

Preparation Time-15 minutes | Cook Time-10 minutes | Servings-2 | Difficulty-Easy

Nutritional Facts- Calories-163 | Fats-4.8g |Carbohydrates-10.8g |Proteins-21.9g

Ingredients

- Half pound of asparagus ends trimmed, cut into 2-inch pieces
- One cup of sugar snap peas
- One pound sea scallops
- One tablespoon of lemon juice
- Two teaspoons of olive oil
- Half teaspoon of dried thyme
- Pinch salt
- Freshly ground black pepper

Instructions

- Bring the asparagus and sugar snap peas to the air fryer basket. Cook for 2 to 3 minutes or until the vegetables are just starting to get tender.
- Meanwhile, check the scallops for a small muscle attached to the side, and pull it off and discard.
- In a medium bowl, toss the scallops with lemon juice, olive oil, thyme, salt, and pepper. Place into the air fryer basket on top of the vegetables.
- Steam for 5 to 7 minutes, tossing the basket once during the cooking time until the scallops are just firm when tested with your finger and are opaque in the center, and the vegetables are tender. Serve immediately.

Sesame Carrots

Preparation Time-10 minutes | Cook Time-8 minutes | Servings-2 | Difficulty-Easy

Nutritional Facts- Calories-95 | Fats-7.8g |Carbohydrates-7.8g |Proteins-1.5g

Ingredients

- Two cups of sliced carrots
- One teaspoon of sesame seeds
- One tablespoon of chopped scallions
- One teaspoon of minced garlic
- One tablespoon of soy sauce
- One tablespoon of minced ginger
- Two tablespoons of sesame oil

Instructions

- In a medium bowl, mix together carrots, garlic, soy sauce, ginger, and sesame oil.
- Add carrots mixture into the air fryer basket and cook at 375 for 7 minutes. Shake basket halfway through.
- Garnish with scallions and sesame seeds and serve.

Simple Potato Chips

Preparation Time-30 minutes | Cook Time-30 minutes | Servings-2 | Difficulty-Hard

Nutritional Facts- Calories-201 | Fats-4.8g |Carbohydrates-18g |Proteins-4.8g

Ingredients

- Four scrubbed, peeled into thin chips potatoes, soaked in water for 30 minutes, drained and pat dried
- Salt the taste
- One tablespoon of olive oil
- Two teaspoons of chopped rosemary

Instructions

- In a bowl, mix potato chips with salt and oil, toss to coat, place them in your air fryer's basket and cook at 330 degrees F for 30 minutes.
- Divide among plates, sprinkle rosemary all over and serve as a side dish.
- Enjoy!

Snapper Scampi

Preparation Time-5 minutes | Cook Time-15 minutes | Servings-2 | Difficulty-Easy

Nutritional Facts- Calories-265 | Fats-10.8g |Carbohydrates-1.5g |Proteins-37.8g

Ingredients

- Four (Six-ounce) skinless snapper or arctic char fillets
- One tablespoon of olive oil
- Three tablespoons of lemon juice, divided
- Half teaspoon of dried basil
- Pinch salt
- Freshly ground black pepper
- Two tablespoons of butter
- Two minced cloves of garlic

Instructions

- Olive oil and one tablespoon of lemon juice are massaged into the fish fillets. Place in the air fryer basket and season with salt, basil, and pepper.
- Grill for 7–8 minutes, or until the salmon flakes easily when examined with a fork. Place the fish on a serving plate after removing it from the basket. To remain warm, cover.
- Combine the remaining two tablespoons of lemon juice, butter, and garlic in a 6-by-6-by-2-inch pan. Cook for 1 to 2 minutes in the air fryer, or until the garlic is sizzling. Serve with this sauce poured over the fish.

Spiced Tempeh

Preparation Time-15 minutes | Cook Time-20 minutes | Servings-2 | Difficulty-Easy

Nutritional Facts- Calories-308 | Fats-8.1g |Carbohydrates-18g |Proteins-17g

Ingredients

Tempeh Bits

- A quarter cup of vegetable oil
- Eight ounces of tempeh
- One teaspoon of lemon pepper
- One teaspoon of chili powder
- Two teaspoons of sweet paprika
- Two teaspoons of garlic powder
- Two teaspoons of onion powder
- A quarter teaspoon of sea salt
- 1/8 teaspoon of cayenne pepper or more to taste

Salad

- Fifteen and a half ounces can of chickpeas
- One lb. of chopped kale
- One cup of shredded carrots
- Two tablespoons of toasted sesame seeds

Dressing

- One tablespoon of freshly grated ginger
- Two tablespoons of toasted sesame oil
- A quarter cup of low sodium soy sauce
- 1/3 cup of seasoned rice vinegar

Instructions

- Blanch kale in a pot of salted boiling water for about 30 seconds and immediately run under cold water; drain and squeeze out excess water. Set aside.
- Preheat your air fryer toast oven to 425 degrees F.
- In a small bowl, combine all the spices for tempeh.
- Add oil to a separate bowl. Slice tempeh into thin pieces.
- Dip each tempeh slice into the oil and arrange them on a paper-lined baking sheet; generously sprinkle with the spices until well covered and bake for about 20 minutes or until crispy and golden brown, then remove from air fryer toast oven. In a large bowl, combine all the salad ingredients and set them aside.
- In a jar, combine all the dressing ingredients, close and shake until well blended; pour the dressing over salad and toss to coat well.
- Crumble the crispy tempeh on top of the salad to serve. Enjoy!

Spicy Chicken Wings

Preparation Time-5 minutes | Cook Time-15 minutes | Servings-2 | Difficulty-Easy

Nutritional Facts- Calories-184 | Fats-10.8g |Carbohydrates-4.8g |Proteins-15g

Ingredients

- Eight to sixteen chicken wings
- Three tablespoons of hot sauce
- Cooking spray

Instructions

- Spritz the air fry basket with cooking spray.
- Arrange the chicken wings in the air fry basket.
- Place the basket on the air fry position.
- Select Air Fry, set the temperature to 360 degrees F (182C) and set time to 15 minutes. Flip the wings at least three times during cooking.
- When cooking is complete, the chicken wings will be well browned. Remove the pan from the air fryer grill.
- Transfer the air-fried wings to a plate and serve with hot sauce.

Spicy Edamame

Preparation Time-10 minutes | Cook Time-18 minutes | Servings-2 | Difficulty-Easy

Nutritional Facts- Calories-172 | Fats-8.1g |Carbohydrates-2.1g |Proteins-13g

Ingredients

- Sixteen ounces of defrosted frozen edamame in the shell
- Juice and zest of one lemon
- One tablespoon of sliced garlic
- Two teaspoons of olive oil
- Half teaspoon of chili powder
- Half teaspoon paprika
- Salt

Instructions

- Toss edamame with lemon zest, garlic, oil, chili powder, paprika, and salt.
- Add edamame into the air fryer basket and cook at 400 F for 18 minutes. Shake basket twice.
- Drizzle lemon juice over edamame and serve.

Steamed Broccoli

Preparation Time-10 minutes | Cook Time-5 minutes | Servings-2 | Difficulty-Easy

Nutritional Facts- Calories-160 | Fats-10.8g |Carbohydrates-6.9g |Proteins-13.8g

Ingredients

- One pound of broccoli florets
- One and a half cups of water
- Salt and pepper to taste
- One teaspoon of extra virgin olive oil

Instructions

- Add water to the bottom of your air fryer toast oven and set the basket on top.
- Toss the broccoli florets with salt, pepper and olive oil until evenly combined, then transfer to the basket of your air fryer toast oven.
- Select keep warm for 10 minutes.
- Remove the basket and serve the broccoli.

Sweet Potato Fries

Preparation Time-10 minutes | Cook Time-20 minutes | Servings-2 | Difficulty-Easy

Nutritional Facts- Calories-201 | Fats-6g |Carbohydrates-18g |Proteins-6.9g

Ingredients

- Two peeled and chopped sweet potatoes
- Salt and black pepper to the taste
- Two tablespoons of olive oil
- Half teaspoon of curry powder
- A quarter teaspoon of ground coriander
- A quarter cup of ketchup
- Two tablespoons of mayonnaise
- Half teaspoon of ground cumin
- A pinch of ginger powder
- A pinch of cinnamon powder

Instructions

- In your air fryer's basket, mix sweet potato fries with salt, pepper, coriander, curry powder and oil, toss well and cook at 370 degrees F for 20 minutes, flipping them once.
- Meanwhile, in a bowl, mix ketchup with mayo, cumin, ginger and cinnamon and whisk well.
- Divide fries among plates, drizzle ketchup mix over them and serve as a side dish.
- Enjoy!

Thai Salad

Preparation Time-10 minutes | Cook Time-5 minutes | Servings-2 | Difficulty-Easy

Nutritional Facts- Calories-172 | Fats-4.8g |Carbohydrates-7.8g |Proteins-12.9g

Ingredients

- One cup of grated carrots
- One cup of shredded red cabbage

- A pinch of salt and black pepper
- A handful of chopped cilantro
- One small chopped cucumber
- Juice from one lime
- Two teaspoons of red curry paste
- Twelve big cooked, peeled and deveined shrimp

Instructions

- In a pan that fits your, mix cabbage with carrots, cucumber and shrimp, toss,
- introduce in your air fryer and cook at 360 degrees F for 5 minutes.
- Add salt, pepper, cilantro, lime juice and red curry paste, toss again, divide among plates and serve right away.

Tortilla Chips

Preparation Time-10 minutes | Cook Time-7 minutes | Servings-2 | Difficulty-Easy

Nutritional Facts- Calories-61 | Fats-1.5g |Carbohydrates-6.9g |Proteins-4.8g

Ingredients

- Eight corn tortillas, cut into triangles
- Salt and black pepper to the taste
- One tablespoon of olive oil
- A pinch of garlic powder
- A pinch of sweet paprika

Instructions

- In a bowl, mix tortilla chips with oil, add salt, pepper, garlic powder and paprika, toss well, place them in your air fryer's basket and cook them at 400 degrees F for 6 minutes.
- Serve them as a side for a fish dish.
- Enjoy!

Veggie Fries

Preparation Time-10 minutes | Cook Time-30 minutes | Servings-2 | Difficulty-Moderate

Nutritional Facts- Calories-102 | Fats-1g |Carbohydrates-10.8g |Proteins-4g

Ingredients

- Four parsnips, cut into medium sticks
- Four mixed carrots cut into medium sticks
- Two sweet potatoes cut into medium sticks

- Salt and black pepper to the taste
- Two tablespoons of chopped rosemary
- Two tablespoons of olive oil
- One tablespoon of flour
- Half teaspoon of garlic powder

Instructions

- Put veggie fries in a bowl, add oil, garlic powder, salt, pepper, flour and rosemary and toss to coat.
- Put sweet potatoes in your preheated air fryer, cook them for 10 minutes at 350 degrees F and transfer them to a platter.
- Put parsnip fries in your air fryer, cook for 5 minutes and transfer over potato fries.
- Put carrot fries in your air fryer, cook for 15 minutes at 350 degrees F and transfer to the platter with the other fries.
- Divide veggie fries among plates and serve them as a side dish.
- Enjoy!

Vermouth Mushrooms

Preparation Time-10 minutes | Cook Time-25 minutes | Servings-2 | Difficulty-Easy

Nutritional Facts- Calories-121 | Fats-1g |Carbohydrates-7.8g |Proteins-4.8g

Ingredients

- One tablespoon of olive oil
- Two pounds white mushrooms
- Two tablespoons of white vermouth
- Two teaspoons of herbs de Provence
- Two minced cloves of garlic

Instructions

- In your air fryer, mix oil with mushrooms, herbs de Provence and garlic, toss and cook at 350 degrees F for 20 minutes.
- Add vermouth, toss and cook for 5 minutes more.
- Divide among plates and serve as a side dish.
- Enjoy!

Wild Rice Pilaf

Preparation Time-10 minutes | Cook Time-25 minutes | Servings-2 | Difficulty-Easy

Nutritional Facts- Calories-144 | Fats-4g |Carbohydrates-15.9g |Proteins-4g

Ingredients

- One chopped shallot
- One teaspoon of minced garlic
- A drizzle of olive oil
- One cup of farro
- 3/4 cup of wild rice
- Four cups of chicken stock
- Salt and black pepper to the taste
- One tablespoon of chopped parsley
- Half cup of toasted and chopped hazelnuts
- 3/4 cup of dried cherries
- Chopped chives for serving

Instructions

- In a dish that fits your air fryer, mix shallot with garlic, oil, faro, wild rice, stock, salt, pepper, parsley, hazelnuts and cherries, stir, place in your air fryer's basket and cook at 350 degrees F for 25 minutes.
- Divide among plates and serve as a side dish.
- Enjoy!

Yellow Squash and Zucchinis Side Dish

Preparation Time-10 minutes | Cook Time-35 minutes | Servings-2 | Difficulty-Easy

Nutritional Facts- Calories-167 | Fats-1.5g |Carbohydrates-6.9g |Proteins-4.8g

Ingredients

Six teaspoons of olive oil
- One pound of sliced zucchinis
- Half pound of cubed carrots
- One halved, deseeded and cut into chunks yellow squash
- Salt and white pepper to the taste
- One tablespoon of chopped tarragon

Instructions

- In your air fryer's basket, mix zucchinis with carrots, squash, salt, pepper and oil, toss well and cook at 400 degrees F for 25 minutes.
- Divide them among plates and serve as a side dish with tarragon sprinkled on top.
- Enjoy!

Zucchini Croquettes

Preparation Time-10 minutes | Cook Time-10 minutes | Servings-2 | Difficulty-Easy

Nutritional Facts- Calories-110 | Fats-4.8g |Carbohydrates-7.8g |Proteins-4g

Ingredients

- One grated carrot
- One grated zucchini
- Two crumbled slices of bread
- One egg
- Salt and black pepper to the taste
- Half teaspoon of sweet paprika
- One teaspoon of minced garlic
- Two tablespoons of grated parmesan cheese
- One tablespoon of cornflour

Instructions

- Put zucchini in a bowl, add salt, leave aside for 10 minutes, squeeze excess water and transfer them to another bowl.
- Add carrots, salt, pepper, paprika, garlic, flour, parmesan, egg and bread crumbs, stir well, shape eight croquettes, place them in your air fryer and cook at 360 degrees F for 10 minutes.
- Divide among plates and serve as a side dish
- Enjoy!

Zucchini Fries

Preparation Time-10 minutes | Cook Time-13 minutes | Servings-2 | Difficulty-Easy

Nutritional Facts- Calories-178 | Fats-6g |Carbohydrates-10.8g |Proteins-17g

Ingredients

- One zucchini, chopped into sticks
- A drizzle of olive oil
- Black pepper and salt as per taste
- Two whisked eggs
- One cup of bread crumbs
- Half cup of flour

Instructions

- In a mixing bowl, combine salt, flour, and pepper, and toss to combine.
- Place breadcrumbs in a separate bowl.

- Mix eggs with a teaspoon of pepper and salt in a separate bowl.
- Dredge the zucchini fries in flour, then in eggs, and last in bread crumbs.
- Cook zucchini fries for 12 minutes in an air fryer greased with olive oil and heated to 400 degrees F.
- As a side dish, serve them.
- Enjoy!

Zucchini Garlic Bites

Preparation Time-15 minutes | Cook Time-25 minutes | Servings-2 | Difficulty-Moderate

Nutritional Facts- Calories-192 | Fats-4.8g |Carbohydrates-6.9g |Proteins-15.9g

Ingredients

- Two bags of Salt and Vinegar Chips crushed
- One cup of zucchini grated and drained
- Half cup of parmesan cheese
- One tablespoon of parsley
- One teaspoon of oregano
- Marinara Sauce
- Two whisked eggs
- Two teaspoons of garlic
- One teaspoon of basil

Instructions

Preheat the oven to 400 degrees Fahrenheit. Spray a baking sheet lightly with nonstick spray, or use your air fryer!

- Grate zucchini on a cheese grater. Using a paper towel, wipe away the excess water.
- Place all ingredients, except the marinara sauce, in a medium mixing dish and stir well.
- Using about a tablespoon of the mix, form small balls and set them on a baking sheet.
- In the oven or your air fryer, bake for 15-18 minutes, or until golden brown.
- Marinara sauce is served on the side.

Zucchini Mix and Herbed Eggplant

Preparation Time-10 minutes | Cook Time-10 minutes | Servings-2 | Difficulty-Easy

Nutritional Facts- Calories-67 | Fats-1.5g |Carbohydrates-12.9g |Proteins-17g

Ingredients

- One teaspoon of dried thyme
- Three tablespoons of olive oil
- One eggplant
- Two tablespoons of lemon juice
- One teaspoon of dried oregano
- Three cubed zucchinis
- Black pepper and salt

Instructions

- Place the eggplants on the Air Fryer Grill Pan, add thyme, zucchinis, olive oil, salt.
- Add pepper, oregano, and lemon juice.
- Set the Air Fryer Grill to the air fry function.
- Cook for 8 minutes at 360 degrees F.
- Serve immediately.

Chapter 6~Air Fried Vegetable Recipes

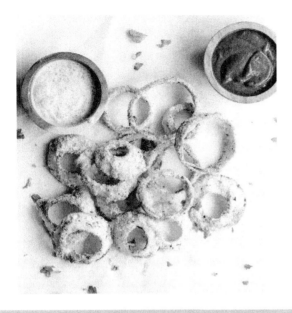

Almond Flour Battered and Crisped Onion Rings

Preparation Time~5 minutes | Cook Time~15 minutes | Servings~2 | Difficulty~Easy

Nutritional Facts~ Calories~217 | Fats~16.8g |Carbohydrates~4.8g |Proteins~4g

Ingredients

- Half cup of almond flour
- 1/3 cup of coconut milk
- One big white onion, sliced into rings
- One beaten egg
- One tablespoon of baking powder
- One tablespoon of smoked paprika
- Salt and pepper to taste

Instructions

- Preheat the air fryer for 5 minutes.
- In a mixing bowl, mix the almond flour, baking powder, smoked paprika, salt and pepper.
- In another bowl, combine the eggs and coconut milk.
- Soak the onion slices into the egg mixture.
- Dredge the onion slices in the almond flour mixture.
- Pour into the air fryer rack/basket. Set temperature to 325°F, and set time to 15 minutes.

Press start. Shake the fryer basket for even cooking.

Aloo Tikka

Preparation Time~10 minutes | Cook Time~30 minutes | Servings~2 to 4| Difficulty~Moderate

Nutritional Facts~ Calories~332 | Fats~9.9g |Carbohydrates~30g |Proteins~15g

Ingredients

- Four medium potatoes, cut into cubes
- One big capsicum, cut into cubes
- One onion, cut into quarters
- Five tablespoons of gram flour
- A pinch of salt to taste

For chutney

- Two cups of fresh green coriander
- Half cup of mint leaves
- Four teaspoons of fennel
- Two tablespoons of ginger-garlic paste
- One small onion
- Six flakes of garlic (optional)
- Salt to taste
- Three tablespoons of lemon juice

Instructions

- Take a clean and dry container. Put into it the coriander, mint, fennel, and ginger, onion/garlic, salt and lemon juice. Mix them. Pour the mixture into a grinder and blend until you get a thick paste.
- Now move on to the potato pieces. Slit these pieces almost till the end and leave them aside. Now stuff all the pieces with the paste that was obtained from the previous step. Now leave the stuffed potato aside.
- Take the chutney and add to it the gram flour and some salt. Mix them together properly. Rub this mixture all over the stuffed potato pieces. Now leave the cottage cheese aside.
- Now, to the leftover chutney, add the capsicum and onions. Apply the chutney generously on each of the pieces of capsicum and onion. Now take satay sticks and arrange the potato pieces and vegetables on separate sticks.
- Preheat the Air Fryer at 290 Fahrenheit for around 5 minutes. Open the basket. Arrange the

satay sticks properly. Close the basket. Keep the sticks with the cottage cheese at 180 degrees for around half an hour while the sticks with the vegetables are to be kept at the same temperature for only 7 minutes.

- Turn the sticks in between so that one side does not get burnt and also to provide a uniform cook.

Apricot Kebab

Preparation Time-10 minutes | Cook Time-40 minutes | Servings-2 | Difficulty-Moderate

Nutritional Facts- Calories-212 | Fats-9.9g |Carbohydrates-21g |Proteins-4g

Ingredients

- Two cups of fresh apricots
- Three chopped onions
- Five roughly chopped green chilies
- One and a half tablespoons of ginger paste
- One and a half teaspoons of garlic paste
- One and a half teaspoons of salt
- Three teaspoons of lemon juice
- Two teaspoons of garam masala
- Three eggs
- Two and a half tablespoons of white sesame seeds

Instructions

- Grind the ingredients except for the egg and form a smooth paste. Coat the apricots in the paste. Now, beat the eggs and add a little salt to them.
- Dip the coated apricots in the egg mixture and then transfer them to the sesame seeds and coat the apricots well. Place the vegetables on a stick.
- Preheat the Air fryer at 160 degrees Fahrenheit for around 5 minutes. Place the sticks in the basket and let them cook for another 25 minutes at the same temperature.
- Turn the sticks over in between the cooking process to get a uniform cook.

Asparagus Pancakes

Preparation Time-10 minutes | Cook Time-10 minutes | Servings-2 | Difficulty-Easy

Nutritional Facts- Calories-189 | Fats-6g |Carbohydrates-12g |Proteins-7.8g

Ingredients

- One shredded asparagus

- One and a half cups of almond flour
- Three eggs
- Two teaspoons of dried basil
- Two teaspoons of dried parsley
- Salt and Pepper to taste
- Three tablespoons of Butter

Instructions

- Preheat the air fryer to 250 Fahrenheit.
- In a small bowl, mix the ingredients together. Ensure that the mixture is smooth and well-balanced.
- Take a pancake mold and grease it with butter. Add the batter to the mold and place it in the air fryer basket.
- Cook till both the sides of the pancake have browned on both sides and serve with maple syrup.

Asparagus Strata

Preparation Time-10 minutes | Cook Time-20 minutes | Servings-2 | Difficulty-Easy

Nutritional Facts- Calories-166 | Fats-4g |Carbohydrates-1g |Proteins-12g

Ingredients

- Six asparagus spears, cut into 2-inch pieces
- Two slices of whole-wheat bread, cut into 1/2-inch cubes
- Four eggs
- Three tablespoons of whole milk
- Half cup of grated Havarti or Swiss cheese
- Two tablespoons of chopped flat-leaf parsley
- Pinch salt
- Freshly ground black pepper

Instructions

- Place the asparagus spears and One tablespoon of water in a 6-inch baking pan and place in the Air fryer basket Oven.
- Bake until crisp and tender. Detach the asparagus from the pan and drain it. Spray the pan with nonstick cooking spray. Arrange the bread cubes and asparagus into the pan and set them aside. In a medium bowl, beat the eggs with the milk until combined.
- Add the cheese, parsley, salt, and pepper. Pour into the baking pan. Set temperature to 360°F,

and set time to 14 minutes or until the eggs are set, and the top starts to brown. Press start, and you are done.

Avocado Egg Rolls

Preparation Time-10 minutes | Cook Time-10 minutes | Servings-2 | Difficulty-Easy

Nutritional Facts- Calories-99 | Fats-4g |Carbohydrates-4g |Proteins-9g

Ingredients

- Four egg roll wrappers
- One peeled and pitted avocado
- Half sliced tomato
- Salt and ground black pepper, to taste
- Cooking spray

Instructions

- Set the air fryer basket with cooking spray.
- Put the tomato and avocados in a food processor. Sprinkle with salt and ground black pepper. Pulse to mix and coarsely mash until smooth.
- Unfold the wrappers on a clean work surface, and then divide the mixture in the center of each wrapper. Roll the wrapper up and press to seal.
- Transfer the rolls to the basket and spritz with cooking spray.
- Slide the basket into the air fryer. Cook at the corresponding preset mode or Air Fry at 356 degrees Fahrenheit for 5 minutes.
- Set the rolls halfway through the cooking time.
- When cooked, the rolls should be golden brown.
- Serve immediately.

Baked Cheesy Eggplant with Marinara

Preparation Time-5 minutes | Cook Time-45 minutes | Servings-2 | Difficulty-Moderate

Nutritional Facts- Calories-405 | Fats-20g |Carbohydrates-4g |Proteins-12.9g

Ingredients

- One sliced clove of garlic
- One large eggplant
- One tablespoon of olive oil
- Salt as per taste
- A quarter cup and two tablespoons of bread crumbs
- A quarter cup and two tablespoons of ricotta cheese
- A quarter cup grated Parmesan cheese
- A quarter cup water, plus more as needed
- A quarter teaspoon of red pepper flakes
- One and a half cups of prepared marinara sauce
- One and a half teaspoons of olive oil
- Two tablespoons of shredded pepper jack cheese
- Salt and black pepper

Instructions

- Cut the eggplant in five sections crosswise. Two sections should be peeled and cut into 1/2-inch cubes.
- Lightly butter the air fryer's baking pan. Heat one tablespoon of olive oil at 390°F for 5 minutes. Cook for 2 minutes per side with half eggplant strips. Place on a plate to cool.
- Add garlic and one and a half teaspoons of olive oil. Allow for a minute of cooking time. Toss in the diced eggplants. Season with pepper flakes and salt. Cook for 4 minutes in the oven. Reduce the heat to 330 degrees Fahrenheit. Continue to cook the eggplants for another 8 minutes or until they are tender.
- Combine the marinara sauce and water in a mixing bowl. Cook for 7 minutes, or until thoroughly heated. Every now and again, there's a sway. Place in a mixing basin.
- Whisk together Parmesan cheese, pepper, pepper jack cheese, salt, and ricotta in a mixing bowl. Spread the cheese evenly over the eggplant slices, then fold them in half.
- In a baking pan, place the folded eggplant. On top, pour the marinara sauce.
- Whisk together the bread crumbs and olive oil in a small bowl. Sprinkle evenly throughout the sauce.
- Place the baking dish in the cooking basket of the Air fryer oven. Cook at 390°F for 15 minutes, or until the tops are gently browned.
- Serve and enjoy.

Baked Potatoes

Preparation Time-20 minutes | Cook Time-45 minutes | Servings-2 | Difficulty-Moderate

Nutritional Facts- Calories-302 | Fats-20g |Carbohydrates-7.8g |Proteins-24g

Ingredients

- Two potatoes
- One tablespoon of olive oil
- Salt to taste
- Half cup of butter
- A quarter cup of milk
- A quarter cup of sour cream
- Half cup of shredded cheddar, divided

Instructions

- Poke the potatoes using a fork.
- Add to the air fryer.
- Set it to bake.
- Cook at 400 F for 40 minutes.
- Take out of the oven.
- Slice the potato in half
- Scoop out the potato flesh.
- Mix potato flesh with the remaining ingredients.
- Put the mixture back to the potato shells.
- Bake in the air fryer for 5 minutes.

Balsamic Potatoes

Preparation Time-10 minutes | Cook Time-20 minutes | Servings-2 | Difficulty-Easy

Nutritional Facts- Calories-301 | Fats-6g |Carbohydrates-18g |Proteins-6g

Ingredients

- One and a half pounds of halved baby potatoes
- Two chopped garlic cloves
- Two chopped red onions
- Nine ounces of cherry tomatoes
- Three tablespoons of olive oil
- One and a half tablespoons of balsamic vinegar
- Two chopped thyme springs
- Salt and black pepper to the taste

Instructions

- In your food processor, mix garlic with onions, oil, vinegar, thyme, salt and pepper and pulse really well.
- In a bowl, mix potatoes with tomatoes and balsamic marinade, toss well, transfer to your air fryer and cook at 380 degrees F for 20 minutes.
- Divide among plates and serve.
- Enjoy!

Bell Pepper-Corn Wrapped in Tortilla

Preparation Time-5 minutes | Cook Time-15 minutes | Servings-2 | Difficulty-Easy

Nutritional Facts- Calories-458 | Fats-18g |Carbohydrates-12g |Proteins-31.8g

Ingredients

- One chopped small red bell pepper
- One diced small yellow onion
- One tablespoon of water
- Two cobs of grilled corn kernels
- Four large tortillas
- Four pieces of chopped commercial vegan nuggets
- Mixed greens for garnish

Instructions

- Preheat the air fryer oven to 400F.
- In a skillet heated over medium heat, sauté the vegan nuggets together with the onions, bell peppers, and corn kernels. Set aside.
- Place filling inside the corn tortillas.
- Pour the tortillas into the Oven rack/basket. Place the rack on the middle shelf of the Air fryer oven. Set temperature to 400F, and set time to 15 minutes until the tortilla wraps are crispy.
- Serve with mixed greens on top.

Black Bean and Sweet Potato Burritos

Preparation Time-15 minutes | Cook Time-30 minutes | Servings-2 to 4 | Difficulty-Moderate

Nutritional Facts- Calories-260 | Fats-12.9g |Carbohydrates-4.8g |Proteins-28.9g

Ingredients

Two sweet potatoes
- One tablespoon of vegetable oil
- Kosher salt and black pepper, to taste
- Two to four large flour tortillas
- One (16-ounce) can of refried black beans, divided
- One and a half cups of baby spinach, divided
- Four scrambled eggs
- 1/3 cup of grated Cheddar cheese, divided
- A quarter cup of salsa
- A quarter cup of sour cream
- Cooking spray

Instructions

- Set the sweet potatoes in a large bowl, then drizzle with vegetable oil and sprinkle with salt and black pepper. Toss to coat well.
- Put the potatoes in the air fryer basket.
- Slide the basket into the air fryer. Cook at the corresponding preset mode or Air Fry at 400F (205C) for 10 minutes.
- Set the potatoes halfway through the cooking time.
- When done, the potatoes should be lightly browned. Remove the potatoes from the air fryer.
- Unfold the tortillas on a clean work surface. Divide the black beans, spinach, air-fried sweet potatoes, scrambled eggs, and cheese on top of the tortillas.
- Fold the long side of the tortillas over the filling, and then fold in the shorter side to wrap the filling to make the burritos.
- Wrap the burritos in aluminum foil and put them in the basket.
- Slide the basket into the air fryer. Cook at the corresponding preset mode or Air Fry at 356 degrees Fahrenheit for 20 minutes. Flip the burritos halfway through the cooking time.
- Remove the burritos from the air fryer and spread with sour cream and salsa. Serve immediately.

Broccoli Momos

Preparation Time-10 minutes | Cook Time-25 minutes | Servings-2 | Difficulty-Easy

Nutritional Facts- Calories-210 | Fats-9.9g |Carbohydrates-21g|Proteins-12.9g

Ingredients

For dough

- One and a half cups of all-purpose flour
- Half teaspoon of salt
- Five tablespoons of water

For filling

- Two cups of grated broccoli
- Two tablespoons of oil
- Two teaspoons of ginger-garlic paste
- Two teaspoons of soya sauce
- Two teaspoons of vinegar

Instructions

- Knead the dough and cover it with plastic wrap, and set it aside. Next, cook the ingredients for the filling and try to ensure that the broccoli is covered well with the sauce.
- Roll the dough and cut it into a square. Place the filling in the center. Now, wrap the dough to cover the filling and pinch the edges together.
- Preheat the Air fryer at 200° F for 5 minutes. Place the momos in the fry basket and close it. Let them cook at the same temperature for another 20 minutes.
- Recommended sides are chili sauce or ketchup.

Brown Rice, Spinach and Tofu Frittata

Preparation Time-5 minutes | Cook Time-55 minutes | Servings-2 | Difficulty-Hard

Nutritional Facts- Calories-226 | Fats-7.8g |Carbohydrates-4.8g |Proteins-10.8g

Ingredients

- Half cup of chopped baby spinach
- Half cup of chopped kale
- Half chopped onion
- Half teaspoon of turmeric
- One and 1/3 cup of cooked brown rice
- One flax egg
- One package firm tofu
- One tablespoon of olive oil
- One chopped yellow pepper
- Two tablespoons of soy sauce
- Two teaspoons of arrowroot powder
- Two teaspoons of Dijon mustard
- 2/3 cup of almond milk
- Three chopped big mushrooms
- Three tablespoons of nutritional yeast
- Four crushed cloves of garlic
- Four chopped spring onions
- A handful of chopped basil leaves

Instructions

- Preheat the air fryer oven to 375F. Grease a pan that will fit inside the air fryer oven.
- Prepare the frittata crust by mixing the brown rice and flax egg. Press the rice onto the baking dish until you form a crust. Brush with a little oil and cook for 10 minutes.

- Meanwhile, heat olive oil in a skillet over medium flame and sauté the garlic and onions for 2 minutes.
- Add the pepper and mushroom and continue stirring for 3 minutes.
- Stir in the kale, spinach, spring onions, and basil. Remove from the pan and set aside.
- In a food processor, press together the tofu, turmeric, mustard, soy sauce, vegan milk, nutritional yeast, and arrowroot powder. Pour in a mixing bowl and stir in the sautéed vegetables.
- Pour the vegan frittata mixture over the rice crust and cook in the air fryer oven for 40 minutes.

Brussels sprouts with Balsamic Oil

Preparation Time-5 minutes | Cook Time-15 minutes | Servings-2 | Difficulty-Easy

Nutritional Facts- Calories-92 | Fats-6.9g |Carbohydrates-4.8g |Proteins- 1.5g

Ingredients

- A quarter teaspoon of salt
- One tablespoon of balsamic vinegar
- Two cups of halved Brussels sprouts
- One tablespoon of olive oil

Instructions

- Preheat the air fryer oven for 5 minutes.
- Mix all ingredients in a bowl until the Brussel sprouts are well coated.
- Place in the air fryer oven basket.
- Close and cook for 15 minutes at 350 degrees F.

Butter Toasted Cremini Mushrooms

Preparation Time-10 minutes | Cook Time-30 minutes | Servings-2 | Difficulty-Moderate

Nutritional Facts- Calories-350 | Fats-15g |Carbohydrates-1g|Proteins-42g

Ingredients

- One pound button or cremini mushrooms washed stems trimmed, and cut into quarters or thick slices
- A quarter cup of water
- One teaspoon of kosher salt
- Three tablespoons of unsalted butter

Instructions

- Bring a large piece of aluminum foil to the sheet pan. Bring the mushroom pieces in the middle of the foil. Scatter them out into an even layer. Set the water over them, season with the salt, and add the butter. Wrap the mushrooms in the foil.
- Place the pan on the toast position.
- Select Toast, set the temperature to 325 degrees F (163C).
- After 15 minutes, detach the pan from the air fryer grill. Bring the foil packet to a cutting board and carefully unwrap it. Set the mushrooms and cooking liquid from the foil onto the sheet pan.
- Place the basket on the toast position.
- Select Toast, set the temperature to 356 degrees Fahrenheit, and set the time for 15 minutes.
- After about 10 minutes, detach the pan from the air fryer grill and stir the mushrooms. Return the pan to the air fryer grill and continue cooking for anywhere from 5 to 15 more minutes, or until the liquid is mostly gone and the mushrooms start to brown.
- Serve immediately.

Buttered Corn

Preparation Time-10 minutes | Cook Time-20 minutes | Servings-2 | Difficulty-Easy

Nutritional Facts- Calories-268 | Fats-16.8g |Carbohydrates-27.9g |Proteins-6g

Ingredients

Two fresh whole corn on the cob
Half cup of butter, melted
Salt, as required

Instructions

- Husk the corn and detach all the silk.
- Brush each corn with melted butter and sprinkle with salt.
- Place the water tray in the bottom of your air fryer grill.
- Place about two cups of lukewarm water into the water tray.
- Place the drip pan over the water tray and then arrange the heating element.
- Now, place the grilling pan over the heating element.

- Plug in the grill and press the 'Power' button to turn it on.
- Then press the "Fan" button.
- Set the temperature settings according to the manufacturer's directions.
- Cover the grill with a lid and let it preheat.
- After preheating, remove the lid and grease the grilling pan.
- Place the corn over the grilling pan.
- Cover with the lid and cook for about 20 minutes, rotating after every 5 minutes and brushing with butter once halfway through.
- Serve warm.

Carrots, Yellow Squash and Zucchini Mix

Preparation Time-5 minutes | Cook Time-35 minutes | Servings-2 | Difficulty-Easy

Nutritional Facts- Calories-122 | Fats-9g |Carbohydrates-4.8g |Proteins-6g

Ingredients

- Half tablespoon of chopped tarragon leaves
- A quarter teaspoon of white pepper
- Half teaspoon of salt
- Half pound of yellow squash
- Half pound of zucchini
- Three teaspoons of olive oil
- A quarter-pound of carrots

Instructions

- Stem and root the end of squash and zucchini and cut in 1/3-inch half-moons. Peel and cut carrots into 1-inch cubes
- Merge carrot cubes with Two teaspoons of olive oil, tossing to combine.
- Pour into the air fryer oven basket, set temperature to 400F, and set time to 5 minutes.
- As carrots cook, drizzle remaining olive oil over squash and zucchini pieces, then season with pepper and salt. Toss well to coat.
- Add squash and zucchini when the timer for carrots goes off. Cook 30 minutes, making sure to toss 2-3 times during the cooking process.
- Once done, take out veggies and toss with tarragon. Serve up warm.

Cauliflower Bites

Preparation Time-15 minutes | Cook Time-10 minutes | Servings-2 to 4 | Difficulty-Easy

Nutritional Facts- Calories-285 | Fats-12.9g |Carbohydrates-7.8g |Proteins-39g

Ingredients

Cauliflower bites

Four cups of cauliflower rice

- One beaten egg
- One cup of grated Parmesan cheese
- One cup of shredded cheddar
- Two tablespoons of chopped chives
- A quarter cup of breadcrumbs
- Salt and pepper to taste

Sauce

- Half cup of ketchup
- Two tablespoons of hot sauce

Instructions

Combine cauliflower bites ingredients in a bowl.
Mix well.
Form balls from the mixture.
Choose air fry setting.
Add cauliflower bites to the air fryer.
Cook at 375 F for 10 minutes.
Mix ketchup and hot sauce.
Serve cauliflower bites with dip.

Cauliflower Kebab

Preparation Time-10 minutes | Cook Time-35 minutes | Servings-2 | Difficulty-Moderate

Nutritional Facts- Calories-199 | Fats-10.8g |Carbohydrates-18g |Proteins-7.8g

Ingredients

- Two cups of cauliflower florets
- Three chopped onions
- Five roughly chopped green chilies
- One and a half tablespoons of ginger paste
- One and a half teaspoons of garlic paste
- One and a half teaspoons of salt
- Three teaspoons of lemon juice
- Two teaspoons of garam masala
- Three eggs
- Two and a half tablespoons of white sesame seeds

Instructions

- Grind the ingredients except for the egg and form a smooth paste. Coat the florets in the paste. Now, beat the eggs and add a little salt to them.
- Dip the coated florets in the egg mixture and then transfer them to the sesame seeds and coat the florets well. Place the vegetables on a stick.
- Preheat the Air fryer at 160 degrees Fahrenheit for around 5 minutes. Place the sticks in the basket and let them cook for another 25 minutes at the same temperature.
- Turn the sticks over in between the cooking process to get a uniform cook.

Cauliflower Momos

Preparation Time-15 minutes | Cook Time-25 minutes | Servings-2 | Difficulty-Easy

Nutritional Facts- Calories-178 | Fats-6g |Carbohydrates-24g |Proteins-6.9g

Ingredients

For dough

- One and a half cups of all-purpose flour
- Half teaspoon of salt
- Five tablespoons of water

For filling

- Two cups of grated cauliflower
- Two tablespoons of oil
- Two teaspoons of ginger-garlic paste
- Two teaspoons of soya sauce
- Two teaspoons of vinegar

Instructions

- Knead the dough and cover it with plastic wrap, and set it aside. Next, cook the ingredients for the filling and try to ensure that the cauliflower is covered well with the sauce.
- Roll the dough and cut it into a square. Place the filling in the center. Now, wrap the dough to cover the filling and pinch the edges together.
- Preheat the Air fryer at 200° F for 5 minutes. Place the momos in the fry basket and close it. Let them cook at the same temperature for another 20 minutes.
- Recommended sides are chili sauce or ketchup.

Cauliflower Rice

Preparation Time-5 minutes | Cook Time-20 minutes | Servings-2 | Difficulty-Easy

Nutritional Facts- Calories-70 | Fats-7.8g |Carbohydrates-1g |Proteins-17g

Ingredients

- One teaspoon of turmeric
- Half cup of diced carrot
- A quarter cup of diced onion
- One tablespoon of low-sodium soy sauce
- Half block of extra firm tofu
- A quarter cup of frozen peas
- One minced clove of garlic
- A quarter cup of chopped broccoli
- Half tablespoon of minced ginger
- Half tablespoon of rice vinegar
- One teaspoon of toasted sesame oil
- Two tablespoons of reduced-sodium soy sauce
- Two cups of riced cauliflower

Instructions

- Crumble tofu in a large bowl and toss with all the round one ingredients.
- Preheat the air fryer oven to 370 degrees, place the baking dish in the Air fryer oven
- cooking basket, set the temperature to 370 degrees F, and set the time to 10 minutes and cook 10 minutes, making sure to shake once.
- In another bowl, toss ingredients from Round 2 together.
- Add Round 2 mixture to air fryer and cook another 10 minutes, ensuring to shake 5 minutes in.
- Enjoy!

Cheesy Bean and Salsa Tacos

Preparation Time-12 minutes | Cook Time-8 minutes | Servings-2 to 4 | Difficulty-Easy

Nutritional Facts- Calories-373 | Fats-21g |Carbohydrates-12.9g |Proteins-34g

Ingredients

- One can of drained and rinsed black beans
- Half cup of prepared salsa
- One and a half teaspoons of chili powder

- Four ounces of grated cheese
- Two tablespoons of minced onion
- Eight flour tortillas
- Two tablespoons of vegetable or extra-virgin olive oil
- Shredded lettuce, for serving

Instructions

- In a medium bowl, add the beans, chili powder and salsa. Coarsely mash them with a potato masher. Fold in the onion and cheese and stir until combined.
- Set the flour tortillas on a cutting board and spoon 2 to Three tablespoons of the filling into each tortilla. Set the tortillas over, pressing lightly to even out the filling. Garnish the tacos on one side with half the olive oil and put them, oiled side down, on the sheet pan. Garnish the top side with the remaining olive oil.
- Place the pan into the air fryer grill.
- Select Air Fry, set the temperature to 400 degrees F (205C), and set time to 7 minutes. Set the tacos halfway through the cooking time.
- Remove the pan from the air fryer grill and allow it to cool. Serve.

Cherry Tomatoes Skewers

Preparation Time-30 minutes | Cook Time-10 minutes | Servings-2 | Difficulty-Moderate

Nutritional Facts- Calories-155 | Fats-1g |Carbohydrates-1g|Proteins-7.8g

Ingredients

- Three tablespoons of balsamic vinegar
- Twenty-four cherry tomatoes
- Two tablespoons of olive oil
- Three minced garlic cloves
- One tablespoon of chopped thyme
- Salt and black pepper to the taste

For the dressing

- Two tablespoons of balsamic vinegar
- Salt and black pepper to the taste
- Four tablespoons olive oil

Instructions

- In a bowl, mix two tablespoons of oil with three tablespoons of vinegar, three garlic cloves, thyme,

salt and black pepper and whisk well.
- Add tomatoes, toss to coat and leave aside for 30 minutes.
- Arrange six tomatoes on one skewer and repeat with the rest of the tomatoes.
- Introduce them in your air fryer and cook at 360 degrees F for 6 minutes.
- In another bowl, mix two tablespoons of vinegar with salt, pepper and four tablespoons of oil and whisk well.
- Arrange tomato skewers among plates and serve with the dressing drizzled on top.
- Enjoy!

Cottage Cheese Kebab

Preparation Time-10 minutes | Cook Time-30 minutes | Servings-2 | Difficulty-Moderate

Nutritional Facts- Calories-305 | Fats-13.8g |Carbohydrates-14g |Proteins-12g

Ingredients

- Two cups of cubed cottage cheese
- Three chopped onions
- Five roughly chopped green chilies
- One and a half tablespoons of ginger paste
- One and a half teaspoons of garlic paste
- One and a half teaspoons of salt
- Three teaspoons of lemon juice
- Two tablespoons of coriander powder
- Three tablespoons of chopped capsicum
- Two tablespoons of peanut flour
- Three eggs

Instructions

- Coat the cottage cheese cubes with the cornflour and mix the other ingredients in a bowl. Make the mixture into a smooth paste and coat the cheese cubes with the mixture. Beat the eggs in a bowl and add a little salt to them.
- Dip the cubes in the egg mixture and coat them with sesame seeds and leave them in the refrigerator for an hour.
- Preheat the Air fryer at 290 Fahrenheit for around 5 minutes. Place the kebabs in the basket and let them cook for another 25 minutes at the same temperature. Turn the kebabs over in between the cooking process to get a uniform cook.

- Serve the kebabs with mint chutney.

Creamy Spinach Quiche

Preparation Time-10 minutes | Cook Time-20 minutes | Servings-2 | Difficulty-Easy

Nutritional Facts- Calories-254 | Fats-13.8g |Carbohydrates-5.7g |Proteins-37.8g

Ingredients

- Premade quiche crust, chilled and rolled flat to a 7-inch round
- Two eggs
- A quarter cup of milk
- Pinch of salt and pepper
- One clove of garlic
- Half cup of cooked, drained and coarsely chopped spinach
- A quarter cup of shredded mozzarella cheese
- A quarter cup of shredded cheddar cheese

Instructions

- Preheat the air fryer oven to 360 degrees F.
- Press the premade crust into a 7-inch pie tin or any appropriately sized glass or ceramic heat-safe dish. Press and trim at the edges if necessary. With a fork, pierce several holes in the dough to allow air circulation and prevent cracking of the crust while cooking.
- In a mixing bowl, beat the eggs until fluffy and until the yolks and white are evenly combined.
- Add milk, garlic, spinach, salt and pepper, and half the cheddar and mozzarella cheese to the eggs. Set the rest of the cheese aside for now, and stir the mixture until completely blended. Make sure the spinach is not clumped together but rather spread among the other ingredients.
- Pour the mixture into the pie crust slowly and carefully to avoid splashing. The mixture should almost fill the crust, but not completely – leaving a quarter-inch of crust at the edges.
- Place the baking dish in the Air fryer oven cooking basket. Set the air fryer oven timer for 15 minutes. After15 minutes, the air fryer will shut off, and the quiche will already be firm, and the crust begins to brown. Sprinkle the rest of the cheddar and mozzarella cheese on top of the quiche filling. Reset the air fryer oven at 360 degrees for 5 minutes. After 5 minutes, when the air fryer shuts off, the cheese will have formed an exquisite crust on top, and the quiche will be golden brown and perfect. Remove from the air fryer using oven mitts or tongs, and set on a heat-safe surface to cool for a few minutes before cutting.

Crisp Avocado and Slaw Tacos

Preparation Time-20 minutes | Cook Time-7 minutes | Servings-2 | Difficulty-Easy

Nutritional Facts- Calories-348 | Fats-15g |Carbohydrates-1g |Proteins-42g

Ingredients

- A quarter cup of all-purpose flour
- A quarter teaspoon of salt
- A quarter teaspoon of ground black pepper
- Two large egg whites
- One and a quarter cups of panko bread crumbs
- Two tablespoons of olive oil
- Two peeled and halved avocados, cut into 1/2-inch-thick slices
- Half thinly sliced small red cabbage
- One thinly sliced deseeded jalapeño
- Two thinly sliced green onions
- Half cup of cilantro leaves
- A quarter cup of mayonnaise
- Juice and zest of one lime
- Four warmed corn tortillas
- Half cup of sour cream
- Cooking spray

Instructions

- Set the air fryer basket with cooking spray.
- Pour the flour in a large bowl and sprinkle with salt and black pepper, and then stir to mix well.
- Whisk the egg whites in a separate bowl. Combine the panko with olive oil on a shallow dish.
- Dredge the avocado slices in the bowl of flour, then into the egg to coat. Shake the excess off, and then roll the slices over the panko.
- Set the avocado slices in a single layer in the basket and spritz the cooking spray.
- Slide the basket into the air fryer. Cook at the corresponding preset mode or Air Fry at 400F (205C) for 6 minutes.

- Flip the slices halfway through with tongs.
- When cooking is complete, the avocado slices should be tender and lightly browned.
- Combine the cabbage, jalapeño, onions, cilantro leaves, mayo, lime juice and zest, and a touch of salt in a separate large bowl. Toss to mix well.
- Unfold the tortillas on a clean work surface, then spread with cabbage slaw and air-fried avocados. Top with sour cream and serve.

Crispy Cheesy Broccoli Tots

Preparation Time-20 minutes | Cook Time-15 minutes | Servings-2 | Difficulty-Easy

Nutritional Facts- Calories-304 | Fats-7.8g |Carbohydrates-1g |Proteins-20g

Ingredients

- Twelve ounces of frozen broccoli, thawed, drained, and patted dry
- One large, lightly beaten egg
- Half cup of seasoned whole-wheat bread crumbs
- A quarter cup of shredded cheese
- A quarter cup of grated Parmesan cheese
- One and a half teaspoons of minced garlic
- Salt and freshly ground black pepper
- Cooking spray

Instructions

- Spritz the air fry basket lightly with cooking spray.
- Bring the remaining ingredients into a food processor and process until the mixture resembles a coarse meal. Transfer the mixture to a bowl.
- Using a tablespoon of, scoop out the broccoli mixture and form it into 24 oval "tater tot" shapes with your hands.
- Put the tots in the prepared basket in a single layer, spacing them 1 inch apart. Mist the tots lightly with cooking spray.
- Place the air fry basket on the air fry position.
- Select Air Fry, set the temperature to 375 degrees F (190C), and set time to 15 minutes. Flip the tots halfway through the cooking time.
- When done, the tots will be lightly browned and crispy. Remove from the air fryer grill and serve on a plate.

Dal Mint Kebab

Preparation Time-15 minutes | Cook Time-40 minutes | Servings-2 | Difficulty-Moderate

Nutritional Facts- Calories-299 | Fats-10.8g |Carbohydrates-9g |Proteins-21.9g

Ingredients

- One cup of chickpeas
- Half inch ginger grated or one and a half teaspoon of ginger-garlic paste
- Two finely chopped green chilies
- A quarter teaspoon of red chili powder
- A pinch of salt to taste
- Half teaspoon of roasted cumin powder
- Two teaspoons of coriander powder
- One and a half tablespoons of chopped coriander
- Half teaspoon of dried mango powder
- One cup of dry breadcrumbs
- A quarter teaspoon of black salt
- Two tablespoons of all-purpose flour for coating purposes
- Two tablespoons of finely chopped mint
- One finely chopped onion
- Half cup of milk

Instructions

- Take an open vessel. Boil the chickpeas in the vessel until their texture becomes soft. Make sure that they do not become soggy.
- Now take this chickpea into another container. Add the grated ginger and the cut green chilies. Grind this mixture until it becomes a thick paste. Keep adding water as and when required. Now add the onions, mint, breadcrumbs and all the various masalas required. Mix this well until you get a soft dough.
- Now make small balls of this mixture (about the size of a lemon) and mold them into the shape of flat and round kebabs.
- Here is where the milk comes into play. Pour a very small amount of milk onto each kebab to wet it. Now roll the kebab in the dry breadcrumbs.
- Preheat the Air Fryer for 5 minutes at 300 Fahrenheit. Take out the basket. Arrange the kebabs in the basket, leaving gaps between them so that no two kebabs are touching each other. Keep the fryer at 340 Fahrenheit for around half

an hour. Halfway through the cooking process, turn the kebabs over so that they can be cooked properly.

- Recommended sides for this dish are mint chutney, tomato ketchup or yogurt chutney.

Delicious Creamy Green Beans

Preparation Time-10 minutes | Cook Time-15 minutes | Servings-2 | Difficulty-Easy

Nutritional Facts- Calories-231 | Fats-6.9g |Carbohydrates-15g |Proteins-7.8g

Ingredients

- Half cup of heavy cream
- One cup of shredded mozzarella
- 2/3 cup of grated parmesan
- Salt and black pepper to the taste
- Two pounds green beans
- Two teaspoons of grated lemon zest
- A pinch of red pepper flakes

Instructions

- Put the beans in a dish that fits your air fryer, add heavy cream, salt, pepper, lemon zest, pepper flakes, mozzarella and parmesan, toss, introduce in your air fryer and cook at 350 degrees F for 15 minutes.
- Divide among plates and serve right away.

Easy Green Beans and Potatoes

Preparation Time-10 minutes | Cook Time-15 minutes | Servings-2 | Difficulty-Easy

Nutritional Facts- Calories-374 | Fats-15g |Carbohydrates-27.9g |Proteins-12g

Ingredients

- Two pounds green beans
- Sox halved new potatoes
- Salt and black pepper to the taste
- A drizzle of olive oil
- Six cooked and chopped bacon slices

Instructions

- In a bowl, mix green beans with potatoes, salt, pepper and oil, toss, transfer to your air fryer and cook at 390 degrees F for 15 minutes.
- Divide among plates and serve with bacon sprinkled on top.

- Enjoy!

Easy Roasted Vegetables

Preparation Time-10 minutes | Cook Time-18 minutes | Servings-2 | Difficulty-Easy

Nutritional Facts- Calories-61 | Fats-1g|Carbohydrates-6g |Proteins-17g

Ingredients

- Half cup of sliced mushrooms
- Half cup of sliced zucchini
- Half cup of sliced yellow squash
- Half cup of baby carrots
- One cup of cauliflower florets
- One cup of broccoli florets
- A quarter cup of grated parmesan cheese
- One teaspoon of red pepper flakes
- One tablespoon of minced garlic
- One tablespoon of olive oil
- A quarter cup of balsamic vinegar
- One small sliced onion
- One teaspoon of sea salt

Instructions

- Preheat the air fryer to 400 degrees F.
- In a large mixing bowl, mix together olive oil, garlic, vinegar, red pepper flakes, pepper, and salt.
- Add vegetables and toss until well coated.
- Add vegetables into the air fryer basket and cook for 8 minutes. Shake basket and cook for 8 minutes more.
- Add parmesan cheese and cook for 2 minutes more.
- Serve and enjoy.

Easy Spicy Toasted Asparagus

Preparation Time-10 minutes | Cook Time-15 minutes | Servings-2 | Difficulty-Easy

Nutritional Facts- Calories-298 | Fats-7.8g |Carbohydrates-4g |Proteins-21g

Ingredients

- Two pounds of trimmed asparagus
- Three tablespoons of extra-virgin olive oil, divided
- One teaspoon of kosher salt, divided

- One pint cherry tomatoes
- Four large eggs
- A quarter teaspoon of freshly ground black pepper

Instructions

- Put the asparagus on the sheet pan and drizzle with two tablespoons of olive oil, tossing to coat. Season with a half teaspoon of kosher salt.
- Place the pan on the toast position.
- Select Toast, set temperature to 375 degrees F (190C), and set time to 12 minutes.
- Meanwhile, set the cherry tomatoes with the remaining One tablespoon of olive oil in a medium bowl until well coated.
- After 6 minutes, detach the pan and toss the asparagus. Evenly scatter the asparagus in the middle of the sheet pan. Attach the tomatoes around the perimeter of the pan. Return the pan to the air fryer grill and continue cooking.
- After 2 minutes, remove the pan from the air fryer grill.
- Gently crack the eggs, one at a time, over the asparagus, spacing them out. Flavor with the remaining half teaspoon of kosher salt and pepper. Return the pan to the air fryer grill and continue cooking. Cook until the eggs are cooked to your desired doneness.
- When done, set the asparagus and eggs among four plates. Set each plate evenly with the tomatoes and serve.

Eggplant and Garlic Sauce

Preparation Time-10 minutes | Cook Time-10 minutes | Servings-2 | Difficulty-Easy

Nutritional Facts- Calories-145 | Fats-1g|Carbohydrates-7.8g |Proteins-9.9g

Ingredients

- Two tablespoons of olive oil
- Two minced cloves of garlic
- Three halved and sliced eggplants
- One chopped red chili pepper
- One chopped green onion stalk
- One tablespoon of grated ginger
- One tablespoon of soy sauce
- One tablespoon of balsamic vinegar

Instructions

- Heat up a pan that fits your air fryer with the oil over medium-high heat, add eggplant slices and cook for 2 minutes.
- Add chili pepper, garlic, green onions, ginger, soy sauce and vinegar, introduce in your air fryer and cook at 320 degrees F for 7 minutes.
- Divide among plates and serve.

Eggplant Subs

Preparation Time-15 minutes | Cook Time-15 minutes | Servings-2 | Difficulty-Easy

Nutritional Facts- Calories-256 | Fats-12.9g |Carbohydrates-13g |Proteins-23g

Ingredients

- Six peeled and chopped eggplant slices
- A quarter cup of jarred pizza sauce
- Six tablespoons of grated Parmesan cheese
- Three Italian sub rolls split open lengthwise, warmed
- Cooking spray

Instructions

- Set the air fryer basket with cooking spray.
- Arrange the eggplant slices in the basket and spritz with cooking spray.
- Slide the basket into the air fryer. Cook at the corresponding preset mode or Air Fry at 356 degrees Fahrenheit for 10 minutes.
- Flip the slices halfway through the cooking time.
- When cooked, the eggplant slices should be slightly wilted and tender.
- Divide and spread the pizza sauce and cheese on top of the eggplant slice
- Slide the basket into the air fryer. Cook at the corresponding preset mode or Air Fry at 375F (190C) for 2 minutes. When cooked, the cheese will be melted.
- Assemble each sub roll with two slices of eggplant and serve immediately.

Fast Spicy Kung Pao Tofu

Preparation Time-10 minutes | Cook Time-10 minutes | Servings-2 | Difficulty-Easy

Nutritional Facts- Calories-356 | Fats-8.7g |Carbohydrates-1.5g |Proteins-61.8g

Ingredients

- 1/3 cup of Asian-Style sauce
- One teaspoon of cornstarch
- Half teaspoon of red pepper flakes,
- One pound of extra-firm tofu, cut into 1-inch cubes
- One small peeled and sliced carrot
- One small green bell pepper
- Three scallions
- Three tablespoons of Toasted unsalted peanuts

Instructions

- In a large bowl, merge together the sauce, red pepper flakes, and cornstarch. Fold in the tofu, pepper, carrot, and the white parts of the scallions and toss to coat. Spread the mixture evenly on the sheet pan.
- Place the pan on the toast position in the air fryer grill.
- Select Toast, set temperature to 375F (190C), and set time to 10 minutes. Merge the ingredients once halfway through the cooking time.
- When done, remove the pan from the air fryer grill. Serve.

Flavored Fennel

Preparation Time-10 minutes | Cook Time-10 minutes | Servings-2 | Difficulty-Easy

Nutritional Facts- Calories-120 | Fats-4g | Carbohydrates-9.9g | Proteins-4.8g

Ingredients

- Two quarter-cut fennel bulbs
- Three tablespoons of olive oil
- Salt and black pepper to the taste
- One minced garlic clove
- One chopped red chili pepper
- 3/4 cup of veggie stock
- Juice from half lemon
- A quarter cup of white wine
- A quarter cup of grated parmesan

Instructions

- Heat up a pan that fits your air fryer with the oil over medium-high heat, add garlic and chili pepper, stir and cook for 2 minutes.

- Add fennel, salt, pepper, stock, wine, lemon juice, and parmesan, toss to coat, introduce in your air fryer and cook at 350 degrees F for 6 minutes.
- Divide among plates and serve right away.

Flavored Green Beans

Preparation Time-10 minutes | Cook Time-15 minutes | Servings-2 | Difficulty-Easy

Nutritional Facts- Calories-211 | Fats-6g | Carbohydrates-15g | Proteins-4.8g

Ingredients

- One pound of red potatoes, cut into wedges
- One pound of green beans
- Two minced cloves of garlic
- Two tablespoons of olive oil
- Salt and black pepper to the taste
- Half teaspoon of dried oregano

Instructions

- In a pan that fits your air fryer, combine potatoes with green beans, garlic, oil, salt, pepper and oregano,
- toss, introduce in your air fryer and cook at 380 degrees F for 15 minutes.
- Divide among plates and serve.
- Enjoy!

Garlicky Mixed Veggies

Preparation Time-15 minutes | Cook Time-10 minutes | Servings-2 | Difficulty-Easy

Nutritional Facts- Calories-147 | Fats-7.8g | Carbohydrates-15g | Proteins-5.7g

Ingredients

- One bunch of trimmed fresh asparagus
- Six ounces of fresh halved mushrooms
- Six halved Campari tomatoes
- One red onion
- Three minced garlic cloves
- Two tablespoons of olive oil
- Salt and ground black pepper, as required

Instructions

- In a large bowl, merge all ingredients and toss to coat well.

- Place the water tray in the bottom of the Air Fryer Grill.
- Place about two cups of lukewarm water into the water tray.
- Place the drip pan over the water tray.
- Now, place the grilling pan overheating element.
- Plugin the Grill and press the 'Power' button to turn it on.
- Then press the 'Fan' button.
- Set the temperature settings according to the manufacturer's directions.
- Cover the grill with a lid and let it preheat.
- After preheating, remove the lid and grease the grilling pan.
- Place the vegetables over the grilling pan.
- Cover with the lid and cook for about 8 minutes, flipping occasionally.

Green Bean, Mushroom, and Chickpea Wraps

Preparation Time-15 minutes | Cook Time-10 minutes | Servings-2 | Difficulty-Easy

Nutritional Facts- Calories-145 | Fats-10.8g |Carbohydrates-4g |Proteins-9.9g

Ingredients

- Eight ounces of green beans
- Two sliced portobello mushroom caps
- One sliced large red pepper
- Two tablespoons of olive oil, divided
- A quarter teaspoon of salt
- One (Fifteen-ounce) can of drained chickpeas
- Three tablespoons of lemon juice
- A quarter teaspoon of ground black pepper
- Four whole-grain wraps
- Four ounces of crumbled fresh herb or garlic goat cheese
- One lemon, cut into wedges

Instructions

- Add the green beans, mushrooms, red pepper to a large bowl. Set with One tablespoon of olive oil and season with salt. Toss until well coated.
- Transfer the vegetable mixture to a baking pan.
- Slide the pan into the air fryer. Cook at the corresponding preset mode or Air Fry at 400F (205C) for 9 minutes.

- Stir the vegetable mixture three times during cooking.
- When cooked, the vegetables should be tender.
- Meanwhile, mash the chickpeas with lemon juice, pepper and the remaining One tablespoon of oil until well blended
- Unfold the wraps on a clean work surface. Spoon the chickpea mash on the wraps and spread it all over.
- Divide the cooked veggies among wraps. Sprinkle 1 ounce of crumbled goat cheese on top of each wrap. Fold to wrap. Squeeze the lemon wedges on top and serve.

Green Beans and Parmesan

Preparation Time-10 minutes | Cook Time-10 minutes | Servings-2 | Difficulty-Easy

Nutritional Facts- Calories-121 | Fats-7.8g |Carbohydrates-9g |Proteins-4.8g

Ingredients

- Twelve ounces of green beans
- Two teaspoons of minced garlic
- Two tablespoons of olive oil
- Salt and black pepper to the taste
- One whisked egg
- 1/3 cup of grated parmesan

Instructions

- In a bowl, mix oil with salt, pepper, garlic and egg and whisk well.
- Add green beans to this mix, toss well and sprinkle parmesan all over.
- Transfer green beans to your air fryer and cook them at 390 degrees F for 8 minutes.
- Divide green beans between plates and serve them right away.

Green Beans and Tomatoes

Preparation Time-10 minutes | Cook Time-15 minutes | Servings-2 | Difficulty-Easy

Nutritional Facts- Calories-173 | Fats-6g |Carbohydrates-12.9g |Proteins-9g

Ingredients

- One pint of cherry tomatoes
- One pound of green beans

- Two tablespoons of olive oil
- Salt and black pepper to the taste

Instructions

- In a bowl, mix cherry tomatoes with green beans, olive oil, salt and pepper, toss, transfer to your air fryer and cook at 400 degrees F for 15 minutes.
- Divide among plates and serve right away.

Guacamole

Preparation Time-15 minutes | Cook Time-8 minutes | Servings-2 | Difficulty-Easy

Nutritional Facts- Calories-230 | Fats-20g |Carbohydrates-9.9g |Proteins-17g

Ingredients

- Two halved and pitted ripe avocados
- Two teaspoons of vegetable oil
- Three tablespoons of fresh lime juice
- One crushed garlic clove
- A quarter teaspoon of ground chipotle chili
- Salt, as required
- A quarter cup of finely chopped red onion
- A quarter cup of fresh finely chopped cilantro

Instructions

- Brush the cut sides of each avocado half with oil.
- Place the water tray in the bottom of Air fryer grill.
- Place about two cups of lukewarm water into the water tray.
- Place the drip pan over the water tray and then arrange the heating element.
- Now, place the grilling pan over the heating element.
- Plugin the Grill and press the 'Power' button to turn it on.
- Then press the 'Fan" button.
- Set the temperature settings according to the manufacturer's directions.
- Cover the grill with a lid and let it preheat.
- After preheating, remove the lid and grease the grilling pan.
- Place the avocado halves over the grilling pan, cut side down.
- Cook, uncovered for about 2-4 minutes.

- Transfer the avocados onto the cutting board and let them cool slightly.
- Remove the peel and transfer the flesh into a bowl.
- Add the lime juice, garlic, chipotle and salt and with a fork, mash until almost smooth.
- Stir in onion and cilantro and refrigerate, covered for about 1 hour before serving.

Healthy Squash & Zucchini

Preparation Time-10 minutes | Cook Time-25 minutes | Servings-2 | Difficulty-Easy

Nutritional Facts- Calories-67 | Fats-4g |Carbohydrates-7.8g |Proteins-17g

Ingredients

- One lb. of zucchini, cut into 1/2-inch half-moons
- One lb. of yellow squash, cut into 1/2-inch half-moons
- One tablespoon of olive oil
- Pepper
- Salt

Instructions

- In a mixing bowl, add zucchini, squash, oil, pepper, and salt and toss well.
- Add zucchini and squash mixture into the air fryer basket and cook at 400 F for 20 minutes. Shake basket halfway through.
- Shake basket well and cook for 5 minutes more.
- Serve and enjoy.

Herbed Eggplant and Zucchini Mix

Preparation Time-10 minutes | Cook Time-10 minutes | Servings-2 | Difficulty-Easy

Nutritional Facts- Calories-152 | Fats-4.8g |Carbohydrates-19g |Proteins-4.8g

Ingredients

- One roughly cubed eggplant
- Three roughly cubed zucchinis
- Two tablespoons of lemon juice
- Salt and black pepper to the taste
- One teaspoon of dried thyme
- One teaspoon of dried oregano
- Three tablespoons of olive oil

Instructions

- Put eggplant in a dish that fits your air fryer, add zucchinis, lemon juice, salt, pepper, thyme, oregano and
- olive oil, toss, introduce in your air fryer and cook at 360 degrees F for 8 minutes.
- Divide among plates and serve right away.

Jalapeño Poppers

Preparation Time-10 minutes | Cook Time-10 minutes | Servings-2 | Difficulty-Easy

Nutritional Facts- Calories-244 | Fats-12g |Carbohydrates-4.8g |Proteins-12g

Ingredients

- Twelve to eighteen whole fresh jalapeños
- One cup of nonfat refried beans
- One cup of shredded Monterey Jack cheese
- One sliced scallion
- One teaspoon of salt, divided
- A quarter cup of all-purpose flour
- Two large eggs
- Half cup of fine cornmeal
- Olive oil or canola oil cooking spray

Instructions

- Start by slicing each jalapeño lengthwise on one side. Place the jalapeños side by side in a microwave-safe bowl and microwave them until they are slightly soft, usually around 5 minutes.
- While your jalapeños are cooking, mix refried beans, scallions, half a teaspoon of salt, and cheese in a bowl.
- Once your jalapeños are softened, you can scoop out the seeds and add one tablespoon of your refried bean mixture. Press the jalapeño closed around the filling.
- Set your eggs in a small bowl and place your flour in a separate bowl. In a third bowl, mix your cornmeal and the remaining salt in a third bowl.
- Roll each pepper in the flour, then dip it in the egg, and finally roll it in the cornmeal, making sure to coat the entire pepper.
- Place the peppers on a flat surface and coat them with a cooking spray; olive oil cooking spray is suggested.

- Pour into the Air Fryer Oven rack/basket. Place the rack on the middle shelf of the Air fryer oven. Set temperature to 400°F, and set time to 5 minutes. Select START/STOP to begin. Turn each pepper and then cook for another 5 minutes; serve hot.

Marinated Veggie Skewers

Preparation Time-20 minutes | Cook Time-10 minutes | Servings-2 | Difficulty-Easy

Nutritional Facts- Calories-125 | Fats-6.9g |Carbohydrates-12.9g |Proteins-4g

Ingredients

For Marinade

- Two minced cloves of garlic
- Two teaspoons of minced fresh basil
- Two teaspoons of minced fresh oregano
- Half teaspoon of cayenne pepper
- Sea Salt and ground black pepper
- Two tablespoons of fresh lemon juice
- Two tablespoons of olive oil

For Veggies

- Two large zucchinis, cut into thick slices
- Eight large quartered button mushrooms
- One seeded and cubed yellow bell pepper
- One seeded and cubed red bell pepper

Instructions

- For marinade, in a large bowl, attach all the ingredients and mix until well combined.
- Bring the vegetables and toss to coat well.
- Cover and refrigerate to marinate for at least 6-8 hours.
- Remove the vegetables from the bowl and thread onto pre-soaked wooden skewers.
- Place the water tray in the bottom of the Air Fryer Electric Grill.
- Place about two cups of lukewarm water into the water tray.
- Place the drip pan over the water tray and then arrange the heating element.
- Now, place the grilling pan over the heating element.
- Plugin the Grill and press the 'Power' button to turn it on.

- Then press the 'Fan" button.
- Set the temperature settings according to the manufacturer's directions. Cover the grill with a lid and let it preheat.
- After preheating, remove the lid and grease the grilling pan.
- Place the skewers over the grilling pan. Cover with the lid and cook for about 8-10 minutes, flipping occasionally. Serve hot.

Mediterranean Veggies

Preparation Time-10 minutes | Cook Time-10 minutes | Servings-2 | Difficulty-Easy

Nutritional Facts- Calories-161 | Fats-11.1g |Carbohydrates-13g |Proteins-1.5g

Ingredients

- One cup of chopped mixed bell peppers
- One cup of chopped eggplant
- One cup of chopped zucchini
- One cup of chopped mushrooms
- Half cup of chopped onion
- Half cup of sun-dried tomato vinaigrette dressing

Instructions

- In a large bowl, merge all ingredients and toss to coat well.
- Refrigerate to marinate for about 1 hour.
- Place the water tray in the bottom of the Air Fryer Grill.
- Place about two cups of lukewarm water into the water tray.
- Place the drip pan over the water tray and then arrange the heating element.
- Now, place the grilling pan over the heating element.
- Plugin the Grill and press the 'Power' button to turn it on.
- Then press the 'Fan" button.
- Set the temperature settings according to the manufacturer's directions.
- Cover the grill with a lid and let it preheat.
- After preheating, remove the lid and grease the grilling pan.
- Place the vegetables over the grilling pan.
- Cover with the lid and cook for about 8-10 minutes, flipping occasionally.

- Serve hot.

Mushroom and Cabbage Spring Rolls

Preparation Time-20 minutes | Cook Time-15 minutes | Servings-2 | Difficulty-Easy

Nutritional Facts- Calories-325 | Fats-15.9g |Carbohydrates-1g |Proteins-41g

Ingredients

- Two tablespoons of vegetable oil
- Four cups of sliced Napa cabbage
- Five ounces of diced shiitake mushrooms
- Three carrots
- One tablespoon of minced fresh ginger
- One tablespoon of minced garlic
- One bunch of scallions
- Two tablespoons of soy sauce
- One (Four ounces) package of cellophane noodles
- A quarter teaspoon of cornstarch
- One (Twelve ounces) package of thawed frozen spring roll wrappers
- Cooking spray

Instructions

- Warm the olive oil in a nonstick skillet until shimmering.
- Add the cabbage, mushrooms, and carrots and sauté for 3 minutes or until tender.
- Add the ginger, garlic, and scallions and sauté for 1 minute or until fragrant.
- Mix in the soy sauce and turn off the heat. Discard any liquid that remains in the skillet and allow it to cool.
- Bring a pot of water to a boil, then turn off the heat and pour in the noodles. Let sit until the noodles are al dente. Transfer One cup of the noodles to the skillet and toss with the cooked vegetables. Reserve the remaining noodles for other use.
- Set the cornstarch in a small dish of water, and then place the wrappers on a clean work surface. Dab the edges of the wrappers with cornstarch.
- Scoop up three tablespoons of filling in the center of each wrapper, and then fold the corner in front of you over the filling. Tuck the wrapper under the filling, and then fold the corners on both sides into the center. Keep rolling to seal the wrapper. Repeat with remaining wrappers.

- Set the air fryer basket with cooking spray. Arrange the wrappers in the basket and spritz with cooking spray.
- Slide the basket into the air fryer. Cook at the corresponding preset mode or Air Fry at 400F (205C) for 10 minutes.
- Flip the wrappers halfway through the cooking time.
- When cooking is complete, the wrappers will be golden brown.
- Serve immediately.

Mushroom Pasta

Preparation Time-10 minutes | Cook Time-25 minutes | Servings-2 | Difficulty-Easy

Nutritional Facts- Calories-324 | Fats-13.8g |Carbohydrates-1g |Proteins-19g

Ingredients

One cup of pasta
One and a half tablespoons of olive oil
A pinch of salt

For tossing pasta

- One and a half tablespoons of olive oil
- Salt and pepper to taste
- Half teaspoon of oregano
- Half teaspoon of basil

For sauce

- Two tablespoons of olive oil
- Two cups of sliced mushroom
- Two tablespoons of all-purpose flour
- Two cups of milk
- One teaspoon of dried oregano
- Half teaspoon of dried basil
- Half teaspoon of dried parsley
- Salt and pepper to taste

Instructions

- Boil the pasta and sieve it when done. You will need to toss the pasta in the ingredients mentioned above and set it aside.
- For the sauce, add the ingredients to a pan and bring the ingredients to a boil. Stir the sauce and continue to simmer to make a thicker sauce. Add the pasta to the sauce and transfer this into a glass bowl garnished with cheese.

- Preheat the Air Fryer at 160 degrees for 5 minutes. Place the bowl in the basket and close it. Let it continue to cook at the same temperature for 10 minutes more. Keep stirring the pasta in between.

Okra Flat cakes

Preparation Time-10 minutes | Cook Time-35 minutes | Servings-2 | Difficulty-Moderate

Nutritional Facts- Calories-213 | Fats-4g |Carbohydrates-19g |Proteins-6g

Ingredients

- Two tablespoons of garam masala
- Two cups of sliced okra
- Three teaspoons of finely chopped ginger
- Two tablespoons of fresh coriander leaves
- Three finely chopped green chilies
- One and a half tablespoons of lemon juice
- Salt and pepper to taste

Instructions

- Mix the ingredients in a clean bowl and add water to it. Make sure that the paste is not too watery but is enough to apply on the okra.
- Preheat the Air Fryer at 160 degrees Fahrenheit for 5 minutes. Place the galettes in the fry basket and let them cook for another 25 minutes at the same temperature. Keep rolling them over to get a uniform cook.
- Serve either with mint chutney or ketchup.

Onion Rings

Preparation Time-10 minutes | Cook Time-10 minutes | Servings-2 | Difficulty-Easy

Nutritional Facts- Calories-442 | Fats-12g |Carbohydrates-31.8g |Proteins-6.9g

Ingredients

Two sliced white onions
- One cup of flour
- Two beaten eggs
- One cup of breadcrumbs

Instructions

- Cover the onion rings with flour.
- Dip in the egg.
- Dredge with breadcrumbs.

- Add to the air fryer.
- Set it to air fry.
- Cook at 400 F for 10 minutes.

Pineapple and Veggie Skewers

Preparation Time-20 minutes | Cook Time-15 minutes | Servings-2 | Difficulty-Easy

Nutritional Facts- Calories-220 | Fats-12g | Carbohydrates-30g | Proteins-4.5g

Ingredients

- 1/3 cup of olive oil
- One and a half teaspoons of dried basil
- 1/3 teaspoon of dried oregano
- Salt and ground black pepper, as required
- Two zucchinis, cut into 1-inch slices
- Two yellow squashes, cut into 1-inch slices
- Half pound of whole fresh mushrooms
- One chopped red bell pepper
- One chopped red onion
- Twelve cherry tomatoes
- One chopped fresh pineapple

Instructions

- In a bowl, add oil, herbs, salt and black pepper and mix well.
- Thread the veggies and pineapple onto pre-soaked wooden skewers.
- Brush the veggies and pineapple with the oil mixture evenly.
- Place the water tray in the bottom of the Air Fryer Electric Grill.
- Place about two cups of lukewarm water into the water tray.
- Place the drip pan over the water tray and then arrange the heating element.
- Now, place the grilling pan over the heating element.
- Plugin the Grill and press the 'Power' button to turn it on.
- Then press the 'Fan" button.
- Set the temperature settings according to the manufacturer's directions.
- Cover the grill with a lid and let it preheat.
- After preheating, remove the lid and grease the grilling pan.
- Place the skewers over the grilling pan.

- Cover with the lid and cook for about 10-15 minutes, flipping occasionally.
- Serve hot.

Pineapple Kebab

Preparation Time-5 minutes | Cook Time-30 minutes | Servings-2 | Difficulty-Easy

Nutritional Facts- Calories-210 | Fats-7.8g | Carbohydrates-13.8g | Proteins-12g

Ingredients

- Two cups of cubed pineapples
- Three chopped onions
- Five roughly chopped green chilies
- One and a half tablespoons of ginger paste
- One and a half teaspoons of garlic paste
- One and a half teaspoons of salt
- Three teaspoons of lemon juice
- Two teaspoons of garam masala
- Four tablespoons of chopped coriander
- Three tablespoons of cream
- Three tablespoons of chopped capsicum
- Three eggs
- Two and a half tablespoons of white sesame seeds

Instructions

- Grind the ingredients except for the egg and form a smooth paste. Coat the pineapples in the paste. Now, beat the eggs and add a little salt to them.
- Dip the coated vegetables in the egg mixture and then transfer them to the sesame seeds and coat the pineapples well.
- Place the vegetables on a stick.
- Preheat the Air fryer at 160 degrees Fahrenheit for around 5 minutes. Place the sticks in the basket and let them cook for another 25 minutes at the same temperature. Turn the sticks over in between the cooking process to get a uniform cook.

Potatoes and Special Tomato Sauce

Preparation Time-10 minutes | Cook Time-18 minutes | Servings-2 | Difficulty-Easy

Nutritional Facts- Calories-211 | Fats-6g | Carbohydrates-13.8g | Proteins-6g

Ingredients

- Two pounds of cubed potatoes
- Four minced garlic cloves
- One chopped yellow onion
- One cup of tomato sauce
- Two tablespoons of chopped basil
- Two tablespoons of olive oil
- Half teaspoon of dried oregano
- Half teaspoon of dried parsley

Instructions

- Heat up a pan that fits your air fryer with the oil over medium heat, add onion, stir and cook for 1-2 minutes.
- Add garlic, potatoes, parsley, tomato sauce and oregano, stir, introduce in your air fryer and cook at 370egrees F and cook for 16 minutes.
- Add basil, toss everything, divide among plates and serve.

Potatoes and Tomatoes Mix

Preparation Time-10 minutes | Cook Time-16 minutes | Servings-2 | Difficulty-Easy

Nutritional Facts- Calories-182 | Fats-4g |Carbohydrates-30g |Proteins-17g

Ingredients

- One and a half pounds of quartered red potatoes
- Two tablespoons of olive oil
- One pint of cherry tomatoes
- One teaspoon of sweet paprika
- One tablespoon of chopped rosemary
- Salt and black pepper to the taste
- Three minced garlic cloves

Instructions

- In a bowl, mix potatoes with tomatoes, oil, paprika, rosemary, garlic, salt and pepper, toss, transfer to your
- air fryer and cook at 380 degrees F for 16 minutes.
- Divide among plates and serve.

Quick Vegetable Kebabs

Preparation Time-10 minutes | Cook Time-10 minutes | Servings-2 | Difficulty-Easy

Nutritional Facts- Calories-50 | Fats-1g |Carbohydrates-10.8g |Proteins-1.5g

Ingredients

- Two cubed bell peppers
- Half cubed onion
- One cubed zucchini
- One cubed eggplant
- Pepper
- Salt

Instructions

- Thread vegetables onto the skewers and spray them with cooking spray. Season with pepper and salt.
- Preheat the air fryer to 390 F.
- Place skewers into the air fryer basket and cook for 10 minutes. Turn halfway through.
- Serve and enjoy.

Roasted Eggplant, Peppers, Garlic, and Onion

Preparation Time-15 minutes | Cook Time-20 minutes | Servings-2 | Difficulty-Easy

Nutritional Facts- Calories-184 | Fats-10.8g |Carbohydrates-4.8g |Proteins-12g

Ingredients

- One small halved and sliced eggplant
- One yellow bell pepper
- One red bell pepper
- Two quartered garlic cloves
- One sliced red onion
- One tablespoon of extra-virgin oil
- Salt and fresh black pepper
- Half cup of chopped fresh basil for garnish
- Cooking spray

Instructions

- Grease a nonstick baking dish with cooking spray.
- Place the eggplant, garlic, red onion, and bell peppers in the greased baking dish. Set with the olive oil and toss to coat well. Spritz any uncoated

- surfaces with cooking spray.
- Place the baking dish in the bake position.
- Select Bake, set temperature to 356 degrees Fahrenheit, and set time to 20 minutes.
- Set the vegetables halfway through the cooking time.
- When done, remove from the air fryer grill and sprinkle with salt and pepper.
- Sprinkle the basil on top for garnish and serve.

Sesame Mustard Greens

Preparation Time-10 minutes | Cook Time-11 minutes | Servings-2 | Difficulty-Easy

Nutritional Facts- Calories-120 | Fats-1g | Carbohydrates-4g | Proteins-6.9

Ingredients

- Two minced cloves of garlic
- One pound of torn mustard greens
- One tablespoon of olive oil
- Half cup of sliced yellow onion
- Salt and black pepper to the taste
- Three tablespoons of veggie stock
- A quarter teaspoon of dark sesame oil

Instructions

- Heat up a pan that fits your air fryer with the oil over medium heat, add onions, stir and brown them for 5 minutes.
- Add garlic, stock, greens, salt and pepper, stir, introduce in your air fryer and cook at 350 degrees F for 6 minutes.
- Add sesame oil, toss to coat, divide among plates and serve.

Simple Tomatoes and Bell Pepper Sauce

Preparation Time-10 minutes | Cook Time-15 minutes | Servings-2 | Difficulty-Easy

Nutritional Facts- Calories-123 | Fats-1g | Carbohydrates-7.8g | Proteins-9.9g

Ingredients

- Two chopped red bell peppers
- Two minced cloves of garlic
- One pound of halved cherry tomatoes
- One teaspoon of dried rosemary
- Three bay leaves

- Two tablespoons of olive oil
- One tablespoon of balsamic vinegar
- Salt and black pepper to the taste

Instructions

- In a bowl, mix tomatoes with garlic, salt, black pepper, rosemary, bay leaves, half of the oil and half of the vinegar, toss to coat, introduce in your air fryer and roast them at 320 degrees F for 15 minutes.
- Meanwhile, in your food processor, mix bell peppers with a pinch of sea salt, black pepper, the rest of the oil and the rest of the vinegar and blend very well.
- Divide roasted tomatoes between plates, drizzle the bell peppers sauce over them and serve.

Smoked Paprika Cauliflower Florets

Preparation Time-10 minutes | Cook Time-20 minutes | Servings-2 | Difficulty-Easy

Nutritional Facts- Calories-256 | Fats-12g | Carbohydrates-1g | Proteins-31.8g

Ingredients

- One large head cauliflower
- Two teaspoons of smoked paprika
- One teaspoon of garlic powder
- Salt and black pepper, to taste
- Cooking spray

Instructions

- Spray the air fry basket with cooking spray.
- In a medium bowl, merge the cauliflower florets with the smoked paprika and garlic powder until evenly coated. Sprinkle with salt and pepper.
- Place the cauliflower florets in the air fry basket and lightly mist with cooking spray.
- Place the air fry basket on the air fry position.
- Select Air Fry, set temperature to 400F (205C), and set time to 20 minutes. Stir the cauliflower four times during cooking.
- Remove the cauliflower from the air fryer grill and serve hot.

Spicy Sweet Potato Fries

Preparation Time-5 minutes | Cook Time-37 minutes | Servings-2 | Difficulty-Easy

Nutritional Facts- Calories-99 | Fats-12.9g

|Carbohydrates-1g|Proteins-7.8g

Ingredients

- Two tablespoons of sweet potato fry seasoning mix
- Two tablespoons of olive oil
- Two sweet potatoes

Seasoning Mix

- Two tablespoons of salt
- One tablespoon of cayenne pepper
- One tablespoon of dried oregano
- One tablespoon of fennel
- Two tablespoons of coriander

Instructions

- Slice both ends off sweet potatoes and peel. Slice lengthwise in half and again crosswise to make four pieces from each potato.
- Slice each potato piece into 2-3 slices, and then slice into fries.
- Grind together all of the seasoning, mix ingredients and mix in the salt.
- Ensure the air fryer oven is preheated to 350 degrees F.
- Toss potato pieces in olive oil, sprinkling with seasoning mix and tossing well to coat thoroughly.
- Add fries to the air fryer basket. Set temperature to 350 degrees F, and set time to 27 minutes. Select START/STOP to begin.
- Take out the basket and turn the fries. Turn off the air fryer and let cook 10-12 minutes till the fries are golden.

Stuffed Eggplants

Preparation Time-10 minutes | Cook Time-30 minutes | Servings-2 | Difficulty-Moderate

Nutritional Facts- Calories-240 | Fats-4g |Carbohydrates-21g |Proteins-17g

Ingredients

- Four halved small eggplants

- Salt and black pepper to the taste
- Ten tablespoons of olive oil
- Two and a half pounds tomatoes, cut into halves and grated
- One chopped green bell pepper
- One chopped yellow onion
- One tablespoon of minced garlic
- Half cup of chopped cauliflower
- One teaspoon of chopped oregano
- Half cup of chopped parsley
- Three ounces of crumbled feta cheese

Instructions

- Season eggplants with salt, pepper and four tablespoons of oil, toss, put them in your air fryer and cook at 350 degrees F for 16 minutes.
- Meanwhile, heat up a pan with three tablespoons of oil over medium-high heat, add onion, stir and cook for 5 minutes.
- Add bell pepper, garlic and cauliflower, stir, cook for 5 minutes, take off heat, add parsley, tomato, salt, pepper, oregano and cheese, and whisk everything.
- Stuff eggplants with the veggie mix, drizzle the rest of the oil over them, put them in your air fryer and cook at 350 degrees F for 6 minutes more.
- Divide among plates and serve right away.

Stuffed Mushrooms

Preparation Time-8 minutes | Cook Time-8 minutes | Servings-2 | Difficulty-Easy

Nutritional Facts- Calories-260 | Fats-12.9g |Carbohydrates-6g |Proteins-31.8g

Ingredients

- Two diced Rashers Bacon
- Half diced Onion
- Half diced Bell Pepper
- One diced Small Carrot
- Twenty-four Medium Size Mushrooms
- One cup of Shredded Cheddar Plus Extra for the Top
- Half cup of Sour Cream

Instructions

- Chop the mushrooms stalks finely into the Air

fryer Oven rack/basket. Place the rack on the middle shelf of the Air fryer oven. Set temperature to 350F, and set time to 8 minutes and fry them up with the bacon, onion, pepper and carrot. When the veggies are fairly tender, stir in the sour cream and the cheese. Keep on the heat until the cheese has melted and everything is mixed nicely.

- Now grab the mushroom caps and heap a plop of filling on each one.
- Place in the fryer basket and top with a little extra cheese.

Tofu Nuggets

Preparation Time-15 minutes | Cook Time-25 minutes | Servings-2 | Difficulty-Easy

Nutritional Facts- Calories-356 | Fats-8.7g |Carbohydrates-1.5g |Proteins-60g

Ingredients

Tofu

- Sixteen ounces of cube-sliced tofu
- Cooking spray
- A quarter cup of flour
- One teaspoon of garlic powder
- Half teaspoon of paprika
- Half teaspoon of ground cumin
- Salt to taste

Sauce

- One tablespoon of avocado oil
- Two tablespoons of sugar
- Three tablespoons of soy sauce
- Two tablespoons of honey
- One teaspoon of garlic powder
- One tablespoon of grated ginger
- Pepper to taste

Instructions

- Spray tofu cubes with oil.
- Mix remaining ingredients in a bowl.
- Coat tofu evenly with this mixture.
- Add the tofu cubes to the air fryer.
- Set it to air fry.
- Cook at 350 degrees F for 10 minutes.
- Toss and cook for 15 minutes.
- In a bowl, mix the sauce ingredients.

- Toss the tofu in the sauce and serve.

Tomato and Basil Tart

Preparation Time-10 minutes | Cook Time-15 minutes | Servings-2 | Difficulty-Easy

Nutritional Facts- Calories-140 | Fats-1.5g |Carbohydrates-1.5g |Proteins-9.9g

Ingredients

- One bunch of chopped basil
- Four eggs
- One minced clove of garlic
- Salt and black pepper to the taste
- Half cup of halved cherry tomatoes
- A quarter cup of grated cheddar cheese

Instructions

- In a bowl, mix eggs with salt, black pepper, cheese and basil and whisk well.
- Pour this into a baking dish that fits your air fryer, arrange tomatoes on top, introduce in the fryer and cook at 320 degrees F for 14 minutes.
- Slice and serve right away.

Veg Momos

Preparation Time-15 minutes | Cook Time-35 minutes | Servings-2 | Difficulty-Moderate

Nutritional Facts- Calories-210 | Fats-9.9g |Carbohydrates-21g|Proteins-12.9g

Ingredients

For dough

- One and a half cups of all-purpose flour
- Half teaspoon of salt or to taste
- Five tablespoons of water

For filling

- Two cups of grated carrots
- Two cups of grated cabbage
- Two tablespoons of oil
- Two teaspoons of ginger-garlic paste
- Two teaspoons of soya sauce
- Two teaspoons of vinegar

Instructions

- Knead the dough and cover it with plastic wrap, and set it aside. Next, cook the ingredients for the filling and try to ensure that the vegetables are covered well with the sauce.

- Roll the dough and cut it into a square. Place the filling in the center. Now, wrap the dough to cover the filling and pinch the edges together.
- Preheat the Air fryer at 200° F for 5 minutes. Place the momos in the fry basket and close it. Let them cook at the same temperature for another 20 minutes.
- Recommended sides are chili sauce or ketchup.

Winter Vegetarian Frittata

Preparation Time-5 minutes | Cook Time-30 minutes | Servings-2 | Difficulty-Easy

Nutritional Facts- Calories-302 | Fats-20g |Carbohydrates-7.8g |Proteins-24g

Ingredients

- One peeled and thinly sliced leek
- Two finely minced cloves of garlic
- Three finely chopped medium-sized carrots
- Two tablespoons of olive oil
- Six eggs
- Sea salt and ground black pepper
- Half teaspoon of finely minced dried marjoram
- Half cup of yellow cheese of choice

Instructions

- Sauté the leek, garlic, and carrot in hot olive oil until they are tender and fragrant; reserve.
- In the meantime, preheat your air fryer oven to 330 degrees F.
- In a bowl, merge the eggs along with the salt, ground black pepper, and marjoram.
- Then, grease the inside of your baking dish with a nonstick cooking spray. Pour the whisked eggs into the baking dish. Stir in the sautéed carrot mixture. Top with the cheese shreds.
- Place the baking dish in the air fryer oven cooking basket. Cook for about 30 minutes and serve warm.

Zucchini Lasagna

Preparation Time-15 minutes | Cook Time-15 minutes | Servings-2 | Difficulty-Easy

Nutritional Facts- Calories-233 | Fats-7.8g |Carbohydrates-3.18g |Proteins-34.8g

Ingredients

- One sliced thinly lengthwise zucchini, divided
- Half cup of marinara sauce, divided
- A quarter cup of ricotta, divided
- One cup of fresh basil leaves
- A quarter cup of chopped spinach leaves, divided

Instructions

- Set half of the zucchini slices in a small loaf pan.
- Spread with half of marinara sauce and ricotta.
- Top with half of spinach and basil.
- Repeat layers with the remaining ingredients.
- Cover the pan with foil.
- Place inside the air fryer.
- Set it to bake.
- Cook at 400 F
- Remove foil and cook for another 5 minutes.

Zucchini Noodles Delight

Preparation Time-10 minutes | Cook Time-20 minutes | Servings-2 | Difficulty-Easy

Nutritional Facts- Calories-121 | Fats-1.5g |Carbohydrates-4.8g |Proteins-9g

Ingredients

- Two tablespoons of olive oil
- Three zucchinis, cut with a spiralizer
- Sixteen ounces of sliced mushrooms
- A quarter cup of chopped sun-dried tomatoes
- One teaspoon of minced garlic
- Half cup of halved cherry tomatoes
- Two cups of tomatoes sauce
- Two cups of torn spinach
- Salt and black pepper to the taste
- A handful of chopped basil

Instructions

- Put zucchini noodles in a bowl, season salt and black pepper and leave them aside for 10 minutes.
- Heat up a pan that fits your air fryer with the oil over medium-high heat, add garlic, stir and cook for 1 minute.
- Add mushrooms, sun-dried tomatoes, cherry tomatoes, spinach, cayenne, sauce and zucchini noodles, stir, introduce in your air fryer and cook at 320 degrees F for 10 minutes.

- Divide among plates and serve with basil sprinkled on top.

- Recommended sides are tamarind or mint chutney.

Zucchini Samosa

Preparation Time-15 minutes | Cook Time-30 minutes | Servings-2 | Difficulty-Moderate

Nutritional Facts- Calories-250 | Fats-9g |Carbohydrates-16.8g |Proteins-25g

Ingredients

For wrappers

- Two tablespoons of unsalted butter
- One and a half cups of all-purpose flour
- A pinch of salt to taste
- Water as required

For filling

- Three mashed medium zucchinis
- A quarter cup of boiled peas
- One teaspoon of powdered ginger
- Two finely chopped green chilies
- Half teaspoon of cumin
- One teaspoon of coarsely crushed coriander
- One dry red chili broken into pieces
- Salt as per taste
- Half teaspoon of dried mango powder
- Half teaspoon of red chili power
- Two tablespoons of coriander

Instructions

- Mix the dough for the outer covering and make it stiff and smooth. Leave it to rest in a container while making the filling.
- Cook the ingredients in a pan and stir them well to make a thick paste. Roll the paste out.
- Roll the dough into balls and flatten them. Cut them in halves and add the filling. Use water to help you fold the edges to create the shape of a cone.
- Preheat the Air Fryer for around 5 to 6 minutes at 300 Fahrenheit. Place all the samosas in the fry basket and close the basket properly. Keep the Air Fryer at 200 degrees for another 20 to 25 minutes. Around the halfway point, open the basket and turn the samosas over for uniform cooking. After this, fry at 250 degrees for around 10 minutes in order to give them the desired golden-brown color. Serve hot.

Chapter 7~Air Fried Dessert Recipes

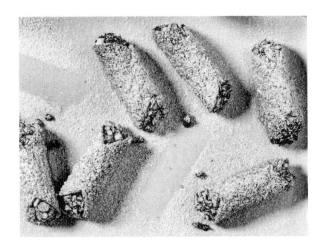

Apple Bread

Preparation Time-10 minutes | Cook Time-40 minutes | Servings-2 | Difficulty-Moderate

Nutritional Facts- Calories-192 | Fats-7.8g |Carbohydrates-15.9g |Proteins-7.8g

Ingredients

- Three cups of cored and cubed apples
- One cup of sugar
- One tablespoon of vanilla
- Two eggs
- One tablespoon of apple pie spice
- Two cups of white flour
- One tablespoon of baking powder
- One stick of butter
- One cup of water

Instructions

- In a bowl, mix egg with one butter stick, apple pie spice and sugar and stir using your mixer.
- Add apples and stir again well.
- In another bowl, mix baking powder with flour and stir.
- Combine the two mixtures, stir and pour into a spring form pan.
- Put spring form pan in your air fryer and cook at 320 degrees F for 40 minutes
- Slice and serve.

Apple Chips with Dip

Preparation Time-10 minutes | Cook Time-13 minutes | Servings-2 | Difficulty-Easy

Nutritional Facts- Calories-253 | Fats-9g |Carbohydrates-12.9g |Proteins-23g

Ingredients

- One apple, thinly slice using a mandolin slicer
- One tablespoon of almond butter
- A quarter cup of plain yogurt
- Two teaspoons of olive oil
- One teaspoon of ground cinnamon
- Drops liquid stevia

Instructions

- Add apple slices, oil, and cinnamon to a large bowl and toss well.
- Spray air fryer basket with cooking spray.
- Place apple slices in an air fryer basket and cook at 375 degrees F for 12 minutes. Turn after every 4 minutes.
- Meanwhile, in a small bowl, mix together almond butter, yogurt, and sweetener.
- Serve apple chips with dip and enjoy.

Apricot and Raisin Cake

Preparation Time-10 minutes | Cook Time-15 minutes | Servings-2 | Difficulty-Easy

Nutritional Facts- Calories-126 | Fats-1g|Carbohydrates-26g |Proteins-4.8g

Ingredients

- ½ cup of dried apricots
- Two tablespoons of orange juice
- ¾ cup of self-raising flour
- 1/3 cup of Sugar
- One egg
- Half cup of Raisins

Instructions

- Preheat the air fryer to 320 degrees Fahrenheit.
- Blend the juice and dried apricots until smooth in a blender or food processor.
- Combine the sugar and flour in a separate bowl.
- The egg should be whisked. Combine the flour and sugar in a mixing bowl. Combine all of the ingredients.

- Combine the apricot puree and raisins in a mixing bowl.
- A small amount of oil should be sprayed into an air fryer-safe baking tin. Turn the mixture over and smooth it out.
- Cook for 12 minutes in the air fryer, checking after 10 minutes. To check if it's done, use a metal skewer. If necessary, return the cake to the air fryer for a few minutes more to brown.
- Allow cooling completely before removing from the pan and slicing.

Baked Apples

Preparation Time-9 minutes | Cook Time-16 minutes | Servings-2 | Difficulty-Easy

Nutritional Facts- Calories-171 | Fats-6g |Carbohydrates-30g |Proteins-17g

Ingredients

One large apple

Filling

- One tablespoon of melted butter
- A quarter teaspoon of ground cinnamon
- One pinch salt
- Three tablespoons of light or golden-brown sugar
- One pinch freshly grated nutmeg, optional
- Two tablespoons of old-fashioned oats

Instructions

For apples

- Wash the apple, pat it dry, then cut it in half from stem to end (choose apples that are slightly flattering on the edges rather than spherical – this will help the apple half stand up straight in the air fryer basket without tumbling over).
- Scoop out the core and seeds, as well as some flesh, with a large ice cream scoop, spoon, or paring knife (to make a cavity, big enough to hold the filling). We left both ends intact for a nicer presentation, but if you're feeding young children, you can chop it out.
- To make less than a half cup of, chop only the scooped-out flesh into quarter-inch pieces (be careful not to include any seeds or core)

For filling

- Stir together the brown sugar, melted butter, cinnamon, nutmeg, and salt until well blended.

- Combine the oats and apple chunks in a mixing bowl.
- Fill the apple halves halfway with the filling (packing lightly into the cavity).

Bake

- Place the apple halves on top of the half cup of water in the bottom pan/air fryer basket, making sure they don't bounce about. The air fryer should be closed.
- Preheat the air fryer to 350°F for 12 to 15 minutes (we recommend testing after 13 minutes because different models cook differently). The apples were excellent in 15 minutes using the Instant Vortex air fryer).
- Allow apples to cool for at least 2 minutes in the air fryer before serving hot with a dollop of vanilla ice cream.

Banana & marshmallow Relish

Preparation Time-5 minutes | Cook Time-6 minutes | Servings-2 | Difficulty-Easy

Nutritional Facts- Calories-153 | Fats-6.9g |Carbohydrates-21g |Proteins-6g

Ingredients

- One and a half ounces of mini marshmallows
- One and a half ounces of graham cracker cereal
- Four medium-sized bananas
- One and a half ounces of mini peanut butter chips
- One and a half ounces of mini semi-sweet chocolate chips

Instructions

- Heat your air fryer to 400°F.
- Using a knife, slice vertically through the inner side of the unpeeled bananas but not to the bottom, piercing the opposite skin. Open up the cut slits.
- Fill the slits with marshmallows, crackers, chocolate and peanut butter chips
- Put the filled bananas into the basket, ensuring they are upright. Cook for 6 minutes until the banana peel is black and the chips are toasted and melted.

Banana Cake

Preparation Time-25 minutes | Cook Time-20 minutes | Servings-2 to 4 | Difficulty-Easy

Nutritional Facts- Calories-147 | Fats-6g |Carbohydrates-13.8g |Proteins-15.9g

Ingredients

- A quarter teaspoon of baking soda
- 1/3 teaspoon of baking powder
- A quarter teaspoon of salt
- Four and a half tablespoons of granulated white sugar
- Three tablespoons of butter
- One and a half-peeled small ripe banana
- One large egg
- Three tablespoons of buttermilk
- One teaspoon of vanilla extract
- Half cup plus One tablespoon of flour
- Cooking spray

Instructions

- Spritz a baking pan with cooking spray.
- Merge the flour, baking soda, baking powder, and salt in a large bowl. Stir to mix well.
- Beat the sugar and butter in a separate bowl with a mixer on medium speed for 3 minutes.
- Beat in the eggs, vanilla extract, buttermilk and bananas into the sugar and butter mix with a mixer.
- Pour in the flour mix and whip with a mixer until smooth.
- Scrape the batter into the pan and level the batter with a spatula.
- Bring the pan into the air fryer oven. Press the Power Button. Cook at 325 degrees F (165C) for 20 minutes.
- After 15 minutes, detach from the air fryer oven. Check the doneness. Bring to the air fryer oven and continue cooking.
- When done, a toothpick inserted in the center should come out clean.
- Set the cake on a cooling rack and allow it to cool for 15 minutes before slicing to serve.

Berries Mix

Preparation Time-5 minutes | Cook Time-8 minutes | Servings-2 | Difficulty-Easy

Nutritional Facts- Calories-163 | Fats-6g |Carbohydrates-13.8g |Proteins-17g

Ingredients

- Two tablespoons of lemon juice
- One and a half tablespoons of maple syrup
- One and a half tablespoons of champagne vinegar
- One tablespoon of olive oil
- One pound of halved strawberries
- One and a half cups of blueberries
- A quarter cup of torn basil leaves

Instructions

- In a pan that fits your air fryer, mix lemon juice with maple syrup and vinegar,
- bring to a boil over medium-high heat, add oil, blueberries and strawberries, stir, introduce in your air fryer and cook at 310 degrees F for 6 minutes.
- Sprinkle basil on top and serve!

Black Tea Cake

Preparation Time-10 minutes | Cook Time-35 minutes | Servings-2 | Difficulty-Moderate

Nutritional Facts- Calories-198 | Fats-7.8g |Carbohydrates-16.8g |Proteins-17g

Ingredients

- Six tablespoons of black tea powder
- Two cups of milk
- Half cup of butter
- Two cups of sugar
- Four eggs
- Two teaspoons of vanilla extract
- Half cup of olive oil
- Three and a half cups of flour
- One teaspoon of baking soda
- Three teaspoons of baking powder

For the cream

- Six tablespoons of honey
- Four cups of sugar

- One cup of softened butter

Instructions

- Put the milk in a pot, heat up over medium heat, add tea, stir well, take off the heat and leave aside to cool down.
- In a bowl, mix a half cup of butter with two cups of sugar, eggs, vegetable oil, vanilla extract, baking powder, baking soda and three and a half cups of flour and stir everything really well.
- Pour this into two greased round pans, introduce each in the fryer at 330 degrees F and bake for 25 minutes.
- In a bowl, mix one cup of butter with honey and 4 cups of sugar and stir really well.
- Arrange one cake on a platter, spread the cream all over, top with the other cake and keep in the fridge until you serve it.

Blackcurrant Pudding

Preparation Time-10 minutes | Cook Time-15 minutes | Servings-2 | Difficulty-Easy

Nutritional Facts- Calories-132 | Fats-9g | Carbohydrates-9.9g | Proteins-6g

Ingredients

- Two cups of milk
- Two cups of almond flour
- Two tablespoons of custard powder
- Three tablespoons of powdered sugar
- One cup of blackcurrant pulp
- Three tablespoons of unsalted butter

Instructions

- Boil the milk and the sugar in a pan and add the custard powder followed by the almond flour and stir till you get a thick mixture. Chop the figs fine and add them to the mixture.
- Preheat the fryer to 300 degrees Fahrenheit for five minutes. Place the dish in the basket and reduce the temperature to 250 degrees Fahrenheit. Cook for ten minutes and set aside to cool.

Blueberry Muffins

Preparation Time-15 minutes | Cook Time-15 minutes | Servings-2 | Difficulty-Easy

Nutritional Facts- Calories-191 | Fats-16.5g

| Carbohydrates-14.5g | Proteins-8g

Ingredients

- A quarter cup of unsweetened coconut milk
- Two large eggs
- Half teaspoon of vanilla extract
- On and a half cups of almond flour
- A quarter cup of Swerve
- One teaspoon of baking powder
- A quarter teaspoon of ground cinnamon
- Pinch of ground cloves
- Pinch of ground nutmeg
- 1/8 teaspoon of salt
- Half cup of fresh blueberries
- A quarter cup of chopped pecans

Instructions

- In a blender, add the almond milk, eggs and vanilla extract and pulse for about 20-30 seconds.
- Add the almond flour, Swerve, baking powder, spices and salt and pulse for about 30-45 seconds until well blended.
- Transfer the mixture into a bowl
- Gently, fold in half of the blueberries and pecans.
- Place the mixture into eight silicone muffin cups and top each with remaining blueberries.
- Select "Air Fry" of Air Fryer Oven and then adjust the temperature to 325 degrees Fahrenheit.
- Set the timer for 15 minutes and press "Start/Stop" to begin cooking.
- When the unit beeps to show that it is preheated, place the cups over the airing rack and insert them in the air fryer.
- When cooking time is complete, remove the cups from the air fryer and place them onto a wire rack to cool for about 10 minutes.
- Carefully invert the muffins onto the wire rack to completely cool before serving.

Blueberry Pudding

Preparation Time-10 minutes | Cook Time-25 minutes | Servings-2 | Difficulty-Easy

Nutritional Facts- Calories-161 | Fats-6g | Carbohydrates-12g | Proteins-4g

Ingredients

- Two cups of flour

- Two cups of rolled oats
- Eight cups of blueberries
- One melted stick of butter
- One cup of chopped walnuts
- Three tablespoons of maple syrup
- Two tablespoons of chopped rosemary

Instructions

- Spread blueberries in a greased baking pan and leave aside.
- In your food processor, mix rolled oats with the flour, walnuts, butter, maple syrup and rosemary, blend well, layer this over blueberries, introduce everything in your air fryer and cook at 350 degrees F for 25 minutes.
- Leave dessert to cool down, cut and serve.

Blueberry Scones

Preparation Time-10 minutes | Cook Time-10 minutes | Servings-2 | Difficulty-Easy

Nutritional Facts- Calories-155 | Fats-6.9g |Carbohydrates-13.8g |Proteins-6g

Ingredients

- One cup of white flour
- One cup of blueberries
- Two eggs
- Half cup of heavy cream
- Half cup of butter
- Five tablespoons of sugar
- Two teaspoons of vanilla extract
- Two teaspoons of baking powder

Instructions

- In a bowl, mix flour, salt, baking powder and blueberries and stir.
- In another bowl, mix heavy cream with butter, vanilla extract, sugar and eggs and stir well.
- Combine the two mixtures, knead until you obtain your dough, shape ten triangles from this mix, place them on a baking sheet (lined) that fits the air fryer and cook them at 320 degrees F for 10 minutes.
- Serve them cold.

Bourbon Glazed Pineapple

Preparation Time-10 minutes | Cook Time-30 minutes | Servings-2 | Difficulty-Moderate

Nutritional Facts- Calories-196 | Fats-6.9g |Carbohydrates-27.9g |Proteins-7.8g

Ingredients

- Two tablespoons of Brown Sugar
- Two tablespoons of bourbon
- Half teaspoon of Vanilla Extract
- One peeled pineapple
- Two tablespoons of melted butter

Instructions

- Place pineapple on the spit of an Air Fryer and secure with the attachments of fork.
- In a small bowl, combine bourbon, melted butter, brown sugar, and vanilla extract; whisk.
- Grill the pineapple at 400 degrees F for 40 minutes by scrubbing with the bourbon coat every 5 minutes.
- Ensure to press the rotate button.
- Take out the pineapple from the grill and chop it into slices.
- Serve with chopped pecans, ice cream, whipped cream and a drizzle of caramel sauce.

Bread Dough and Amaretto Dessert

Preparation Time-10 minutes | Cook Time-12 minutes | Servings-2 | Difficulty-Easy

Nutritional Facts- Calories-200 | Fats-12g |Carbohydrates-21.9g |Proteins-9.9g

Ingredients

- One pound bread dough
- One cup of sugar
- Half cup of melted butter
- One cup of heavy cream
- Twelve ounces of chocolate chips
- Two tablespoons of amaretto liqueur

Instructions

- Roll dough, cut into 20 slices and then cut each slice in halves.
- Brush dough pieces with butter, sprinkle sugar, place them in your air fryer's basket after you've brushed some butter, cook them at 350 degrees F

for 5 minutes, flip them, cook for 3 minutes more and transfer to a platter.

- Heat up a pan with the heavy cream over medium heat, add chocolate chips and stir until they melt.
- Add liqueur, stir again, transfer to a bowl and serve bread dippers with this sauce.
- Enjoy!

Bread Pudding

Preparation Time-10 minutes | Cook Time-One hour and 20 minutes | Servings-2 | Difficulty-Hard

Nutritional Facts- Calories-379 | Fats-10.8g |Carbohydrates-60g |Proteins-9g

Ingredients

- Three eggs
- Two tablespoons of vanilla
- Three cups of whole milk
- Three egg yolks
- Two teaspoons of cinnamon
- Eight tablespoons of butter
- One cup of cubed French bread
- Two cups of granulated sugar
- A quarter Pyrex bowl

Instructions

- Mix milk and butter in a bowl and heat in the microwave.
- Break the egg into another bowl and whisk.
- Add cinnamon, sugar, eggs, and vanilla.
- Add the milk mix.
- Add dried bread; mix until the bread is soaked.
- Put the mixture in a Pyrex bowl
- Place the Pyrex bowl on the Air Fryer Grill pan.
- Set the Air Fryer Grill to bagel/toast.
- Cook 60 minutes at 270F.
- Allow cooling before serving

British Victoria Sponge

Preparation Time-15 minutes | Cook Time-30 minutes | Servings-2 | Difficulty-Moderate

Nutritional Facts- Calories-234 | Fats-13.8g |Carbohydrates-23g |Proteins-4.8g

Ingredients

Victoria Sponge

- Half cup of Plain Flour
- Half cup of Butter
- Half cup of Caster Sugar
- Two Medium Eggs

Cake Filling

- Two tablespoons of Strawberry Jam
- A quarter cup of Butter
- Half cup of Icing Sugar
- One tablespoon of Whipped Cream

Instructions

- Preheat the air fryer to 356°F.
- Grease a baking dish large enough to fit in your Air fryer, but not too small; otherwise, you'll end up with a tiny cake!
- Cream together the butter and sugar until light and creamy.
- Mix in the eggs, one at a time, adding a pinch of flour to each one.
- Fold in the remaining flour with a light touch.
- Place the mixture in the tin and cook for 15 minutes at 356 degrees Fahrenheit, then another 10 minutes at 338 degrees Fahrenheit in the Air fryer.
- Allow it cool completely before slicing in the center to make two equal slices of sponge.
- To make the filling, whip the butter and gradually add the icing sugar and whipped cream until the mixture is thick and creamy.
- Place a layer of strawberry jam on top, followed by a layer of cake filling, and finally, your other sponge on top sponged together.
- Serve!

Brown Butter Cookies

Preparation Time- 10 minutes | Cook Time-10 minutes | Servings-2 | Difficulty-Easy

Nutritional Facts- Calories-144 | Fats-7.8g |Carbohydrates-12.9g |Proteins-1.5g

Ingredients

- One and a half cups of butter
- Two cups of brown sugar
- Two eggs whisked
- Three cups of flour
- 2/3 cup of chopped pecans

- Two teaspoons of vanilla extract
- One teaspoon of baking soda
- Half teaspoon of baking powder

Instructions

- Heat up a pan with the butter over medium heat, stir until it melts, add brown sugar and stir until it dissolves.
- In a bowl, mix flour with pecans, vanilla extract, baking soda, baking powder and eggs and stir well.
- Add brown butter, stir well and arrange spoonfuls of this mix on a baking sheet (lined)that fits the air fryer.
- Introduce in the fryer and cook at 340 degrees F for 10 minutes.
- Leave cookies to cool down and serve.

Brownies

Preparation Time-20 minutes | Cook Time-15 minutes | Servings-2 | Difficulty-Moderate

Nutritional Facts- Calories-195 | Fats-10.8g |Carbohydrates-6g |Proteins-7.8g

Ingredients

- Half cup of granulated sugar
- One-third cup of cocoa powder
- A quarter cup of melted and cooled slightly butter
- One large egg
- A quarter cup of all-purpose flour
- A quarter teaspoon of baking powder
- Pinch kosher salt

Instructions

- Grease a 6-inch diameter cake pan with cooking spray. Whisk in a medium bowl to mix sugar, salt, chocolate powder, flour and baking powder.
- Whisk the melted butter and egg in a small bowl until mixed. To dry ingredients, add wet ingredients and stir till combined.
- Move brownie batter to the prepared cake pan as well as the smooth top. Cook for 16-18 minutes in the air fryer at 350 ° F. Before slicing, let cool for 10 minutes.

Carrot Cake

Preparation Time-10 minutes | Cook Time-30 minutes | Servings-2 | Difficulty-Moderate

Nutritional Facts- Calories-125 | Fats-9.9g |Carbohydrates-9.9g |Proteins-15g

Ingredients

- Five ounces of Soft brown sugar
- Two eggs, beaten
- Five ounces of butter
- One orange, zest & juice
- One cup of self-raising flour
- One teaspoon of ground cinnamon
- One cup of grated carrot
- Three ounces of sultanas

Instructions

- Preheat the air fryer to 175 degrees Celsius.
- Cream the sugar and butter together in a mixing basin.
- Gradually pour in the beaten eggs.
- Fold in the flour a little at a time, mixing well after each addition. Add the sultanas, grated carrots, and orange juice and zest. Gently combine all of the ingredients.
- Pour the mixture into a greased baking tray.
- Cook for 25-30 minutes with the baking tin in the air fryer basket. Use a metal skewer or cocktail stick to poke the cake in the middle to see if it's done. Cook it for a little longer if it comes out wet.
- Remove the baking tin from the air fryer basket and set it aside for 10 minutes to cool before removing the tin.

Cashew Bars

Preparation Time-10 minutes | Cook Time-15 minutes | Servings-2 | Difficulty-Easy

Nutritional Facts- Calories-121 | Fats-4.8g |Carbohydrates-12g |Proteins-6g

Ingredients

- 1/3 cup of honey
- A quarter cup of almond meal
- One tablespoon of almond butter
- One and a half cups of chopped cashews
- Four chopped dates
- 3/4 cup of shredded coconut

- One tablespoon of chia seeds

Instructions

- In a bowl, mix honey with almond meal and almond butter and stir well.
- Add cashews, coconut, dates and chia seeds and stir well again.
- Spread this on a baking sheet (lined) that fits the air fryer and press well.
- Introduce in the fryer and cook at 300 degrees F for 15 minutes.
- Leave the mix to cool down, cut into medium bars and serve.
- Enjoy!

Chocolate and Coconut Macaroons

Preparation Time-10 minutes | Cook Time-10 minutes | Servings-2 | Difficulty-Easy

Nutritional Facts- Calories-325 | Fats-16.5g |Carbohydrates-1g|Proteins-39g

Ingredients

- Three egg whites, at room temperature
- A quarter teaspoon of salt
- 1/3 cup of granulated white sugar
- Four and a half tablespoons of unsweetened cocoa powder
- Two and a quarter cups of unsweetened shredded coconut

Instructions

- Line the air fry basket with parchment paper.
- Whisk the egg whites with salt in a large bowl with a hand mixer on high speed until stiff peaks form.
- Whisk in the sugar with the hand mixer on high speed until the mixture is thick. Mix in the cocoa powder and coconut.
- Scoop two tablespoons of the mixture and shape the mixture in a ball. Set with remaining mixture to make 24 balls in total.
- Arrange the balls in a single layer in the air fry basket and leave a little space between every two balls.
- Place the basket on the air fry position.
- Select Air Fry, set the temperature to 375F (190C) and set time to 8 minutes.

- When cooking is complete, the balls should be golden brown.
- Serve immediately.

Chocolate and Pomegranate Bars

Preparation Time- Two hours| Cook Time-10 minutes | Servings-2 | Difficulty-Easy

Nutritional Facts- Calories-78 | Fats-1.5g |Carbohydrates-10.8g |Proteins-1.5g

Ingredients

- Half cup of milk
- One teaspoon of vanilla extract
- One and a half cups of chopped dark chocolate
- Half cup of chopped almonds
- Half cup of pomegranate seeds

Instructions

- Heat up a pan with the milk over medium-low heat, add chocolate, stir for 5 minutes, take off heat add vanilla extract, half of the pomegranate seeds and half of the nuts and stir.
- Pour this into a lined baking pan, spread, sprinkle a pinch of salt, the rest of the pomegranate arils and nuts, introduce in your air fryer and cook at 300 degrees F for 4 minutes.
- Keep in the fridge for 2 hours before serving.

Chocolate Buttermilk Cake

Preparation Time-20 minutes | Cook Time-20 minutes | Servings-2 | Difficulty-Moderate

Nutritional Facts- Calories-325 | Fats-15.9g |Carbohydrates-1.5g |Proteins-37.8g

Ingredients

- Half cup of all-purpose flour
- A pinch of salt
- Half cup of granulated white sugar
- A quarter cup of unsweetened cocoa powder
- A pinch of baking soda
- 2/3 cup of buttermilk
- Two tablespoons plus two teaspoons of vegetable oil
- One teaspoon of vanilla extract
- Cooking spray

Instructions

- Spritz a baking pan with cooking spray.
- Merge the flour, cocoa powder, baking soda, sugar, and salt in a large bowl. Stir to mix well.
- Mix in the buttermilk, vanilla, and vegetable oil. Keep stirring until it forms a grainy and thick dough.
- Scrape the chocolate batter from the bowl and transfer to the pan; level the batter in an even layer with a spatula.
- Bring the pan into the air fryer oven. Press the Power Button. Cook at 325F (165C) for 20 minutes.
- After 15 minutes, detach from the air fryer oven. Check the doneness. Bring to the air fryer oven and continue cooking.
- When done, a toothpick inserted in the center should come out clean.
- Set the cake on a cooling rack and allow it to cool for 15 minutes before slicing to serve.

Chocolate Cake

Preparation Time-10 minutes | Cook Time-30 minutes | Servings-2 | Difficulty-Moderate

Nutritional Facts- Calories-234 | Fats-7.8g |Carbohydrates-30g |Proteins-6g

Ingredients

- 3⁄4 cup of white flour
- 3⁄4 cup of whole wheat flour
- One teaspoon of baking soda
- 3⁄4 teaspoon of pumpkin pie spice
- 3⁄4 cup of sugar
- One mashed banana
- Half teaspoon of baking powder
- Two tablespoons of canola oil
- Half cup of Greek yogurt
- Eight ounces of canned pumpkin puree
- Cooking spray
- One egg
- Half teaspoon of vanilla extract
- 2/3 cup of chocolate chips

Instructions

- In a bowl, mix white flour with whole wheat flour, salt, baking soda and powder and pumpkin spice and stir.
- In another bowl, mix sugar with oil, banana, yogurt, pumpkin puree, vanilla and egg and stir using a mixer.
- Combine the two mixtures, add chocolate chips, stir, pour this into a greased Bundt pan that fits your air fryer.
- Introduce in your air fryer and cook at 330 degrees F for 30 minutes.
- Leave the cake to cool down before cutting and serving it.

Chocolate Chip Cookies

Preparation Time-15 minutes | Cook Time-10 minutes | Servings-2 | Difficulty-Easy

Nutritional Facts- Calories-198 | Fats-7.5g |Carbohydrates-9.6g |Proteins-16.2g

Ingredients

- One cup of unsalted butter
- 3/4 cup of packed dark brown sugar
- Two large eggs
- One teaspoon of baking soda
- Two cups of chocolate chunks or chips
- 3/4 cup of granulated sugar
- One tablespoon of vanilla extract
- One teaspoon of kosher salt
- Two and 1/3 cups of all-purpose flour
- 3/4 cup of chopped walnuts
- Cooking spray
- Flaky sea salt, for garnish (optional)

Instructions

- Allow two sticks of unsalted butter to soften in the bowl of a stand mixer with the attachment of paddle. (Alternatively, a big mixing bowl and an electric hand mixer can be used.) 3 to 4 minutes on medium speed, beat 3/4 cup of granulated sugar and 3/4 cup of packed dark brown sugar until mixed and frothy.
- Combine two large eggs, one tablespoon of vanilla extract, and one teaspoon of kosher salt in a mixing bowl and whisk just until mixed. In small increments, One teaspoon of baking soda and 2 1/3 cups of all-purpose flour are to be mixed.
- With a rubber spatula, whisk in 3/4 cup of chopped walnuts and two cups of chocolate chunks until barely blended.

- Preheat an Air Fryer Oven to 350degree F and 5 minutes on the BAKE setting. Line the air fryer racks with parchment paper, leaving enough space for air to flow on both sides.
- Place two tablespoons of dough scoops on the racks, spacing them 1-inch apart. To produce a cookie shape, gently flatten each scoop. If used, season with flaky sea salt. Bake for 5 minutes, or until golden brown.
- Remove the racks from the air fryer and lay them aside to cool for 3 to 5 minutes.
- Repeat with the rest of the dough. Warm the dish before serving.

Chocolate Cookies

Preparation Time-10 minutes | Cook Time-25 minutes | Servings-2 | Difficulty-Easy

Nutritional Facts- Calories-240 | Fats-12g |Carbohydrates-7.8g |Proteins-6g

Ingredients

- One teaspoon of vanilla extract
- Half cup of butter
- One egg
- Four tablespoons of sugar
- Two cups of flour
- Half cup of unsweetened chocolate chips

Instructions

- Heat up a pan with the butter over medium heat, stir and cook for 1 minute.
- In a bowl, mix egg with vanilla extract and sugar and stir well.
- Add melted butter, flour and half of the chocolate chips and stir everything.
- Transfer this to a pan that fits your air fryer, spread the rest of the chocolate chips on top, introduce in the fryer at 330 degrees F and bake for 25 minutes.
- Slice when it's cold and serve.

Chocolate Glazed Donuts

Preparation Time-Two hours and 30 minutes | Cook Time-10 minutes | Servings-2 to 4 | Difficulty-Hard

Nutritional Facts- Calories-188 | Fats-9.9g |Carbohydrates-30g |Proteins-1.5g

Ingredients

- Cooking spray
- Two tablespoons of ground cinnamon
- Two tablespoons of melted butter
- Half cup of milk
- A quarter cup of plus one teaspoon of. granulated sugar, divided
- Two and a quarter teaspoons of active dry yeast
- One large egg
- One teaspoon of pure vanilla extract

For the vanilla glaze

- One cup of powdered sugar
- Two cups of all-purpose flour
- A half teaspoon of kosher salt
- Four tablespoons of melted butter
- Two ounces of milk
- A half teaspoon of pure vanilla extract
- 3/4 cup of powdered sugar
- A quarter cup of unsweetened cocoa powder
- Three tablespoons of milk
- Half cup of granulated sugar

Instructions

- Grease a large bowl with cooking oil spray. Add milk into a small, microwave-safe bowl or glass measuring cup of the microwave for 40 seconds until lukewarm. Insert a teaspoon of sugar and stir to dissolve. Then sprinkle with the yeast and leave to rest for around 8 minutes until frothy.
- Whisk the flour and salt together in a medium bowl. Whisk the remaining quarter of a cup of sugar, butter, egg, and vanilla together in a large bowl. Pour in the mixture of yeast, blend to combine, and add to the dry ingredients, stirring until shaggy dough shapes with a wooden spoon.
- Switch to a floured surface and knead until elastic and just slightly tacky, adding a teaspoon of more flour at a time, about 5 minutes if required. Place the dough in an oiled bowl and cover it with a clean dishtowel. Let the dough rise for around 1 hour in a warm place until it has doubled in size.
- Cover a large baking sheet with parchment paper and gently grease it. Punch down the dough, then move it onto a finely floured work surface and stretch it out into a rectangle that is 1/2 inch thick.

- Punch the doughnuts out with a doughnut cutter or 3 inch and 1-inch biscuit cutters. Knead some scraps together and punch more doughnuts or holes out. Put doughnuts and holes on baking sheets, cover with a dishtowel, and let rise again for an additional 40 minutes to 1 hour.

- Grease the air fryer basket with cooking spray and insert two doughnuts and two doughnut holes at a time to ensure the doughnuts do not touch. Cook until deeply golden at 375 ° F for 6 minutes. Put on the cooling rack and repeat for the remaining dough.

- Dip doughnuts in glaze. Return to the rack for cooling and let set before serving for 5 minutes.

- Whisk the powdered sugar, milk, and vanilla together in a medium bowl until smooth.

- Combine the powdered sugar, chocolate powder, and milk in a medium bowl.

- Whisk together cinnamon and sugar in a big shallow cup. Brush doughnuts with melted butter as well as toss in cinnamon sugar.

Chocolate Profiteroles

Preparation Time-15 minutes | Cook Time-20 minutes | Servings-2 | Difficulty-Easy

Nutritional Facts- Calories-246 | Fats-19g |Carbohydrates-21g |Proteins-9g

Ingredients
Profiteroles

- Half cup of Butter
- One cup of Plain Flour
- Six Medium Eggs
- One and a quarter cups of Water

Cream Filling

- Two teaspoons of Vanilla Essence
- Two teaspoons of Icing Sugar
- One and a quarter cup of Whipped Cream

Chocolate Sauce

- Half cup of a chunk of Milk Chocolate
- Two tablespoons of Whipped Cream
- A quarter cup of Butter

Instructions

- Preheat the air fryer to 338°F.

- In a big pan, melt the butter in the water over medium heat, making sure it comes to a boil.

- Remove it from the heat and whisk in the flour (a little at a time) until it forms a huge dough in the center of the pan, then return it to the heat.

- Place the dough to the side to allow it to cool. Mix in the eggs until you get a smooth consistency. Cook for 10 minutes at 356 degrees Fahrenheit in profiterole shapes.

- While the eclairs are baking, prepare the cream filling by whisking together vanilla extract, whipped cream, and icing sugar until smooth.

- Make the chocolate topping while the profiteroles are cooking by combining the chocolate, butter, and cream in a glass bowl set over a pan of simmering water. Mix until the chocolate has melted.

- Finish with melted chocolate on top of your profiteroles.

Chocolate-Glazed Custard Donut Holes

Preparation Time-One hour and 50 minutes | Cook Time-5 minutes | Servings-2 | Difficulty-Hard

Nutritional Facts- Calories-218 | Fats-9g |Carbohydrates-12g |Proteins-26g

Ingredients
Dough

- One

Custard Filling

- One (three and a half ounces) box of French vanilla instant pudding mix
- A quarter cup of heavy cream
- 1/3 cup of whole milk

Chocolate Glaze

- 1/3 cup of heavy cream
- One cup of chocolate chips

Instructions

- Merge the ingredients for the dough in a food processor, then pulse until satiny dough ball forms.

- Transfer the dough on a lightly floured work surface, then knead for 2 minutes by hand and shape the dough back to a ball.

- Spritz a large bowl with cooking spray, and then

transfer the dough ball into the bowl. Set the bowl in plastic and let it rise for 1 1/2 hours or until it doubles in size.

- Transfer the risen dough on a floured work surface, and then shape it into a 24-inch-long log. Cut the log into 24 parts and shape each part into a ball.
- Transfer the balls on two baking sheets and let sit to rise for 30 more minutes.
- Spritz the balls with cooking spray.
- Place the baking sheets on the bake position.
- Select Bake, set temperature to 400F (205C) and set time to 4 minutes. Flip the balls halfway through the cooking time.
- When cooked, the balls should be golden brown.
- Meanwhile, combine the ingredients for the filling in a large bowl and whisk for 2 minutes with a hand mixer until well combined.
- Pour the heavy cream into a saucepan, and then bring to a boil. Put the chocolate chips in a small bowl and pour in the boiled heavy cream immediately. Merge until the chocolate chips are melted and the mixture is smooth.
- Transfer the baked donut holes to a large plate, then pierce a hole into each donut hole and lightly hollow them.
- Pour the filling in a pastry bag with a long tip and gently squeeze the filling into the donut holes. Then top the donut holes with chocolate glaze.
- Set to sit for 10 minutes, and then serve.

Churros

Preparation Time-10 minutes | Cook Time-15 minutes | Servings-2 | Difficulty-Easy

Nutritional Facts- Calories-203 | Fats-7.8g |Carbohydrates-9.9g |Proteins-15.9g

Ingredients

- 3/4 cup of plus two tablespoons of water
- A quarter cup of butter
- One tablespoon of sugar
- A pinch of salt
- 3/4 cup of flour
- Two medium eggs
- Cinnamon sugar
- Half cup of sugar
- One teaspoon of cinnamon

Instructions

- Bring the butter, water, sugar, and a pinch of salt to a boil in a medium saucepan over medium heat. Reduce the heat to low and quickly stir in the flour with a wooden spatula after the mixture has reached a boil. Continue to whisk the mixture until it thickens and no longer sticks to the pot's sides.
- Using a paddle attachment, combine the ingredients in a stand mixer bowl or a heatproof basin. This will allow the churro dough to cool enough for the eggs to be added. This procedure will take approximately 3-5 minutes.
- Once the churro dough has cooled some, add the eggs one at a time, mixing constantly. The mixture will thicken and becomes sticky. Transfer the churro mixture to a piping bag fitted with a star tip at this point.
- Pipe 3-4 inches long churros onto a parchment-lined baking sheet. Using a pair of scissors or a knife, cut the end. Freeze the baking sheet for at least 30 minutes.
- Preheat the air fryer to 360°F 3 minutes before you're ready to bake your churros. Remove the frozen churros from the parchment paper and carefully set them in the air fryer basket, baking for 13-14 minutes. Depending on the size of your air fryer, you may need to bake these churros in several smaller batches. To keep the leftover churros from becoming soggy, place them in the freezer.
- Combine the sugar and cinnamon in a small bowl or plastic bag. As soon as the baked churros are removed from the air fryer, throw them in the cinnamon-sugar mixture to evenly coat them.
- Serve with dulce de leche, sweetened condensed milk, or even Nutella if you're feeling adventurous.

Cinnamon Apple Chips

Preparation Time-10 minutes | Cook Time-10 minutes | Servings-2 | Difficulty-Easy

Nutritional Facts- Calories-170 | Fats-1.5g |Carbohydrates-6.9g |Proteins-4g

Ingredients

- One to two washed, cored and thinly sliced granny smith apples
- One teaspoon of ground cinnamon pinch of salt

Instructions

- Rub apple slices with cinnamon and salt and place them into the air fryer basket.
- Cook at 390 F for 8 minutes. Turn halfway through.
- Serve and enjoy.

Cinnamon Donuts

Preparation Time-15 minutes | Cook Time-8 minutes | Servings-2-4 | Difficulty-Easy

Nutritional Facts- Calories-316 | Fats-9.9g |Carbohydrates-34g |Proteins-4.8g

Ingredients

- Two teaspoons of ground cinnamon
- Half cup of granulated white sugar
- olive or coconut oil spray
- Four tablespoons of butter melted
- Two cups of refrigerated flaky jumbo biscuits

Instructions

- Combine in small bowl cinnamon and sugar; set aside.
- The biscuits are to be divided and placed on a flat surface.
- Cut holes out of the center of each biscuit using an inch round biscuit cutter.
- Cover the basket of air fryer lightly with coconut or olive oil spray. Do not use a non-stick spray.
- Put four donuts in a single layer in the basket. Ensure that they are at a distance.
- Then cook it for five minutes at 360 degrees F or till lightly browned.
- The donuts are to be removed from Air Fryer.
- Dip the donuts in melted butter and coat by rolling in cinnamon sugar.
- Serve immediately.

Cinnamon Pancake

Preparation Time-15 minutes | Cook Time-20 minutes | Servings-2 | Difficulty-Easy

Nutritional Facts- Calories-106 | Fats-1g|Carbohydrates-9.9g |Proteins-9g

Ingredients

- Two eggs
- Two cups of low-fat cream cheese
- Half teaspoon of cinnamon
- One pack of Stevia

Instructions

- Adjust the temperature of your air fryer to 330F.
- Combine cream cheese, cinnamon, eggs, and stevia in a blender.
- Set a quarter of the mixture in the air fryer basket.
- Allow cooking for 2 minutes on both sides.
- Repeat the process with the rest of the mixture. Serve.

Cinnamon Rolls

Preparation Time-15 minutes | Cook Time-15 minutes | Servings-2 | Difficulty-Easy

Nutritional Facts- Calories-210 | Fats-12.9g |Carbohydrates-31.8g |Proteins-7.8g

Ingredients

- One-third cup of packed brown sugar
- One (Eight ounces) tube of refrigerated Crescent rolls
- Kosher salt
- Half cup of powdered sugar
- Two tablespoons of melted butter, plus more for brushing
- All-purpose flour, for surface
- A half teaspoon of ground cinnamon
- Two ounces of softened cream cheese
- One tablespoon of whole milk, plus more if needed

Instructions

- Line the air fryer's bottom with parchment paper and coat with butter. Combine the butter, brown sugar, cinnamon and a large pinch of salt in a medium bowl until it is smooth and fluffy.
- Roll out crescent rolls in one piece on a lightly floured board. Pinch the seams and fold them together in half. Roll into a rectangle of 9"-x-7". Spread the mixture of butter over the dough, leaving a quarter-inch border. Roll up the dough like a jelly roll, starting with a long side, and cut crosswise into six pieces.
- Arrange pieces in a prepared air fryer, cut-side up, evenly spaced.
- Set the air fryer to 350 ° F and cook for about 10 minutes until golden.

- To make the glaze, mix the cream cheese, powdered sugar and milk together in a medium bowl. If required, apply a teaspoon of more milk to the thin glaze.
- Spread the glaze over warm rolls of cinnamon and serve.

Cinnamon Rolls and Cream Cheese Dip

Preparation Time- Two hours | Cook Time-15 minutes | Servings-2 | Difficulty-Easy

Nutritional Facts- Calories-210 | Fats-15g |Carbohydrates-12g |Proteins-7.8g

Ingredients

- One pound bread dough
- 3/4 cup of brown sugar
- One and a half tablespoons of ground cinnamon
- A quarter cup of melted butter

For the cream cheese dip

- Two tablespoons of butter
- Four ounces of cream cheese
- One and a quarter cups of sugar
- Half teaspoon of vanilla

Instructions

- Roll dough on a floured working surface, shape a rectangle and brush with A quarter cup of butter.
- In a bowl, mix cinnamon with sugar, stir, sprinkle this over dough, roll dough into a log, seal well and cut into eight pieces.
- Leave rolls to rise for 2 hours, place them in your air fryer's basket, cook at 350 degrees F for 5 minutes, flip them, cook for 4 minutes more and transfer to a platter.
- In a bowl, mix cream cheese with butter, sugar and vanilla and whisk really well.
- Serve your cinnamon rolls with this cream cheese dip.

Cinnamon Smores

Preparation Time-5 minutes | Cook Time-5 minutes | Servings-2 to 4 | Difficulty-Easy

Nutritional Facts- Calories-234 | Fats-13.8g |Carbohydrates-6g |Proteins-20g

Ingredients

- Twelve whole cinnamon graham crackers halved

- Two (one and a half ounce) chocolate bars, cut into twelve pieces
- Twelve marshmallows

Instructions

- Arrange 12 graham cracker squares in the air fry basket in a single layer.
- Top each square with a piece of chocolate.
- Place the basket on the bake position.
- Select bake set the temperature to 350°F (180°c) and set Time to 3 minutes.
- After 2 minutes, remove the basket and place a marshmallow on each piece of melted chocolate. Return the basket to the air fryer grill and continue to cook for another 1 minute.
- Remove from the air fryer grill to a serving plate.
- Serve topped with the remaining graham cracker squares

Cinnamon Toast with Strawberries

Preparation Time-15 minutes | Cook Time-10 minutes | Servings-2 | Difficulty-Easy

Nutritional Facts- Calories-155 | Fats-1g|Carbohydrates-7.8g |Proteins-24g

Ingredients

- One (Fifteen ounces) refrigerated can of full-fat coconut milk
- Half tablespoon of powdered sugar
- One and a half teaspoons of vanilla extract, divided
- One cup of halved strawberries
- One tablespoon of maple syrup,
- One tablespoon of brown sugar, divided
- 1/3 cup of lite coconut milk
- Two eggs
- Half teaspoon of ground cinnamon
- Two tablespoons of unsalted butter, at room temperature
- Four slices of challah bread

Instructions

- Turn the chilled can of full-fat coconut milk upside down (do not shake the can), open the bottom, and pour out the liquid coconut water. Scoop the remaining solid coconut cream into a medium bowl. Using an electric hand mixer, whip the cream for 3 to 5 minutes, until soft peaks form.

- Add the powdered sugar and half a teaspoon of the vanilla to the coconut cream, and whip it again until creamy. Place the bowl in the refrigerator.
- Place the grill plate on the grill position. Select Grill, set the temperature to 450°F (232°C) and set the time to 15 minutes.
- Merge the strawberries with the maple syrup and toss to coat evenly. Sprinkle evenly with half a tablespoon of the brown sugar.
- In a large shallow bowl, whisk together the lite coconut milk, eggs, the remaining One teaspoon of vanilla, and cinnamon.
- Place the strawberries on the grill plate. Gently press the fruit down to maximize grill marks. Grill for 4 minutes without flipping.
- Meanwhile, butter each slice of bread on both sides. Place one slice in the egg mixture and let it soak for 1 minute. Flip the slice over and soak it for another minute. Repeat with the remaining bread slices. Sprinkle each side of the toast with the remaining 1/Two tablespoons of brown sugar.
- After 4 minutes, remove the strawberries from the grill and set them aside. Decrease the temperature to 400F (204C). Place the bread on the grill plate; Grill for 4 to 6 minutes until golden and caramelized. Check often to ensure the desired doneness.
- Set the toast on a plate and top with the strawberries and whipped coconut cream. Drizzle with maple syrup, if desired.

Clementine Custard

Preparation Time-10 minutes | Cook Time-15 minutes | Servings-2 | Difficulty-Easy

Nutritional Facts- Calories-146 | Fats-6g |Carbohydrates-15.9g |Proteins-6g

Ingredients

- One cup of clementine pulp
- Two cups of milk
- Two tablespoons of custard powder
- Three tablespoons of powdered sugar
- Three tablespoons of unsalted butter

Instructions

- Boil the milk and the sugar in a pan and add the custard powder followed by the clementine pulp and stir till you get a thick mixture.
- Preheat the fryer to 300 Fahrenheit for five minutes. Place the dish in the basket and reduce the temperature to 250 Fahrenheit. Cook for ten minutes and set aside to cool.

Cocoa and Almond Bars

Preparation Time-30 minutes | Cook Time-10 minutes | Servings-2 | Difficulty-Easy

Nutritional Facts- Calories-143 | Fats-6.9g |Carbohydrates-15.9g |Proteins-19g

Ingredients

- A quarter cup of cocoa nibs
- One cup of soaked and drained almonds
- Two tablespoons of cocoa powder
- A quarter cup of hemp seeds
- A quarter cup of goji berries
- A quarter cup of shredded coconut
- Eight pitted and soaked dates

Instructions

- Blend almonds in a food processor, then add cocoa nibs, hemp seeds, goji berries, cocoa powder, and coconut.
- Add the dates, mix well, distribute on a lined baking sheet that fits your air fryer, and cook for 4 minutes at 320 degrees F.
- Before serving, cut into equal portions and chill for 30 minutes.

Cocoa Cake

Preparation Time-10 minutes | Cook Time-18 minutes | Servings-2 | Difficulty-Easy

Nutritional Facts- Calories-340 | Fats-12.9g |Carbohydrates-26g |Proteins-7.8g

Ingredients

- Two ounces of melted butter
- Two eggs
- Two ounces of sugar
- One teaspoon of cocoa powder
- Two ounces of flour
- Half teaspoon of lemon juice

Instructions

- In a bowl, mix one tablespoon of butter with cocoa powder and whisk.
- In another bowl, mix the rest of the butter with sugar, eggs, flour and lemon juice, whisk well and pour half into a cake pan that fits your air fryer.
- Add half of the cocoa mix, spread, add the rest of the butter layer and top with the rest of cocoa.
- Introduce in your air fryer and cook at 360 degrees F for 17 minutes.
- Cool the cake down before slicing and serving.

Cocoa Cookies

Preparation Time-10 minutes | Cook Time-15 minutes | Servings-2 | Difficulty-Easy

Nutritional Facts- Calories-178 | Fats-15g | Carbohydrates-9.9g | Proteins-4.8g

Ingredients

- Six ounces of melted coconut oil
- Six eggs
- Three ounces of cocoa powder
- Two teaspoons of vanilla
- Half teaspoon of baking powder
- Four ounces of cream cheese
- Five tablespoons of sugar

Instructions

- In a blender, mix eggs with coconut oil, cocoa powder, baking powder, vanilla, cream cheese and swerve and stir using a mixer.
- Pour this into a lined baking dish that fits your air fryer, introduce it in the fryer at 320 degrees F and bake for 14 minutes.
- Slice cookie sheet into rectangles and serve.

Coconut Macaroons

Preparation Time-10 minutes | Cook Time- minutes | Servings-2 | Difficulty-Easy

Nutritional Facts- Calories-68 | Fats-7.8g | Carbohydrates-4g | Proteins-1g

Ingredients

- Two tablespoons of sugar
- Four egg whites
- Two cups of shredded coconut
- One teaspoon of vanilla extract

Instructions

- In a bowl, mix egg whites with stevia and beat using your mixer.
- Add coconut and vanilla extract, whisk again, shape small balls out of this mix, introduce them in your air fryer and cook at 340 degrees F for 8 minutes.
- Serve macaroons cold.

Coffee Cheesecakes

Preparation Time-10 minutes | Cook Time-20 minutes | Servings-2 | Difficulty-Easy

Nutritional Facts- Calories-260 | Fats-23g | Carbohydrates-21.9g | Proteins-6.9g

Ingredients

For the cheesecakes

- Two tablespoons of butter
- Eight ounces cream cheese
- Three tablespoons of coffee
- Three eggs
- 1/3 cup of sugar
- One tablespoon of caramel syrup

For the frosting

- Three tablespoons of caramel syrup
- Three tablespoons of butter
- Eight ounces of soft mascarpone cheese
- Two tablespoons of sugar

Instructions

- In your blender, mix cream cheese with eggs, two tablespoons of butter, coffee, One tablespoon of caramel syrup and 1/3 cup of sugar and pulse very well, spoon into a cupcake pan that fits your air fryer, introduce in the fryerand cook at 320 degrees F and bake for 20 minutes.
- Leave aside to cool down, and then keep in the freezer for 3 hours.
- Meanwhile, in a bowl, mix three tablespoons of butter with three tablespoons of caramel syrup, two tablespoons of sugar and mascarpone; blend well, spoon this over cheesecakes and serve them.

Creamy Chocolate Eclairs

Preparation Time-15 minutes | Cook Time-25 minutes | Servings-2 | Difficulty-Easy

Nutritional Facts- Calories-232 | Fats-18g |Carbohydrates-19g |Proteins-7.8g

Ingredients

Éclair Dough

- A quarter cup of Butter
- Half cup of Plain Flour
- Three Medium Eggs
- 3/4 cup of Water

Cream Filling

- One teaspoon of Vanilla Essence
- One teaspoon of Icing Sugar
- 3/4 cup of Whipped Cream

Chocolate Topping

- A quarter cup of chunk-chopped Milk Chocolate
- One tablespoon of Whipped Cream
- One and 1/8 tablespoon of Butter

Instructions

- Preheat the air fryer to 356°F.
- While the temperature rises, Melt the lard in the water in a big pan over medium heat, then bring to a boil.
- Stir in the flour after removing it from the heat.
- Return the pan to heat and stir until a medium ball form in the center.
- Cool the dough by transferring it to a cold plate. After it has cooled, beat in the eggs until the mixture is smooth. Then, using an éclair cutter, cut out éclair shapes and lay them in the air fryer. Cook for 10 minutes at 356 degrees Fahrenheit, then another 8 minutes at 320 degrees Fahrenheit.
- While the dough is baking, make the cream filling by whisking together the vanilla extract, whipped cream, and icing sugar until smooth.
- Allow the eclairs to cool before making the chocolate topping: In a glass bowl, combine the milk chocolate, whipped cream, and butter. Place it over a pan of simmering water and stir until the chocolate has melted.
- Serve by drizzling melted chocolate over the tops of the eclairs.

Delicious Spiced Apples

Preparation Time-10 minutes | Cook Time-10 minutes | Servings-2 | Difficulty-Easy

Nutritional Facts- Calories-234 | Fats-13.8g |Carbohydrates-6g |Proteins-20g

Ingredients

- Small sliced apples
- One teaspoon of apple pie spice
- Half cup of erythritol
- Two tablespoons of coconut oil, melted

Instructions

- Add apple slices in a mixing bowl and sprinkle sweetener, apple pie spice, and coconut oil over the apple and toss to coat.
- Transfer apple slices in an air fryer dish. Place dish in air fryer basket and cook at 350 degrees F for 10 minutes.

Donut Holes

Preparation Time-5 minutes | Cook Time-15 minutes | Servings-2 | Difficulty-Easy

Nutritional Facts- Calories-232 | Fats-8.9g |Carbohydrates-10.8g |Proteins-27.9g

Ingredients

- Half tablespoon of cornstarch
- Water
- One packet of Plant-Based Chocolate Shake
- Half teaspoon of stevia or any sweetener

Instructions

- Except for the stevia, combine all ingredients in a dough-like consistency with just enough water.
- Make balls out of the dough.
- Air fry for 10 minutes or till the exterior is crisp.
- Add a pinch of stevia after cooked.

Easy Chocolate Muffins

Preparation Time-10 minutes | Cook Time-15 minutes | Servings-2 | Difficulty-Easy

Nutritional Facts- Calories-198 | Fats-12.9g |Carbohydrates-10.2g |Proteins-17g

Ingredients

- One cup of Self Raising

- One and 1/8 cup of Caster Sugar
- One and 1/8 tablespoon of Cocoa Powder
- 1/3 cup of Milk Chocolate
- Half cup of Butter
- Two Medium Eggs
- Five tablespoons of Milk
- Water
- Half teaspoon of Vanilla Essence

Instructions

- Preheat the air fryer to 356°F (180°C).
- In a large mixing basin, combine the flour, sugar, and cocoa.
- Rub in the butter until it resembles breadcrumbs.
- In a small mixing dish, crack the eggs, add the milk, and whisk thoroughly.
- In a large mixing basin, whisk together the egg and milk combination.
- Mix in the vanilla extract, then thin with a little water if the mixture is too thick. You should now have a mixture that looks like a bun mix.
- Bash your milk chocolate in a sandwich bag with a rolling pin until it is a mix of sizes. Return it to the mixing bowl and stir it one last time.
- Fill tiny bun cases with the mixture and bake in the air fryer.
- Cook for 9 minutes at 356 degrees Fahrenheit, then 6 minutes at 320 degrees Fahrenheit.
- Serve!

Easy Maple and Pecan Granola

Preparation Time-5 minutes | Cook Time-20 minutes | Servings-2 | Difficulty-Easy

Nutritional Facts- Calories-290 | Fats-9.9g |Carbohydrates-1g|Proteins-37.8g

Ingredients

- One and a half cups of rolled oats
- A quarter cup of maple syrup
- A quarter cup of pecan pieces
- One teaspoon of vanilla extract
- Half teaspoon of ground cinnamon

Instructions

- Line a baking sheet with parchment paper.
- Mix together the oats, pecan pieces, maple syrup, cinnamon, and vanilla in a large bowl and stir

until the oats and pecan pieces are completely coated. Set the mixture evenly on the baking sheet.
- Place the baking sheet on the bake position.
- Select Bake, set temperature to 300F (150C), and set time to 20 minutes. Stir once halfway through the cooking time.
- When done, remove from the air fryer grill and cool before serving.

Fast and Easy Cinnamon Toast

Preparation Time-5 minutes | Cook Time-5 minutes | Servings-2 | Difficulty-Easy

Nutritional Facts- Calories-245 | Fats-15g |Carbohydrates-1g |Proteins-23g

Ingredients

- One and a half teaspoons of cinnamon
- One and a half teaspoons of vanilla extract
- Half cup of sugar
- Two teaspoons of ground black pepper
- Two tablespoons of melted coconut oil
- Six slices of whole wheat bread

Instructions

- Merge all the ingredients, except for the bread, in a large bowl. Stir to mix well.
- Dunk the bread in the bowl of mixture gently to coat and infuse well. Shake the excess off. Arrange the bread slices in the air fryer basket.
- Slide the basket into the air fryer. Cook at the corresponding preset mode or Air Fry at 400F (205C) for 5 minutes.
- Flip the bread halfway through.
- When cooking is complete, the bread should be golden brown.
- Detach the bread slices from the air fryer and slice to serve.

Figs and Coconut Butter Mix

Preparation Time-8 minutes | Cook Time-8 minutes | Servings-2 | Difficulty-Easy

Nutritional Facts- Calories-171 | Fats-7.8g |Carbohydrates-12g |Proteins-9g

Ingredients

- Two tablespoons of coconut butter

- Twelve halved figs
- A quarter cup of sugar
- One cup of toasted and chopped almonds

Instructions

- Put butter in a pan that fits your air fryer and melt over medium-high heat.
- Add figs, sugar and almonds, toss, introduce in your air fryer and cook at 300 degrees F for 4 minutes.
- Divide into bowls and serve cold.

Fluffy Shortbread with Cream

Preparation Time-15 minutes | Cook Time-17 minutes | Servings-2 | Difficulty-Easy

Nutritional Facts- Calories-231 | Fats-19g |Carbohydrates-21g |Proteins-12g

Ingredients

For The Shortbread

- Two and a quarter cups of Plain Flour
- 1/3 cup of Caster Sugar
- One cup of Butter
- Drop Vanilla Essence

For The Cream Filling

- Half cup of Icing Sugar (sieved)
- A quarter cup of Butter
- One Small Lemon (juice and rind)

Instructions

- Preheat the air fryer to 356°F (180°C).
- Combine the flour and sugar in a large mixing basin.
- Add the butter, diced, to the mixing bowl. In a separate bowl, rub the lard into the flour and sugar mixture.
- Add the vanilla extract and mix until a smooth dough forms.
- Roll out and form your dough into 1.5cm tall biscuit shapes with a rolling pin.
- Place them on a baking sheet in the air fryer and cook for 5 minutes at 356 degrees Fahrenheit. Reduce the temperature to 320 degrees Fahrenheit for another 12 minutes to allow them to finish cooking in the center.
- Make the cream while the shortbread is baking. Cream the butter in a mixing dish until light and

creamy. Add the sugar and continue to whip until the mixture is very light. Finally, add the lemon and stir once more. Set aside for now.
- Remove the shortbread from the air fryer when it beeps and set it on a cooling rack to cool for five minutes.
- Place two shortbread biscuits together with a good layer of cream filling in the center once they have cooled (but are not cold).
- Serve!

French toast Sticks with Strawberry Sauce

Preparation Time-5 minutes | Cook Time-15 minutes | Servings-2 | Difficulty-Easy

Nutritional Facts- Calories-161 | Fats-11.1g |Carbohydrates-12.9g |Proteins-17g

Ingredients

- Three slices of low-sodium whole-wheat bread, each cut into four strips
- One tablespoon of melted unsalted butter
- One tablespoon of 2 percent milk
- One tablespoon of sugar
- One whole beaten egg
- One egg white
- One cup of sliced fresh strawberries
- One tablespoon of freshly squeezed lemon juice

Instructions

- Arrange the bread strips on a plate and drizzle with the melted butter.
- In a bowl, whisk together the milk, sugar, egg and egg white.
- Dredge the bread strips into the egg mixture and place them on a wire rack to let the batter drip off. Arrange half the coated bread strips on the sheet pan.
- Slide the pan into the air fryer. Cook at the corresponding preset mode or Air Fry at 380F (193C) for 6 minutes.
- After 3 minutes, remove from the air fryer. Use a tong to turn the strips over. Rotate the pan and return the pan to the air fryer to continue cooking.
- When cooking is processed, the strips should be golden brown. Repeat with the remaining strips.
- In a small bowl, mash the strawberries with a fork

and stir in the lemon juice. Serve the French toast sticks with the strawberry sauce.

German Pancakes

Preparation Time-10 minutes | Cook Time-13 minutes | Servings-2 | Difficulty-Easy

Nutritional Facts- Calories-140 | Fats-9.9g |Carbohydrates-21g |Proteins-15.9g

Ingredients

- A pinch of salt
- Fresh berries
- Maple syrup
- Raw cacao nibs, unsweetened (for antioxidants and crunch)
- One cup of almond milk
- Three whole eggs
- Two heaping tablespoons of unsweetened applesauce
- Swerve confectioner's sugar
- One cup of whole wheat flour
- Greek yogurt

Instructions

- Set the air-fryer to 390°F. As it heats, place the ramekin or an iron tray within the air fryer.
- Add all the batter components to a processor and process until creamy. Also, add applesauce along with a teaspoon of milk to thin it out if the batter appears to be too thick.
- Spray with baking spray(nonstick) on a ramekin or cast-iron tray. After, pour in the batter.
- It is to be air-fried for around 7 to 8 minutes.
- To keep it fresh, put the leftover batter in a lidded airtight jar in the refrigerator.
- Garnish and rejoice.

Glazed Banana

Preparation Time-10 minutes | Cook Time-10 minutes | Servings-2 | Difficulty-Easy

Nutritional Facts- Calories-75 | Fats-4g |Carbohydrates-16.8g |Proteins-1g

Ingredients

- Two peeled and sliced ripe bananas
- One teaspoon of fresh lime juice
- Four teaspoons of maple syrup
- 1/8 teaspoon of ground cinnamon

Instructions

- Coat each banana half with lime juice.
- Arrange the banana halves onto the greased "baking pan" cut sides up.
- Drizzle the banana halves with maple syrup and sprinkle with cinnamon.
- Select "Air Fry" of Air Fryer Oven and then adjust the temperature to 350 degrees Fahrenheit.
- Set the timer for 10 minutes and press "Start/Stop" to begin cooking.
- When the unit beeps to show that it is preheated, insert the baking pan in the air fryer.
- When cooking time is complete, remove the baking pan from the air fryer and serve immediately.

Grape Pudding

Preparation Time-10 minutes | Cook Time-15 minutes | Servings-2 | Difficulty-Easy

Nutritional Facts- Calories-167 | Fats-7.8g |Carbohydrates-10.8g |Proteins-6g

Ingredients

- Two cups of milk
- Two cups of almond flour
- Three tablespoons of grape juice
- Two tablespoons of custard powder
- Three tablespoons of powdered sugar
- Three tablespoons of unsalted butter

Instructions

- Boil the milk and the sugar in a pan and add the custard powder followed by the almond flour and the grape juice and stir till you get a thick mixture.
- Preheat the fryer to 300 degrees Fahrenheit for five minutes. Place the dish in the basket and reduce the temperature to 250 degrees Fahrenheit. Cook for ten minutes and set aside to cool.

Homemade Cannoli

Preparation Time-Two hours and 40 minutes | Cook Time-20 minutes | Servings-2 | Difficulty-Hard

Nutritional Facts- Calories-170 | Fats-10.8g

|Carbohydrates-20g |Proteins-12g

Ingredients

- Half cup of powdered sugar, divided
- 3/4 cup of heavy cream
- Six tablespoons of white wine
- One large egg
- One egg white for brushing
- Vegetable oil for frying
- One teaspoon of pure vanilla extract
- One teaspoon of orange zest
- A quarter teaspoon of kosher salt
- Half cup of mini chocolate chips for garnish
- Two cups of all-purpose flour, plus more for surface
- Sixteen ounces of ricotta
- Half cup of mascarpone cheese
- A quarter cup of granulated sugar
- One teaspoon of kosher salt
- A half teaspoon of cinnamon
- Four tablespoons of cold butter, cut into cubes

Instructions

- By placing a fine-mesh strainer over a wide bowl, drain the ricotta. Let it drain for at
- least an hour in the refrigerator and up to overnight.
- Using a hand mixer, mix heavy cream and a quarter cup of powdered sugar in a large bowl until stiff peaks appear.
- Combine ricotta, mascarpone, a quarter of a cup of powdered sugar, salt, vanilla and orange zest in another large bowl. Fold the whipped cream into it. Refrigerate for at least 1 hour until ready to fill with Cannoli.
- Whisk the flour, sugar, salt, and cinnamon together in a big bowl. Using your hands or pastry cutter, cut butter into the flour mixture until pea-sized. Add the wine and egg and combine until it forms a dough. To make the dough come together, knead a few times in the bowl. Pat into a flat circle, cover and refrigerate for at least 1 hour and up to overnight in plastic wrap.
- Divide the dough into halves on a lightly floured surface. Roll to 1/8" thick. To cut out dough, use a four-circle cookie cutter. Repeat with the dough

that remains. To cut a few extra circles, re-roll the scraps.

- Wrap cannoli molds and brush egg whites around the dough where the dough will join to seal together.
- Working in batches, put molds in air fryer baskets and cook for 12 minutes or until golden at 350 ° F.
- Remove twist shells gently from molds when cool enough to handle or use a kitchen towel to hold them.
- The pipe is filled into shells and then dipped into mini chocolate chips.
- Put filling in a pastry bag. It should be fitted with an open star tip. The filling is to be piped into shells. Next, dip ends in mini chocolate chips and enjoy.

Jaggery Payasam

Preparation Time-10 minutes | Cook Time-15 minutes | Servings-2 | Difficulty-Easy

Nutritional Facts- Calories-189 | Fats-15g |Carbohydrates-12g |Proteins-7.8g

Ingredients

- Two cups of milk
- One cup of melted jaggery
- Two tablespoons of custard powder
- Three tablespoons of powdered sugar
- Three tablespoons of unsalted butter

Instructions

- Boil the milk and the sugar in a pan and add the custard powder followed by the jaggery and stir till you get a thick mixture. You will need to stir continuously.
- Preheat the fryer to 300 Fahrenheit for five minutes. Place the dish in the basket and reduce the temperature to 250 Fahrenheit. Cook for ten minutes and set aside to cool.

Jam Filled Buttermilk Scones

Preparation Time-10 minutes | Cook Time-30 minutes | Servings-2 | Difficulty-Moderate

Nutritional Facts- Calories-384 | Fats-23.1g |Carbohydrates-10.5g |Proteins-34.2g

Ingredients

- Two and a quarter cups of flour
- One teaspoon of salt
- A quarter cup of sugar
- Two teaspoons of Baking Powder
- Twelve tablespoons of butter
- Two large eggs
- 1/3 cup of buttermilk
- One teaspoon of Vanilla Extract
- Half cup of strawberry jams
- Two tablespoons of demerara sugar

Instructions

- Mix baking powder, flour, sugar and salt in a container.
- Grate the butter into the bowl using the larger holes on a box grater.
- Mix the ingredients in the bowl.
- Whisk the patted eggs, vanilla, and buttermilk into the bowl to complete the dough.
- Split the dough in half, form each half of the dough into a disk, cover the disks in plastic wrap and place in the refrigerator for 60 minutes.
- Place a disc in a new sheet of plastic wrap. Roll the disc to 1/2-inch thickness.
- Spread the jam on the disk, leaving a 1/2-inch scab around the edges.
- Roll the other disc in another sheet of plastic wrap to 1/2-inch thickness.
- Place the second discover the first disc and gently press the discs to seal the edges.
- Cut the dough into eight wedges.
- Place shims on two parchment-lined Air Flow racks. Generously brush the wedges with the buttermilk and sprinkle with the demerara sugar. Place the racks on the bottom and center shelves of the appliance.
- Press the power button and increase cook temperature to 375 F and cook time to 18 minutes. Rotate the racks after 10 minutes.

Lemon Bars

Preparation Time-10 minutes | Cook Time-25 minutes | Servings-2 | Difficulty-Easy

Nutritional Facts- Calories-125 | Fats-4.8g |Carbohydrates-15.9g |Proteins-4g

Ingredients

- Four eggs
- Two and a quarter cups of flour
- Juice from two lemons
- One cup of softened butter
- Two cups of sugar

Instructions

- In a bowl, mix butter with Half a cup of sugar and two cups of flour, stir well, press on the bottom of a pan that fits your air fryer, introduce in the fryer and cook at 350 degrees F for 10 minutes.
- In another bowl, mix the rest of the sugar with the rest of the flour, eggs and lemon juice, whisk well and spread over crust.
- Introduce in the fryer at 350 degrees F for 15 minutes more, leave aside to cool down, cut bars and serve them.

Lemon Butterfly Buns with Cherries on Top

Preparation Time-15 minutes | Cook Time-10 minutes | Servings-2 | Difficulty-Easy

Nutritional Facts- Calories-159 | Fats-9g |Carbohydrates-13.8g |Proteins-17g

Ingredients

- Half cup of Butter
- Half cup of Caster Sugar
- Two Medium Eggs
- Half cup of Self Raising Flour
- Half teaspoon of Vanilla Essence
- One teaspoon of Cherries
- A quarter cup of Butter
- Half cup of Icing Sugar
- Juice and rind of half a small Lemon

Instructions

- Preheat the Air fryer to 338 degrees Fahrenheit.
- In a big mixing basin, cream the sugar and butter together until fluffy and light.
- Vanilla essence should be added now.
- One at a time, beat in the eggs, adding a pinch of flour between each one.
- Fold the remaining flour in gently.
- Fill half of the mini bun cases with the ingredients

till you're out. Cook for 8 minutes at 338°F in your Air fryer with the first six.

- Prepare your icing sugar while the buns are baking by creaming the butter and gradually adding the icing sugar. Combine the lemon juice with the rest of the ingredients in a large mixing bowl. Add a splash of water if it's too thick.
- Remove the top slice of the butterfly buns after they have done cooking and cut them in half to
- produce butterfly shapes. To keep it in place, sprinkle icing sugar in the center. Then top with a third of a cherry and icing sugar.
- Serve!

Lemon Cake

Preparation Time-10 minutes | Cook Time-25 minutes | Servings-2 | Difficulty-Easy

Nutritional Facts- Calories-213 | Fats-17g |Carbohydrates-10.8g |Proteins-20g

Ingredients

- Four ounces of flour
- Two and a half ounces of soft butter
- Two ounces of fine granulated sugar
- Two eggs
- Two tablespoons of lemon juice
- One teaspoon of baking powder
- One teaspoon of vanilla extract
- Pinch of salt

Instructions

- Preheat the air fryer for 5 minutes at 320°F.
- In a mixing bowl, using a mixer or whisk, mix butter, vanilla essence, margarine, and sugar until light and creamy, about 5 minutes. Take care not to overmix.
- One by one, beat the eggs into the butter. When the first egg has been fully integrated into the mixture, add the second egg.
- After that, combine the flour, lemon juice, baking powder, and a bit of salt in a mixing bowl. Make a thorough mix.
- Butter the cake pan with some soft butter. To keep the cake from sticking to the pan, cut a circle from parchment paper and place it in the pan.
- Fill the cake pan halfway with batter and level it out with a spatula.

- Slide the fryer basket into the Air Fryer with the cake pan inside. Bake the cake for 20-25 minutes, or until golden brown.
- Make a hole in the center of the cake with a bamboo skewer or a toothpick. When it comes out dry and clean, it's done.
- Allow at least 5 minutes for the cake to cool in the pan. After that, invert the cake pan onto a wire rack to cool.

Lemon Mousse

Preparation Time-10 minutes | Cook Time-12 minutes | Servings-2 | Difficulty-Easy

Nutritional Facts- Calories-369 | Fats-30g |Carbohydrates-20g |Proteins-6g

Ingredients

- Four ounces of softened cream cheese
- Half cup of heavy cream
- Two tablespoons of fresh lemon juice
- Two tablespoons of honey
- Pinch of salt

Instructions

- In a bowl, add all the prepared mix until well combined.
- Transfer the mixture into two ramekins.
- Select "Bake" of Air Fryer Oven and then adjust the temperature to 350 degrees Fahrenheit.
- Set the timer for 12 minutes and press "Start/Stop" to begin cooking.
- When the unit beeps to show that it is preheated, place the ramekins over the airing rack and insert them in the air fryer.
- When cooking time is complete, remove the ramekin from the air fryer and place it onto a wire rack to cool completely.
- Refrigerate the ramekins for at least 3 hours before serving.

Lemon Tart

Preparation Time- One hour | Cook Time-35 minutes | Servings-2 | Difficulty-Easy

Nutritional Facts- Calories-182 | Fats-6.9g |Carbohydrates-7.8g |Proteins-6.9g

Ingredients

For the crust

- Two cups of white flour
- Two tablespoons of sugar
- A pinch of salt
- Twelve tablespoons of cold butter
- Three tablespoons of ice water

For the filling

- One and a quarter cup of sugar
- Juice and zest from two lemons
- Two whisked eggs
- Ten tablespoons of melted and chilled butter

Instructions

- Whisk together two cups of flour, a pinch of salt, and two tablespoons of sugar in a mixing dish.
- Knead in the remaining 12 tablespoons of butter and the water until a dough forms, then roll into a ball, wrap in foil, and chill for 1 hour.
- Transfer dough to a floured surface, flatten it, place it in the bottom of a tart pan, prick with a fork, chill for 20 minutes, then bake for 15 minutes in an air fryer at 360 degrees F.
- Whisk together eggs, one and a quarter cups sugar, lemon juice, ten tablespoons butter, and lemon zest in a mixing dish.
- Pour into pie crust, spread evenly, place in the fryer, and cook for 20 minutes at 360 degrees F.
- Cut it into pieces and serve it.

Lemony-Cheesy Pears

Preparation Time-10 minutes | Cook Time-10 minutes | Servings-2 | Difficulty-Easy

Nutritional Facts- Calories-312 | Fats-23g | Carbohydrates-12.9g | Proteins-23g

Ingredients

- Two large peeled, cored and halved Bartlett pears
- Three tablespoons of melted butter
- Half teaspoon of ground ginger
- A quarter teaspoon of ground cardamom
- Three tablespoons of brown sugar
- Half cup of whole-milk ricotta cheese
- One teaspoon of pure lemon extract
- One teaspoon of pure almond extract
- One tablespoon of honey, plus additional for drizzling

Instructions

- Toss the pears with ginger, butter, sugar, and cardamom in a large bowl. Toss to coat well. Arrange the pears in a baking pan, cut side down.
- Place the pan into the air fryer grill.
- Select Air Fry, set the temperature to 375 degrees F (190C) and set time to 8 minutes.
- After 5 minutes, detach the pan and flip the pears. Return the pan to the air fryer grill and continue cooking.
- When cooking is complete, the pears should be soft and browned. Remove the pan from the air fryer grill.
- In the meantime, combine the remaining ingredients in a separate bowl. Whip for 1 minute with a hand mixer until the mixture is puffed.
- Divide the mixture into four bowls, and then put the pears over the mixture and drizzle with more honey to serve.

Lime Cheesecake

Preparation Time-Four hours and 10 minutes | Cook Time-10 minutes | Servings-2 | Difficulty-Hard

Nutritional Facts- Calories-266 | Fats-23g | Carbohydrates-10.8g | Proteins-7.8g

Ingredients

- Two tablespoons of melted butter
- Two teaspoons of sugar
- Four ounces of flour
- A quarter cup of shredded coconut

For the filling

- One pound cream cheese
- Zest from one lime
- Juice from one lime
- Two cups of hot water
- Two sachets of lime jelly

Instructions

- In a bowl, mix coconut with flour, butter and sugar, stir well and press this on the bottom of a pan that fits your air fryer.
- Meanwhile, put the hot water in a bowl, add jelly sachets and stir until it dissolves.
- Put cream cheese in a bowl, add jelly, lime juice and zest and whisk really well.

- Add this over the crust, spread, introduce in the air fryer and cook at 300 degrees F for 4 minutes.
- Keep in the fridge for 4 hours before serving.

Mandarin Pudding

Preparation Time-20 minutes | Cook Time-40 minutes | Servings-2 | Difficulty-Hard

Nutritional Facts- Calories-172 | Fats-6.9g |Carbohydrates-10.8g |Proteins-6.9g

Ingredients

- Juice from two mandarins
- Four ounces of softened butter
- 3/4 cup of sugar
- 3/4 cup of ground almonds
- One peeled and sliced mandarin
- Two tablespoons of brown sugar
- Two whisked eggs
- 3/4 cup of white flour
- Honey for serving

Instructions

- Butter a loaf pan and sprinkle brown sugar on the bottom. Arrange mandarin slices on top.
- Stir together sugar, butter, eggs, flour, almonds, and mandarin juice in a mixing bowl. Spoon over mandarin slices, place pan in the air fryer, and cook for 40 minutes at 360 degrees F.
- Place the pudding on a platter and drizzle with honey.

Maple Cupcakes

Preparation Time-10 minutes | Cook Time-20 minutes | Servings-2 | Difficulty-Easy

Nutritional Facts- Calories-161 | Fats-10.8g |Carbohydrates-6.9g |Proteins-4g

Ingredients

- Four tablespoons of butter
- Four eggs
- Half cup of pure applesauce
- Two teaspoons of cinnamon powder
- One teaspoon of vanilla extract
- Half cored and chopped apple
- Four teaspoons of maple syrup
- 3/4 cup of white flour
- Half teaspoon of baking powder

Instructions

- Heat the butter in a pan over medium heat, then add the applesauce, eggs, vanilla, and maple syrup, stirring constantly. Remove from the heat and set aside to cool.
- Whisk together the flour, baking powder, cinnamon, and apples, then pour into a cupcake tray and bake for 20 minutes at 350 degrees F in your air fryer.
- Allow cupcakes to cool before transferring to a plate and serving.

Maple Pecan Donuts

Preparation Time-5 minutes | Cook Time-25 minutes | Servings-2 | Difficulty-Easy

Nutritional Facts- Calories-292 | Fats-9.9g |Carbohydrates-12.9g |Proteins-27.9g

Ingredients

- Half Package of Pancakes
- One egg
- One teaspoon of Cinnamon
- Two ounces of Water
- Four chopped Pecans
- Half package of Maple Pecan Shake
- Half teaspoon of Baking Powder
- One teaspoon of Nutmeg
- Half tablespoon of Sugar-free Maple Syrup
- Half teaspoon of Vanilla Extract

Instructions

- Preheat the Air fryer oven to 350 degrees Fahrenheit. Alternatively, use an air fryer.
- Spray a doughnut pan with non-stick oil if using. Roll small sheets of aluminum foil into cylindrical shape and coat with nonstick spray. Then set it aside.
- Whisk together the egg, shake mix, pancake mix, baking powder, nutmeg, cinnamon, and chopped pecans in a medium-sized mixing dish.
- Fill six donut molds or muffin tins with batter.
- Bake for 17-20 minutes in the oven or air fryer.

Milk-Butter Pecan Tart

Preparation Time-Two hours and 25 minutes | Cook Time-30 minutes | Servings-2 | Difficulty-Hard

Nutritional Facts- Calories-312 | Fats-23g |Carbohydrates-12.9g |Proteins-20g

Ingredients

Tart Crust

- A quarter cup of firmly packed brown sugar
- 1/3 cup of softened butter
- One cup of all-purpose flour
- A quarter teaspoon of kosher salt

Filling

- A quarter cup of whole milk
- Four tablespoons of butter
- Half cup of packed brown sugar
- A quarter cup of pure maple syrup
- One and a half cups of finely chopped pecans
- A quarter teaspoon of pure vanilla extract
- A quarter teaspoon of sea salt

Instructions

- Set a baking pan with aluminum foil, and then spritz the pan with cooking spray.
- Stir the brown sugar and butter in a bowl with a hand mixer until puffed, then add the flour and salt and stir until crumbled.
- Set the mixture in the prepared baking pan and tilt the pan to coat the bottom evenly.
- Place the pan on the bake position. Place the pan on the bake position.
- Select Bake, set temperature to 356 degrees Fahrenheit and set time to 13 minutes.
- When done, the crust will be golden brown.
- Meanwhile, pour the milk, butter, sugar, and maple syrup into a saucepan. Stir to mix well. Bring to a simmer, and then cook for one more minute. Stir constantly.
- Turn off the heat and mix the pecans and vanilla into the filling mixture.
- Pour the filling mixture over the golden crust and spread with a spatula to coat the crust evenly.
- Place the pan on the bake position.
- Select Bake and set the time to 12 minutes. When cooked, the filling mixture should be set and frothy.

- Detach the baking pan from the air fryer grill and sprinkle with salt. Set to sit for 10 minutes or until cooled.
- Transfer the pan to the refrigerator to chill for at least 2 hours, then remove the aluminum foil and slice to serve.

Mini Chocolate Peanut Butter Cupcakes

Preparation Time-10 minutes | Cook Time-30 minutes | Servings-2 to 4 | Difficulty-Moderate

Nutritional Facts- Calories-525 | Fats-18g |Carbohydrates-34g |Proteins-39g

Ingredients

- 2/3 cup of flour
- One cup of vegetable oil
- Half cup of whole milk
- One cup of sugar
- Two cups of confectioners' sugar
- A quarter cup of water
- Half teaspoon of salt
- One tablespoon of whole milk
- One large egg
- 3/2 teaspoon of Vanilla Extract
- 1/3 cup of cocoa
- One stick of unsalted butter
- Half teaspoon of baking soda
- Chocolate pearls
- Peanut Butter Frosting
- One teaspoon of Baking Powder

Instructions

- Combine the egg, Half cup of milk, vegetable oil, and vanilla in a bowl and beat to combine.
- Bring together the baking powder, baking soda, flour, sugar, cocoa and salt with the egg mixture and whisk.
- Gradually attach the boiling water to the mixture and toss very well.
- Pour or pour batter into foil cupcake liners until about two-thirds of each is full.
- Place cupcake liners on two Air Flow racks. Position the racks on the bottom and middle shelves of the appliance.
- Press the power button (15 minutes cook time) and decrease cook temperature to 350°F. Turn

- racks halfway through cook time (7 1/2 minutes).
- Let the cupcakes cool for 30 minutes.
- Bring together the peanut butter and butter in a bowl. Add the confectioners' sugar and One tablespoon of milk slowly until frosting is creamy.
- Top cupcakes with frosting and chocolate pearls.

Mini Lava Cakes

Preparation Time-10 minutes | Cook Time-20 minutes | Servings-2 | Difficulty-Easy

Nutritional Facts- Calories-201 | Fats-7.8g |Carbohydrates-24g |Proteins-6g

Ingredients

- Four tablespoons of sugar
- Four tablespoons of milk
- One tablespoon of cocoa powder
- Half teaspoon of orange zest
- One egg
- Two tablespoons of olive oil
- Four tablespoons of flour
- Half teaspoon of baking powder

Instructions

- In a mixing bowl, whisk together the egg, oil, sugar, milk, salt, baking powder, flour, cocoa powder, and orange zest. Pour into buttered ramekins.
- Cook for 20 minutes at 320 degrees F in ramekins in an air fryer.
- Warm lava cakes should be served.

Mini Pumpkin Pie Delights

Preparation Time-15 minutes | Cook Time-15 minutes | Servings-2 | Difficulty-Easy

Nutritional Facts- Calories-178 | Fats-9g |Carbohydrates-16.8g |Proteins-4.8g

Ingredients

- One Pumpkin Pie Filling
- 1/3 cup of Plain Flour
- Two tablespoons of Butter
- One tablespoon of Caster Sugar
- Water

Instructions

- Preheat the Air fryer oven to 356 degrees Fahrenheit.
- For making the pastry, in a mixing bowl, combine the plain flour and butter and rub the fat into the flour. Mix in the sugar thoroughly. Water should be added until the ingredients are moist enough to form a good dough. Knead the dough thoroughly until it is smooth.
- Using butter, grease your pastry casings.
- Cover the cases of your pastry molds with rolled-out pastry.
- Fill to the brim with pumpkin pie filling, about 80 percent full.
- Cook for 15 minutes at 356 degrees Fahrenheit in your air fryer.
- Allow for five minutes of resting time before removing the pies from the casings with a butter knife and placing them on a cooling rack to cool.
- Serve!

Orange Chocolate Fondant

Preparation Time-15 minutes | Cook Time-30 minutes | Servings-2 | Difficulty-Moderate

Nutritional Facts- Calories-169 | Fats-16.8g |Carbohydrates-12.9g |Proteins-12g

Ingredients

- Two tablespoons of Self Raising Flour
- Four tablespoons of Caster Sugar
- Four tablespoons of Dark Chocolate
- Four tablespoons of Butter
- Rind and juice of one Medium Orange
- Two Medium Eggs

Instructions

- Preheat the Air fryer oven to 356 degrees Fahrenheit.
- Oil four ramekins.
- In a glass dish, melt the chocolate and butter over a big pan of simmering water. Stir until the mixture is smooth and creamy.
- Whisk the eggs and sugar together until pale and foamy.
- In the chocolate, combine the orange, egg, and sugar combination. Finally, add the flour and mix everything together evenly.

- Bake for 12 minutes after filling the ramekins 75% full with the mixture.
- Remove the ramekins from the air fryer and cook for 2 minutes in ramekins. To release the edges, turn the ramekins upside down (gently) onto a serving platter and tap the bottom with a blunt knife.
- The fondant will release from the center, leaving you with a wonderful soft-centered pudding.
- Serve with a scoop of vanilla ice cream or a drizzle of caramel sauce.

Orange Frosted Carrot Cake

Preparation Time-15 minutes | Cook Time-10 minutes | Servings-2 | Difficulty-Easy

Nutritional Facts- Calories-176 | Fats-12g | Carbohydrates-16.8g | Proteins-7.8g

Ingredients

- One and a half cups of Self Raising
- 3/4 cup of Brown Sugar
- One teaspoon of Mixed Spice
- Two Large peeled and grated Carrots
- Two Medium Eggs
- 3/4 cup of Olive Oil
- Two tablespoons of Milk
- A quarter cup of Butter
- Rind and juice of one small orange
- One and a quarter cup of Icing Sugar
- Water

Instructions

- Preheat the air fryer for 10 minutes at 356 degrees Fahrenheit.
- Set aside a baking pan that has been lined with a baking sheet.
- In a mixing basin, combine the flour, spices, grated carrots, and sugar. Combine all of the ingredients thoroughly.
- To make a well in the center of the mixture, add the eggs, milk, and oil and beat with a wooden spoon until all of your ingredients are completely combined.
- Cook for 5 minutes at 356 degrees Fahrenheit in your preheated baking tin. Reduce the temperature to 320 degrees Fahrenheit and cook for another 5 minutes.

- Make the icing while the carrot cake is baking. Melt the butter, orange juice, and rind together in a mixing bowl, then whisk in the icing sugar until smooth.
- When the carrot cake is done and has cooled slightly, sprinkle the icing sugar on top.
- Serve by chopping into squares.

Oreos

Preparation Time-10 minutes | Cook Time-10 minutes | Servings-2 to 4 | Difficulty-Easy

Nutritional Facts- Calories-88 | Fats-7.8g | Carbohydrates-9.9g | Proteins-6.9g

Ingredients

- Two to four chocolate sandwich cookies (such as Oreo)
- A quarter cup of water
- A quarter cup of complete pancake mix
- One tablespoon of confectioners' sugar, or to taste
- Cooking spray

Instructions

- Mix the pancake mixture and water until well mixed.
- Line the basket of an air fryer with parchment paper. With nonstick cooking oil, spray the parchment paper.
- In the pancake mixture, dip each cookie and put it in the basket. Make sure they don't touch them; if possible, cook in batches.
- The air fryer is preheated to 400 degrees F (200 degrees C). Add the basket and cook for 5 - 6 minutes; flip and cook 2 to 3 more minutes until golden brown. Sprinkle with confectioner's sugar.

Passion Fruit Pudding

Preparation Time-10 minutes | Cook Time-40 minutes | Servings-2 | Difficulty-Moderate

Nutritional Facts- Calories-320 | Fats-18g | Carbohydrates-6.9g | Proteins-7.8g

Ingredients

- One cup of Paleo passion fruit curd
- Pulp and seeds of four passion fruits
- Three and a half ounces maple syrup
- Three eggs

- Two ounces of melted ghee
- Three and a half ounces of almond milk
- Half cup of almond flour
- Half teaspoon of baking powder

Instructions

- In a bowl, mix half of the fruit curd with passion fruit seeds and pulp, stir and divide into six heatproof ramekins.
- In a bowl, whisk eggs with maple syrup, ghee, the rest of the curd, baking powder, milk and flour and stir well.
- Divide this into the ramekins as well, introduce them in the fryer and cook at 200 degrees F for 40 minutes.
- Leave puddings to cool down and serve!

Peach Pie

Preparation Time-10 minutes | Cook Time-35 minutes | Servings-2 | Difficulty-Moderate

Nutritional Facts- Calories-231 | Fats-6g |Carbohydrates-15.9g |Proteins-4.8g

Ingredients

- One pie dough
- Two and a quarter pounds of pitted and chopped peaches
- Two tablespoons of cornstarch
- Half cup of sugar
- Two tablespoons of flour
- A pinch of ground nutmeg
- One tablespoon of dark rum
- One tablespoon of lemon juice
- Two tablespoons of melted butter

Instructions

- Roll out the pie dough and push it into a pie pan that fits your air fryer.
- Combine peaches, lemon juice, sugar, cornstarch, flour, rum, nutmeg, and butter in a mixing bowl and stir well.
- Pour into a pie plate and spread evenly. Place in your air fryer and cook for 35 minutes at 350 degrees F. Serve either warm or cold.

Pears and Espresso Cream

Preparation Time-10 minutes | Cook Time-30 minutes | Servings-2 | Difficulty-Moderate

Nutritional Facts- Calories-201 | Fats-6.9g |Carbohydrates-15g |Proteins-7.8g

Ingredients

- Four halved and cored pears
- Two tablespoons of lemon juice
- One tablespoon of sugar
- Two tablespoons of water
- Two tablespoons of butter

For the cream

- One cup of whipping cream
- One cup of mascarpone
- 1/3 cup of sugar
- Two tablespoons of cold espresso

Instructions

- In a bowl, mix pears halves with lemon juice, One tablespoon of sugar, butter and water, toss well, transfer them to your air fryer and cook at 360 degrees F for 30 minutes.
- Meanwhile, in a bowl, mix whipping cream with mascarpone, 1/3 cup of sugar and espresso, whisk really well and keep in the fridge until pears are done.
- Divide pears among plates, top with espresso cream and serve them.

Pignoli Cookies

Preparation Time-10 minutes | Cook Time-30 minutes | Servings-2 | Difficulty-Moderate

Nutritional Facts- Calories-170 | Fats-4.8g |Carbohydrates-1g |Proteins-25g

Ingredients

- Two cups of pine nuts
- Four large egg whites
- One cup of confectioners' sugar
- Half cup of sugar
- Ten ounces of almond paste

Instructions

- Whisk together the almond paste and sugar in a bowl until just combined.

- Pat 2 egg whites into the almond mixture.
- Gradually add the confectioner's sugar to the almond mixture and mix well to make a dough.
- Beat the remaining two egg whites in a separate bowl until the whites are foamy.
- Dip your fingers in the flour to prevent the dough from sticking to your fingers. Shape the dough into 1 inch. Balls, dip the balls in the egg whites and cover each ball with the pine nuts.
- Place the balls on two parchment-lined Air Flow Racks and flatten each ball lightly.
- Position the racks on the bottom and center shelves of the appliance.
- Press the power button, reduce the cooking temperature to 325F and raise the cooking time to 18 minutes. Turn racks midway through cook time (9 minutes).

Pistachio Pancakes

Preparation Time-10 minutes | Cook Time-10 minutes | Servings-2 | Difficulty-Easy

Nutritional Facts- Calories-156 | Fats-7.8g |Carbohydrates-15.9g |Proteins-6.9g

Ingredients

- Two tablespoons of sliced pistachio
- One and a half cups of almond flour
- Three eggs
- Two teaspoons of dried basil
- Two teaspoons of dried parsley
- Salt and Pepper to taste
- Three tablespoons of Butter

Instructions

- Preheat the air fryer to 250 Fahrenheit.
- In a small bowl, mix the ingredients together. Ensure that the mixture is smooth and well-balanced.
- Take a pancake mold and grease it with butter. Add the batter to the mold and place it in the air fryer basket.
- Cook till both the sides of the pancake have browned on both sides and serve with maple syrup.

Plum and Currant Tart

Preparation Time-30 minutes | Cook Time-35 minutes | Servings-2 | Difficulty-Hard

Nutritional Facts- Calories-202 | Fats-4.8g |Carbohydrates-12g |Proteins-6g

Ingredients

For the crumble

- A quarter cup of almond flour
- A quarter cup of millet flour
- One cup of brown rice flour
- Half cup of cane sugar
- Ten tablespoons of softened butter
- Three tablespoons of milk

For the filling

- One pound of pitted and halved small plums
- One cup of white currants
- Two tablespoons of cornstarch
- Three tablespoons of sugar
- Half teaspoon of vanilla extract
- Half teaspoon of cinnamon powder
- A quarter teaspoon of ginger powder
- One teaspoon of lime juice

Instructions

- In a bowl, mix brown rice flour with half a cup of sugar, millet flour, almond flour, butter and milk and stir until you obtain a sand-like dough.
- Reserve 1/4 of the dough, press the rest of the dough into a tart pan that fits your air fryer and keep in the fridge for 30 minutes.
- Meanwhile, in a bowl, mix plums with currants, three tablespoons of sugar, cornstarch, vanilla extract, cinnamon, ginger and lime juice and stir well.
- Pour this over tart crust, crumble reserved dough on top, introduce in your air fryer and cook at 350 degrees F for 35 minutes.
- Leave the tart to cool down, slice and serve.

Plum Bars

Preparation Time-10 minutes | Cook Time-18 minutes | Servings-2 | Difficulty-Easy

Nutritional Facts- Calories-112 | Fats-6g |Carbohydrates-18g |Proteins-6.9g

Ingredients

- Two cups of dried plums
- Six tablespoons of water
- Two cups of rolled oats
- One cup of brown sugar
- Half teaspoon of baking soda
- One teaspoon of cinnamon powder
- Two tablespoons of melted butter
- One whisked egg
- Cooking spray

Instructions

- In your food processor, mix plums with water and blend until you obtain a sticky spread.
- In a bowl, mix oats with cinnamon, baking soda, sugar, egg and butter and whisk really well.
- Press half of the oats mix in a baking pan that fits your air fryer sprayed with cooking oil, spread plums mix and top with the other half of the oats mix.
- Introduce in your air fryer and cook at 350 degrees F for 16 minutes.
- Leave mix aside to cool down, cut into medium bars and serve.

Plum Cake

Preparation Time- One hour and 20 minutes | Cook Time-40 minutes | Servings-2 | Difficulty-Hard

Nutritional Facts- Calories-192 | Fats-9g |Carbohydrates-13.8g |Proteins-6.9g

Ingredients

- Seven ounces of flour
- One package of dried yeast
- One ounce of softened butter
- One whisked egg
- Five tablespoons of sugar
- Three ounces of warm milk
- One and 3⁄4 pounds of pitted and quartered plums
- Zest from one lemon
- One ounce of almond flakes

Instructions

- In a bowl, mix yeast with butter, flour and Three tablespoons of sugar and stir well.

- Add milk and egg and whisk for 4 minutes until y our obtain a dough.
- Arrange the dough in a springform pan that fits your air fryer and which you've greased with some butter, cover and leave aside for 1 hour.
- Arrange plumps on top of the butter, sprinkle the rest of the sugar, introduce in your air fryer at 350 degrees F, bake for 36 minutes, cool down, sprinkle almond flakes and lemon zest on top, slice and serve.

Poppyseed Cake

Preparation Time-10 minutes | Cook Time-30 minutes | Servings-2 | Difficulty-Moderate

Nutritional Facts- Calories-212 | Fats-7.8g |Carbohydrates-19g |Proteins-6g

Ingredients

- One and a quarter cups of flour
- One teaspoon of baking powder
- 3⁄4 cup of sugar
- One tablespoon of orange zest
- Two teaspoons of lime zest
- Half cup of softened butter
- Two whisked eggs
- Half teaspoon of vanilla extract
- Two tablespoons of poppy seeds
- One cup of milk

For the cream

- One cup of sugar
- Half cup of passion fruit puree
- Three tablespoons of melted butter
- Four egg yolks

Instructions

- In a bowl, mix flour with baking powder, 3⁄4 cup of sugar, orange zest and lime zest and stir.
- Add half a cup of butter, eggs, poppy seeds, vanilla and milk, stir using your mixer, pour into a cake pan that fits your air fryer and cook at 350 degrees F for about 30 minutes.
- Meanwhile, heat up a pan with three tablespoons of butter over medium heat, add sugar and stir until it dissolves.
- Take off heat, add passion fruit puree and egg yolks gradually and whisk really well.

- Take the cake out of the fryer, cool it down a bit and cut it into halves horizontally.
- Spread 1/4 of passion fruit cream over one half, top with the other cake half and spread 1/4 of the cream on top.
- Serve cold.

Pumpkin Cookies

Preparation Time-10 minutes | Cook Time-15 minutes | Servings-2 | Difficulty-Easy

Nutritional Facts- Calories-153 | Fats-4g |Carbohydrates-7.8g |Proteins-9.9g

Ingredients

- Two and a half cups of flour
- Half teaspoon of baking soda
- One tablespoon of ground flax seed
- Three tablespoons of water
- Half cup of mashed pumpkin flesh
- A quarter cup of honey
- Two tablespoons of butter
- One teaspoon of vanilla extract
- Half cup of dark chocolate chips

Instructions

- In a bowl, mix flaxseed with water, stir and leave aside for a few minutes.
- In another bowl, mix flour with salt and baking soda.
- In a third bowl, mix honey with pumpkin puree, butter, vanilla extract and flaxseed.
- Combine flour with honey mix and chocolate chips and stir.
- Scoop One tablespoon of cookie dough on a baking sheet (lined) that fits your air fryer, repeat with the rest of the dough, introduce them in your air fryer and cook at 350 degrees F for 15 minutes.
- Leave cookies to cool down and serve.

Pumpkin parcels

Preparation Time-5 minutes | Cook Time-12 minutes | Servings-2 | Difficulty-Easy

Nutritional Facts- Calories-182 | Fats-7.8g |Carbohydrates-19g |Proteins-6g

Ingredients

- Three tablespoons of Pumpkin Filling
- One Sheet of Puff Pastry
- One small beaten egg

Instructions

- Preheat the Air fryer oven to 356 degrees Fahrenheit.
- Preheat oven to 350°F. Roll out a sheet of puff pastry and top it with pumpkin pie filling, leaving a 1cm space around the borders.
- It should be cut into nine squares.
- Fill in the spaces with beaten egg to give it that wonderful egg glow.
- Place on a baking sheet in the air fryer for 12 minutes at 356 degrees Fahrenheit.
- Serve!

Pumpkin Pie

Preparation Time-10 minutes | Cook Time-15 minutes | Servings-2 | Difficulty-Easy

Nutritional Facts- Calories-193 | Fats-12g |Carbohydrates-12.9g |Proteins-7.8g

Ingredients

- One tablespoon of sugar
- Two tablespoons of flour
- One tablespoon of butter
- Two tablespoons of water

For the pumpkin pie filling

- Three ounces of chopped pumpkin flesh
- One teaspoon of mixed spice
- One teaspoon of nutmeg
- Three ounces of water
- One whisked egg
- One tablespoon of sugar

Instructions

- Put 3 ounces of water in a pot, bring to a boil over medium-high heat, add pumpkin, egg, One tablespoon of sugar, spice and nutmeg, stir, boil for 20 minutes, take off the heat and blend using an immersion blender.

- In a bowl, mix flour with butter, one tablespoon of sugar and two tablespoons of water and knead your dough well.
- Grease a pie pan that fits your air fryer with butter, press dough into the pan, fill with pumpkin pie filling, place in your air fryer's basket and cook at 360 degrees F for 15 minutes.
- Slice and serve warm.

Raspberry Danish

Preparation Time-20 minutes | Cook Time-25 minutes | Servings-2 | Difficulty-Moderate

Nutritional Facts- Calories-335 | Fats-9.9g |Carbohydrates-40g |Proteins-4.8g

Ingredients

- One tube full-sheet crescent roll dough
- Four ounces of softened cream cheese
- A quarter cup of raspberry jam
- Half cup of chopped fresh raspberries
- One cup of powdered sugar
- Three tablespoons of heavy whipping cream

Instructions

- Place the sheet of crescent roll dough onto a flat surface and unroll it.
- In a microwave-safe bowl, add the cream cheese and microwave for about 20-30 seconds.
- Remove from microwave and stir until creamy and smooth.
- Spread the cream cheese over the dough sheet, followed by the strawberry jam.
- Now, place the raspberry pieces evenly across the top.
- From the short side, roll the dough and pinch the seam to seal.
- Arrange a greased parchment paper onto the steak tray of the oven.
- Carefully curve the rolled pastry into a horseshoe shape and arrange it onto the prepared tray.
- Select "Air Fry" of Air Fryer Oven and then adjust the temperature to 350 degrees Fahrenheit.
- Set the timer for 25 minutes and press "Start/Stop" to begin cooking.
- When the unit beeps to show that it is preheated, insert the tray in the air fryer.
- When cooking time is complete, remove the tray from the air fryer and place it onto a rack to cool.
- Meanwhile, in a bowl, mix together the powdered sugar and cream.
- Drizzle the cream mixture over cooled Danish and serve.

Rhubarb Pie

Preparation Time-30 minutes | Cook Time-45 minutes | Servings-2 | Difficulty-Hard

Nutritional Facts- Calories-210 | Fats-12g |Carbohydrates-12g |Proteins-7.8g

Ingredients

- One and a quarter cups of almond flour
- Eight tablespoons of butter
- Five tablespoons of cold water
- One teaspoon of sugar

For the filling

- Three cups of chopped rhubarb
- Three tablespoons of flour
- One and a half cups of sugar
- Two eggs
- Half teaspoon of ground nutmeg
- One tablespoon of butter
- Two tablespoons of low-fat milk

Instructions

- In a bowl, mix one and a quarter cups of flour with one teaspoon of sugar, eight tablespoons of butter and cold water; stir and knead until you obtain a dough.
- Transfer dough to a floured working surface, shape a disk, flatten, wrap in plastic, keep in the fridge for about 30 minutes, roll and press on the bottom of a pie pan that fits your air fryer.
- In a bowl, mix rhubarb with One and a half cups of sugar, nutmeg, Three tablespoons of flour and whisk.
- In another bowl, whisk eggs with milk, add to rhubarb mix, pour the whole mix into the pie crust, introduce in your air fryer and cook at 390 degrees F for 45 minutes.
- Cut and serve it cold.

Rice pudding

Preparation Time-10 minutes | Cook Time-15 minutes | Servings-2 | Difficulty-Easy

Nutritional Facts- Calories-153 | Fats-6.9g |Carbohydrates-21g |Proteins-6g

Ingredients

- Two cups of milk
- Two tablespoons of custard powder
- Three tablespoons of powdered sugar
- Two tablespoons of rice
- Three tablespoons of unsalted butter

Instructions

- Boil the milk and the sugar in a pan and add the custard powder and stir till you get a thick mixture. Add the rice to the bowl and ensure that the mixture becomes slightly thicker.
- Preheat the fryer to 300 Fahrenheit for five minutes. Place the dish in the basket and reduce the temperature to 250 Fahrenheit. Cook for ten minutes and set aside to cool.

Ricotta and Lemon Cake

Preparation Time-10 minutes | Cook Time-One and 10 minutes | Servings-2 | Difficulty-Hard

Nutritional Facts- Calories-112 | Fats-1g|Carbohydrates-12g |Proteins-6g

Ingredients

- Eight whisked eggs
- Three pounds of ricotta cheese
- Half pound sugar
- Zest from one lemon
- Zest from one orange
- Butter for the pan

Instructions

- In a bowl, mix eggs with sugar, cheese, lemon and orange zest and stir very well.
- Grease a baking pan that fits your air fryer with some batter, spread ricotta mixture, introduce in the fryer at 390 degrees F and bake for 30 minutes.
- Reduce heat to 380 degrees F and bake for 40 more minutes.
- Take out of the oven, leave the cake to cool down and serve!

Semolina pudding

Preparation Time-10 minutes | Cook Time-15 minutes | Servings-2 | Difficulty-Easy

Nutritional Facts- Calories-146 | Fats-6g |Carbohydrates-15.9g |Proteins-6g

Ingredients

- Two cups of milk
- Two tablespoons of custard powder
- Three tablespoons of powdered sugar
- Two tablespoons of semolina
- Three tablespoons of unsalted butter

Instructions

- Boil the milk and the sugar in a pan and add the custard powder and stir till you get a thick mixture. Add the semolina to the bowl and ensure that the mixture becomes slightly thicker.
- Preheat the fryer to 300 Fahrenheit for five minutes. Place the dish in the basket and reduce the temperature to 250 Fahrenheit. Cook for ten minutes and set aside to cool.

Simple Cheesecake

Preparation Time-10 minutes | Cook Time-15 minutes | Servings-2 | Difficulty-Easy

Nutritional Facts- Calories-245 | Fats-12g |Carbohydrates-21g |Proteins-17g

Ingredients

- One pound of cream cheese
- Half teaspoon of vanilla extract
- Two eggs
- Four tablespoons of sugar
- One cup of crumbled graham crackers
- Two tablespoons of butter

Instructions

- In a bowl, mix crackers with butter.
- Press crackers mix on the bottom of a lined cake pan, introduce in your air fryer and cook at 350 degrees F for 4 minutes.
- Meanwhile, in a bowl, mix sugar with cream cheese, eggs and vanilla and whisk well.
- Spread filling over crackers crust and cook your cheesecake in your air fryer at 310 degrees F for 15 minutes.

- Leave cake in the fridge for 3 hours, slice and serve.
- Enjoy!

Soft & creamy chocolate cookie dough

Preparation Time-5 minutes | Cook Time-20 minutes | Servings-2 | Difficulty-Easy

Nutritional Facts- Calories-201 | Fats-13.8g |Carbohydrates-12.9g |Proteins-7.8g

Ingredients

- Half cup of Butter
- 1/3 cup of Brown Sugar
- One cup of Self Raising Flour
- Half cup of Chocolate
- Four tablespoons of Honey
- One tablespoon of Milk

Instructions

- Preheat the air fryer for 10 minutes at 320 degrees F.
- In a large mixing basin, soften the butter, then add the sugar and cream together until fluffy and light.
- Mix in the honey and flour thoroughly.
- Smash the chocolate with a rolling pin until you have a mixture of medium and small chocolate chunks.
- Toss in the chocolate.
- Also, add the milk and mix thoroughly.
- In the air fryer, spoon the cookie batter onto a tin that has been layered with a baking sheet.
- Cook for 20 minutes at 320 degrees Fahrenheit.
- Serve!

Soft chocolate brownies with homemade caramel sauce

Preparation Time-20 minutes | Cook Time-18 minutes | Servings-2 | Difficulty-Easy

Nutritional Facts- Calories-232 | Fats-16.8g |Carbohydrates-15g |Proteins-7.8g

Ingredients

- One cup of Caster Sugar
- Two tablespoons of Water
- 3/4 cup of Milk
- One cup of Butter

- A quarter cup of Chocolate
- One cup of Brown Sugar
- Two Medium beaten eggs
- Half cup of Self Raising Flour
- Two teaspoons of Vanilla Essence

Instructions

- Preheat the Air fryer oven to 356 degrees Fahrenheit.
- Prepare the chocolate brownies first – In a bowl above a pan, melt half of the butter and chocolate over medium heat. Combine the brown sugar, medium eggs, and vanilla extract in a mixing bowl. Mix in the self-rising flour thoroughly.
- Pour the mixture into a greased baking dish that is large enough to fit your air fryer.
- Cook for 15 minutes at 356 degrees Fahrenheit in your air fryer.
- It's time to make the caramel sauce while the brownies are baking. In a small saucepan, melt the caster sugar with the water over medium heat. Then increase the heat to high and cook for another three minutes, or until it turns a light brown color. Remove the pan from the heat and, after 2 minutes, add the butter, constantly stirring until it is completely melted. Then gradually pour in the milk.
- Allow the caramel sauce to cool before using.
- When the brownies are done, cut them into squares and arrange them on a platter with sliced banana and caramel sauce on top.
- Serve!

Special Brownies

Preparation Time-10 minutes | Cook Time-17 minutes | Servings-2 | Difficulty-Easy

Nutritional Facts- Calories-223 | Fats-28.9g |Carbohydrates-7.8g |Proteins-6g

Ingredients

- One egg
- 1/3 cup of cocoa powder
- 1/3 cup of sugar
- Seven tablespoons of butter
- Half teaspoon of vanilla extract
- A quarter cup of white flour
- A quarter cup of chopped walnuts

- Half teaspoon of baking powder
- One tablespoon of peanut butter

Instructions

- Heat up a pan with six tablespoons of butter and the sugar over medium heat, stir, cook for 5 minutes, transfer this to a bowl.
- Add salt, vanilla extract, cocoa powder, egg, baking powder, walnuts and flour, stir the whole thing really well and pour into a pan that fits your air fryer.
- In a bowl, mix one tablespoon of butter with peanut butter, heat up in your microwave for a few seconds, stir well and drizzle this over brownies mix.
- Introduce in your air fryer and bake at 320 degrees F and bake for 17 minutes.
- Leave brownies to cool down, cut and serve.

Sponge Cake

Preparation Time-10 minutes | Cook Time-20 minutes | Servings-2 | Difficulty-Easy

Nutritional Facts- Calories-246 | Fats-4.8g |Carbohydrates-7.8g |Proteins-4g

Ingredients

- Three cups of flour
- Three teaspoons of baking powder
- Half cup of cornstarch
- One teaspoon of baking soda
- One cup of olive oil
- One and a half cups of milk
- One and 2/3 cup of sugar
- Two cups of water
- A quarter cup of lemon juice
- Two teaspoons of vanilla extract

Instructions

- In a bowl, mix flour with cornstarch, baking powder, baking soda and sugar and whisk well.
- In another bowl, mix oil with milk, water, vanilla and lemon juice and whisk.
- Combine the two mixtures, stir, pour in a greased baking dish that fits your air fryer, introduce in the fryer and cook at 350 degrees F for 20 minutes.
- Leave the cake to cool down, cut and serve.

Strawberry Cobbler

Preparation Time-10 minutes | Cook Time-25 minutes | Servings-2 | Difficulty-Easy

Nutritional Facts- Calories-211 | Fats-12.9g |Carbohydrates-12g |Proteins-9g

Ingredients

- 3/4 cup of sugar
- Six cups of halved strawberries
- 1/8 teaspoon of baking powder
- One tablespoon of lemon juice
- Half cup of flour
- A pinch of baking soda
- Half cup of water
- Three and a half tablespoons of olive oil
- Cooking spray

Instructions

- In a bowl, mix strawberries with half of the sugar, sprinkle some flour, add lemon juice, whisk and pour into the baking dish that fits your air fryer and greased with cooking spray.
- In another bowl, mix flour with the rest of the sugar, baking powder and soda and stir well.
- Add the olive oil and mix until the whole thing with your hands.
- Add half a cup of water and spread over strawberries.
- Introduce in the fryer at 355 degrees F and bake for 25 minutes.
- Leave cobbler aside to cool down, slice and serve.

Strawberry Cupcakes with Creamy Strawberry Frosting

Preparation Time-15 minutes | Cook Time-10 minutes | Servings-2 | Difficulty-Easy

Nutritional Facts- Calories-174 | Fats-10.8g |Carbohydrates-18g |Proteins-7.8g

Ingredients

- Half cup of Butter
- Half cup of Caster Sugar
- Two Medium Eggs
- Half cup of Self Raising Flour
- Half teaspoon of Vanilla Essence
- A quarter cup of Butter

- Half cup of Icing Sugar
- Half teaspoon of Pink Food Colouring
- One tablespoon of Whipped Cream
- A quarter cup of blended Fresh Strawberries

Instructions

- Preheat the air fryer to 338°F.
- In a big mixing bowl, cream the butter and sugar while it's heating up. This should be repeated until the mixture is light and fluffy.
- Stir the vanilla extract and the eggs one by one, beating well after each addition. After each egg, stir in a small amount of flour. Fold in the remaining flour gently.
- Fill small bun casings to the top with them, about 80 percent full.
- Place them in the air fryer and cook for 8 minutes at 338°F.
- Make the topping while the cupcakes are baking. To get a creamy mixture, cream the butter and gradually add the icing sugar. Mix well with the whipped cream, food coloring, and pureed strawberries.
- After the cupcakes have been baked, use a piping bag to add your topping in circular motions to give them that gorgeous cupcake look.
- Serve!

Strawberry Donuts

Preparation Time-10 minutes | Cook Time-15 minutes | Servings-2 | Difficulty-Easy

Nutritional Facts- Calories-243 | Fats-12g |Carbohydrates-31.8g |Proteins-7.8g

Ingredients

- Eight ounces of flour
- One tablespoon of brown sugar
- One tablespoon of white sugar
- One egg
- Two and a half tablespoons of butter
- Four ounces of whole milk
- One teaspoon of baking powder

For the strawberry icing

- Two tablespoons of butter
- Three ounces of icing sugar
- Half teaspoon of pink coloring

- A quarter cup of chopped strawberries
- One tablespoon of whipped cream

Instructions

- In a bowl, mix butter, One tablespoon of brown sugar, One tablespoon of white sugar and flour and stir.
- In a second bowl, mix egg with One and a half tablespoons of butter and milk and stir well.
- Combine the two mixtures, stir, shape donuts from this mix, place them in your air fryer's basket and cook at 360 degrees F for 15 minutes.
- Put One tablespoon of butter, icing sugar, food coloring, whipped cream and strawberry puree and whisk well.
- Arrange donuts on a platter and serve with strawberry icing on top.

Strawberry Jam Tarts

Preparation Time-10 minutes | Cook Time-10 minutes | Servings-2 | Difficulty-Easy

Nutritional Facts- Calories-168 | Fats-9.9g |Carbohydrates-13.8g |Proteins-7.8g

Ingredients

- One and a half cups of Plain Flour
- Half cup of Butter
- One and 1/8 tablespoon of Caster Sugar
- Strawberry Jam
- Water

Instructions

- Preheat the air fryer to 356°F (180°C).
- In a large mixing basin, combine the flour, sugar, and butter. To make breadcrumbs, rub the butter into the sugar and flour until it resembles breadcrumbs.
- Pour in enough water to make a firm pastry dough.
- Place pastry in the bottom and around the edges of 9 little pastry boxes that have been greased.
- Place two teaspoons of strawberry jam in the bottom of each one before placing it in the air fryer.
- Cook at 356 degrees Fahrenheit for 10 minutes or until pastry is done.
- Serve!

Strawberry Pie

Preparation Time-10 minutes | Cook Time-20 minutes | Servings-2 | Difficulty-Easy

Nutritional Facts- Calories-235 | Fats-21.9g |Carbohydrates-7.8g |Proteins-6.9g

Ingredients

For the crust

- One cup of shredded coconut
- One cup of sunflower seeds
- A quarter cup of butter

For the filling

- One teaspoon of gelatin
- Eight ounces of cream cheese
- Four ounces of strawberries
- Two tablespoons of water
- Half tablespoon of lemon juice
- A quarter teaspoon of stevia
- Half cup of heavy cream
- Eight ounces of chopped strawberries for serving

Instructions

- In your food processor, mix sunflower seeds with coconut, a pinch of salt and butter, pulse and press this on the bottom of a cake pan that fits your air fryer.
- Heat up a pan with the water over medium heat, add gelatin, stir until it dissolves, leave aside to cool down, add this to your food processor, mix with 4 ounces strawberries, cream cheese, lemon juice and stevia and blend well.
- Add heavy cream, stir well and spread this over crust.
- Top with 8 ounces strawberries, introduce in your air fryer and cook at 330 degrees F for 15 minutes. Keep in the fridge until you serve it.

Strawberry Shortcakes

Preparation Time-20 minutes | Cook Time-45 minutes | Servings-2 | Difficulty-Hard

Nutritional Facts- Calories-173 | Fats-6g |Carbohydrates-10.8g |Proteins-4.8g

Ingredients

- Cooking spray
- A quarter cup plus four tablespoons of sugar
- One and a half cups of flour
- One teaspoon of baking powder
- A quarter teaspoon of baking soda
- 1/3 cup of butter
- One cup of buttermilk
- One whisked egg
- Two cups of sliced strawberries
- One tablespoon of rum
- One tablespoon of chopped mint
- One teaspoon of grated lime zest
- Half cup of whipping cream

Instructions

- In a bowl, mix flour with a quarter cup of sugar, baking powder and baking soda and stir.
- In another bowl, mix buttermilk with egg, stir, add to the flour mix and whisk.
- Spoon this dough into six jars greased with cooking spray, cover with tin foil, arrange them in your air fryer, cook at 360 degrees F for 45 minutes.
- Meanwhile, in a bowl, mix strawberries with Three tablespoons of sugar, rum, mint and lime zest, stir and leave aside in a cold place.
- In another bowl, mix whipping cream with one tablespoon of sugar and stir.
- Take jars out, divide strawberry mix and whipped cream on top and serve.

Strawberry Toast

Preparation Time-5 minutes | Cook Time-10 minutes | Servings-2 | Difficulty-Easy

Nutritional Facts- Calories-155 | Fats-1g|Carbohydrates-6g |Proteins-20g

Ingredients

- Four slices of bread
- One cup of sliced strawberries
- One teaspoon of sugar
- Cooking spray

Instructions

- On a clean work surface, lay the bread slices and spritz one side of each slice of bread with cooking spray.

- Put the bread slices in the air fryer basket, sprayed side down. Top with the strawberries and a sprinkle of sugar.
- Slide the basket into the air fryer. Cook at the corresponding preset mode or Air Fry at 375F (190C) for 8 minutes.
- When cooking is complete, the toast should be well browned on each side. Detach from the air fryer to a plate and serve.

Super simple shortbread chocolate balls

Preparation Time-5 minutes | Cook Time-15 minutes | Servings-2 | Difficulty-Easy

Nutritional Facts- Calories-189 | Fats-9g |Carbohydrates-16.8g |Proteins-7.8g

Ingredients

- One cup of Butter
- 1/3 cup of Caster Sugar
- Two and a quarter cups of Plain Flour
- One teaspoon of Vanilla Essence
- Nine Chocolate chunks
- Two tablespoons of Cocoa

Instructions

- Preheat your air fryer to 356 degrees Fahrenheit before you begin.
- In a mixing basin, combine the flour, sugar, and cocoa.
- Rub in the butter and knead the dough until it is smooth.
- Make balls out of the dough and add a chocolate chunk in the center of each, making sure none of the chocolate chunk shows.
- In your air fryer, place the chocolate shortbread balls on a baking sheet. Cook them for 8 minutes at 356 degrees Fahrenheit, then 5 minutes at 320 degrees Fahrenheit to ensure they are done in the center.
- Serve!

Sweet Banana Bread Pudding

Preparation Time-10 minutes | Cook Time-18 minutes | Servings-2 | Difficulty-Easy

Nutritional Facts- Calories-461 | Fats-21.9g |Carbohydrates-45g |Proteins-27.9g

Ingredients

- Two mashed medium ripe bananas
- Half cup of low-fat milk
- Two tablespoons of maple syrup
- Two tablespoons of peanut butter
- One teaspoon of vanilla extract
- One teaspoon of ground cinnamon
- Two slices of whole-grain bread
- A quarter cup of quick oats
- Cooking spray

Instructions

- Spritz the sheet pan with cooking spray.
- In a large bowl, merge the bananas, milk, maple syrup, peanut butter, vanilla extract and cinnamon with an immersion blender to mix until well combined.
- Set in the bread pieces to coat well. Attach the oats and stir until everything is combined.
- Transfer the mixture to the sheet pan. Cover with aluminum foil.
- Bring the pan into the air fryer oven. Press the Power Button. Cook at 375F (190C) for 18 minutes.
- After 10 minutes, detach the foil and continue to cook for 8 minutes.
- Serve immediately.

Sweet Bananas

Preparation Time-10 minutes | Cook Time-15 minutes | Servings-2 | Difficulty-Easy

Nutritional Facts- Calories-174 | Fats-6g |Carbohydrates-30g |Proteins-17g

Ingredients

- Three tablespoons of butter
- Two eggs
- Eight peeled and halved bananas
- Half cup of cornflour
- Three tablespoons of cinnamon sugar
- One cup of panko

Instructions

- Heat up a pan with the butter over medium-high heat, add panko, stir and cook for 4 minutes and then transfer to a bowl.

- Roll each in flour, eggs and panko mix, arrange them in your air fryer's basket, dust with cinnamon sugar and cook at 280 degrees F for 10 minutes.
- Serve right away.

Sweet Cinnamon Toast

Preparation Time-5 minutes | Cook Time-5 minutes | Servings-2 | Difficulty-Easy

Nutritional Facts- Calories-245 | Fats-15g |Carbohydrates-1g |Proteins-24g

Ingredients

- Half teaspoon of cinnamon
- Half teaspoon of vanilla extract
- A quarter cup of sugar
- One teaspoon of ground black pepper
- One tablespoon of melted coconut oil
- Four slices of whole wheat bread

Instructions

- Merge all the ingredients, except for the bread, in a large bowl. Stir to mix well.
- Dunk the bread in the bowl of mixture gently to coat and infuse well. Shake the excess off. Arrange the bread slices in the air fry basket.
- Place the basket on the air fry position.
- Select Air Fry, set the temperature to 400 degrees F (205C) and set time to 5 minutes. Flip the bread halfway through.
- When cooking is complete, the bread should be golden brown.
- Detach the bread slices from the air fryer grill and slice to serve.

Sweet Potato Cheesecake

Preparation Time-10 minutes | Cook Time-5 minutes | Servings-2 | Difficulty-Easy

Nutritional Facts- Calories-167 | Fats-4g |Carbohydrates-13.8g |Proteins-17g

Ingredients

- Four tablespoons of melted butter
- Six ounces of soft mascarpone
- Eight ounces of soft cream cheese
- 2/3 cup of crumbled graham crackers
- 3/4 cup of milk
- One teaspoon of vanilla extract
- 2/3 cup of sweet potato puree
- A quarter teaspoon of cinnamon powder

Instructions

- In a bowl, mix butter with crumbled crackers, stir well, press on the bottom of a cake pan that fits your air fryer and keep in the fridge for now.
- In another bowl, mix cream cheese with mascarpone, sweet potato puree, milk, cinnamon and vanilla and whisk really well.
- Spread this over crust, introduce it in your air fryer, cook at 300 degrees F for 4 minutes and keep it in the fridge for a few hours before serving.

Sweet Potato Dessert Fries

Preparation Time-10 minutes | Cook Time-30 minutes | Servings-2 to 4 | Difficulty-Moderate

Nutritional Facts- Calories-130 | Fats-4.8g |Carbohydrates-7.8g |Proteins-9g

Ingredients

- Two teaspoons of melted butter (for coating) (Optional)
- One to Two tablespoons of cinnamon
- Dessert Hummus
- Half a tablespoon of coconut oil
- Two medium sweet potatoes or yams peeled
- A quarter cup of coconut sugar or raw sugar
- Optional powdered sugar for dusting
- Vanilla Greek Yogurt
- One tablespoon of arrowroot starch or cornstarch
- Maple Frosting {vegan}

Instructions

- Peel and wash your sweet potatoes with clean water, then dry.
- Slice peeled sweet potatoes 1/2 inch deep, lengthwise.
- Toss 1/Two tablespoons of coconut oil and arrowroot starch in your sweet potato slices.
- Place the air fryer at 370F for 18 minutes. Shake for 8-9 minutes halfway through.
- Take the fries from the fryer and put them in a wide bowl. Drizzle on top of the fries with Two teaspoons of optional butter. Then mix the sugar and cinnamon and toss the fries once again.

- Place it on a serving plate and sprinkle it with powdered sugar.
- Serve fries with the preferred dipping sauce. Hold the fries wrapped in foil and in a fridge to stock. Then reheat to warm again in the oven before serving. You should stay for 2-3 days.

Sweet Squares

Preparation Time-10 minutes | Cook Time-30 minutes | Servings-2 | Difficulty-Moderate

Nutritional Facts- Calories-121 | Fats-4.8g |Carbohydrates-12.9g |Proteins-1.5g

Ingredients

- One cup of flour
- Half cup of softened butter
- One cup of sugar
- A quarter cup of powdered sugar
- Two teaspoons of lemon peel
- Two tablespoons of lemon juice
- Two whisked eggs
- Half teaspoon of baking powder

Instructions

- In a bowl, mix flour with powdered sugar and butter, stir well, press on the bottom of a pan that fits your air fryer, introduce in the fryer and bake at 350 degrees F for 14 minutes.
- In another bowl, mix sugar with lemon juice, lemon peel, eggs and baking powder, stir using your mixer and spread over baked crust.
- Bake for 15 minutes more, leave aside to cool down, cut into medium squares and serve cold.

Sweetened Plantains

Preparation Time-5 minutes | Cook Time-10 minutes | Servings-2 | Difficulty-Easy

Nutritional Facts- Calories-125 | Fats-1.2g |Carbohydrates-31.8g |Proteins-1.5g

Ingredients

- Two ripe sliced plantains
- Two teaspoons of avocado oil
- Salt to taste
- Maple syrup

Instructions

- Toss the plantains in oil.
- Season with salt.
- Cook in the air fryer basket at 400 degrees F for 10 minutes, shaking after 5 minutes. Drizzle with maple syrup before serving.

Tangerine Cake

Preparation Time-10 minutes | Cook Time-20 minutes | Servings-2 | Difficulty-Easy

Nutritional Facts- Calories-189 | Fats-6g |Carbohydrates-10.8g |Proteins-6.9g

Ingredients

- 3/4 cup of sugar
- Two cups of flour
- A quarter cup of olive oil
- Half cup of milk
- One teaspoon of cider vinegar
- Half teaspoon of vanilla extract
- Juice and zest from two lemons
- Juice and zest from one tangerine
- Tangerine segments, for serving

Instructions

- In a bowl, mix flour with sugar and stir.
- In another bowl, mix oil with milk, vinegar, vanilla extract, lemon juice and zest and tangerine zest and whisk very well.
- Add flour, stir well, pour this into a cake pan that fits your air fryer, introduce in the fryer and cook at 360 degrees F for 20 minutes.
- Serve right away with tangerine segments on top.

Tasty Cheese Bites

Preparation Time-10 minutes | Cook Time-10 minutes | Servings-2 | Difficulty-Easy

Nutritional Facts- Calories-383 | Fats-19g |Carbohydrates-27.9g |Proteins-23g

Ingredients

- Four ounces of softened cream cheese
- One tablespoon of erythritol
- A quarter cup of almond flour
- Half teaspoons of vanilla
- Two tablespoons of heavy cream

- A quarter cup of erythritol

Instructions

- Add cream cheese, vanilla, a half cup of

erythritol, and two tablespoons of heavy cream in a stand mixer and mix until smooth.

- Scoop cream cheese mixture onto the parchment-lined plate and place in the refrigerator for 1 hour.
- In a small bowl, mix together almond flour and two tablespoons of erythritol.
- Dip cheesecake bites in remaining heavy cream and coat with almond flour mixture.
- Place the prepared cheesecake bites in the air fryer basket and air fry for 2 minutes at 350 degrees F.
- Make sure cheesecake bites are frozen before air fry; otherwise, they will melt.
- Drizzle with chocolate syrup and serve.

Tasty Orange Cake

Preparation Time-10 minutes | Cook Time-33 minutes | Servings-2 | Difficulty-Moderate

Nutritional Facts- Calories-202 | Fats-13.8g |Carbohydrates-10.8g |Proteins-7.8g

Ingredients

- Six eggs
- One peeled and quartered orange
- One teaspoon of vanilla extract
- One teaspoon of baking powder
- Nine ounces of flour
- Two ounces plus two tablespoons of sugar
- Two tablespoons of orange zest
- Four ounces of cream cheese
- Four ounces of yogurt

Instructions

- In your food processor, pulse orange very well.
- Add flour, two tablespoons of sugar, eggs, baking powder, vanilla extract and pulse well again.
- Transfer this into two springform pans, introduce each in your fryer and cook at 330 degrees F for 16 minutes.
- Meanwhile, in a bowl, mix cream cheese with orange zest, yogurt and the rest of the sugar and stir well.

- Place one cake layer on a plate, add half of the cream cheese mix, add the other cake layer and top with the rest of the cream cheese mix.
- Spread it well, slice and serve.

Tasty Orange Cookies

Preparation Time-10 minutes | Cook Time-12 minutes | Servings-2 | Difficulty-Easy

Nutritional Facts- Calories-131 | Fats-4.8g |Carbohydrates-12.9g |Proteins-4.8g

Ingredients

- Two cups of flour
- One teaspoon of baking powder
- Half cup of softened butter
- 3/4 cup of sugar
- One whished egg
- One teaspoon of vanilla extract
- One tablespoon of orange zest

For the filling

Four ounces of soft cream cheese
Half cup of butter
Two cups of powdered sugar

Instructions

- In a bowl, mix cream cheese with half a cup of butter and two cups of powdered sugar, stir well using your mixer and leave aside for now.
- In another bowl, mix flour with baking powder.
- In a third bowl, mix half a cup of butter with 3/4 cup of sugar, egg, vanilla extract and orange zest and whisk well.
- Combine flour with the orange mix, stir well and scoop One tablespoon of the mix on a baking sheet (lined) that fits your air fryer.
- Repeat with the rest of the orange batter, introduce in the fryer and cook at 340 degrees F for 12 minutes.
- Leave cookies to cool down, spread cream filling on half of the top with the other cookies and serve.

Ten minutes smartie cookies

Preparation Time-5 minutes | Cook Time-5 minutes | Servings-2 | Difficulty-Easy

Nutritional Facts- Calories-152 | Fats-7.8g |Carbohydrates-15.9g |Proteins-5.4g

Ingredients

- Half cup of Butter
- Half cup of Caster Sugar
- One and a half cups of Self Raising Flour
- One teaspoon of Vanilla Essence
- Five tablespoons of Milk
- Three tablespoons of Cocoa
- 1/3 Tube Of Smarties
- A quarter cup of White Chocolate

Instructions

- Preheat the air fryer to 356°F (180°C).
- In a large mixing basin, combine the flour, cocoa, and sugar.
- Rub in the butter, then add the vanilla extract and stir thoroughly.
- Smash the white chocolate with a rolling pin until you have a mixture of medium and small chocolate chips.
- Mix the chocolate and milk into the cookie dough thoroughly.
- Knead the dough until it is nice and soft, adding a bit more milk if necessary.
- Roll out your dough and cut out biscuit shapes with a cookie cutter.
- Place the Smarties half inside the cookie and half out in the open at the top of the cookies.
- Cook the cookies for ten minutes at 356 degrees Fahrenheit in an air fryer on a baking sheet.
- Serve with a glass of warm milk.

Three ingredient shortbread fingers

Preparation Time-5 minutes | Cook Time-15 minutes | Servings-2 | Difficulty-Easy

Nutritional Facts- Calories-131 | Fats-4.8g |Carbohydrates-15g |Proteins-1.5g

Ingredients

- One cup of Butter
- 1/3 cup of Caster Sugar
- Two and a quarter cups of Plain Flour

Instructions

- Preheat the Air fryer oven to 356 degrees Fahrenheit.
- In a mixing basin, combine flour and sugar.
- Rub the butter into the flour and sugar mixture.

- Knead the mixture thoroughly until it is smooth and gorgeous.
- Make finger shapes with the dough and embellish with fork lines.
- Cook for 12 minutes on a baking sheet in the air fryer.

Tomato Cake

Preparation Time-10 minutes | Cook Time-30 minutes | Servings-2 | Difficulty-Moderate

Nutritional Facts- Calories-153 | Fats-1g|Carbohydrates-25g |Proteins-4g

Ingredients

- One and a half cups of flour
- One teaspoon of cinnamon powder
- One teaspoon of baking powder
- One teaspoon of baking soda
- 3/4 cup of maple syrup
- One cup of chopped tomatoes
- Half cup of olive oil
- Two tablespoons of apple cider vinegar

Instructions

- In a bowl, mix flour with baking powder, baking soda, cinnamon and maple syrup and stir well.
- In another bowl, mix tomatoes with olive oil and vinegar and stir well.
- Combine the two mixtures, stir well, pour into a greased round pan that fits your air fryer, introduce in the fryer and cook at 360 degrees F for 30 minutes.
- Leave the cake to cool down, slice and serve.

Vanilla Granola

Preparation Time-10 minutes | Cook Time-40 minutes | Servings-2 | Difficulty-Moderate

Nutritional Facts- Calories-279 | Fats-7.8g |Carbohydrates-26g |Proteins-6g

Ingredients

- One cup of rolled oats
- Three tablespoons of maple syrup
- One tablespoon of sunflower oil
- One tablespoon of coconut sugar
- A quarter teaspoon of vanilla
- A quarter teaspoon of cinnamon

- A quarter teaspoon of sea salt

Instructions

- Mix the oats, maple syrup, sunflower oil, coconut sugar, vanilla, cinnamon, and sea salt in a medium bowl and stir to combine. Transfer the mixture to a baking pan.
- Bring the pan into the air fryer oven. Press the Power Button. Cook at 248°F (120°C) for 40 minutes.
- Stir the granola four times during cooking.
- When cooking is complete, the granola will be mostly dry and lightly browned.
- Let the granola stand for 5 to 10 minutes before serving.

Wrapped Pears

Preparation Time-10 minutes | Cook Time-15 minutes | Servings-2 | Difficulty-Easy

Nutritional Facts- Calories-198 | Fats-9g |Carbohydrates-13.8g |Proteins-7.8g

Ingredients

- Four puff pastry sheets
- Fourteen ounces of vanilla custard
- Two halved pears
- One whisked egg
- Half teaspoon of cinnamon powder
- Two tablespoons of sugar

Instructions

- Place puff pastry slices on a working surface, add spoonfuls of vanilla custard in the center of each, top with pear halves and wrap.
- Brush pears with egg, sprinkle sugar and cinnamon, place them in your air fryer's basket and cook at 320 degrees F for 15 minutes.
- Divide parcels among plates and serve.

Conclusion

The use of air fryers, rather than deep-frying foods, is recommended by a number of authorities. As a result of this increased public awareness of the need for healthfulness, as well as the continuous desire for fried meals, air fryers have experienced a significant increase in popularity. Potatoes are consumed in greater quantities in the United States than any other vegetable, with frozen items such as French fries accounting for 40% of total consumption. Fried dishes can be prepared and cooked in air fryers without the health dangers associated with deep frying in oil. Because air-fried foods have less fat than deep-fried foods, they have the potential to be more nutritious.

In order to provide a better alternative to deep-fried foods, air fryers were developed rather than being used to replace traditional, healthy food preparation methods such as grilling and roasting. Deep-fried foods include a higher percentage of fat than dishes that are prepared in any other method of cooking, including baking. Almost all individuals genuinely prefer the flavor and texture of fried chicken, despite the fact that one hundred grams of the battered and fried chicken breast appear to contain 13.2 grams of fat, compared to 0.39 grams of fat in one hundred grams of oven-roasted chicken breast.

People may enjoy a healthy dinner that has similar flavors and textures because air fryers only use a small amount of oil to fry the food, allowing them to consume fewer calories. Taking precautions is important because lowering one's oil intake could be incredibly advantageous to one's overall health. According to studies, dietary fat derived from vegetable oils has been linked to the majority of health concerns, including increased rates of inflammation and a greater risk of heart disease. Compared to grilled, slow-cooked, roasted, or pan-fried foods, air-fried foods are more nutritious.

Printed in Great Britain
by Amazon

76168137R00167